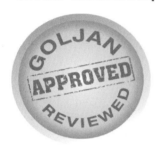

Rapid Review Series

RAPID REVIEW

MICROBIOLOGY
AND IMMUNOLOGY

THIRD EDITION

Ken S. Rosenthal, PhD
Professor
Department of Microbiology and Immunology
Northeastern Ohio Universities Colleges of Medicine and Pharmacy
Rootstown, Ohio

Adjunct Professor
FIU Herbert Wertheim College of Medicine
Florida International University
Miami, Florida

Michael J. Tan, MD, FACP
Assistant Professor of Internal Medicine
Northeastern Ohio Universities Colleges of Medicine and Pharmacy
Rootstown, Ohio

Clinical Physician
Infectious Diseases and HIV
Summa Health System
Akron, Ohio

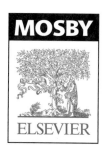

MOSBY

ELSEVIER

MOSBY
ELSEVIER

1600 John F. Kennedy Blvd.
Ste 1800
Philadelphia, PA 19103-2899

RAPID REVIEW MICROBIOLOGY AND IMMUNOLOGY,
THIRD EDITION

ISBN: 978-0-323-06938-0

Notices

Knowledge and best practice in this field are constantly changing. As new research and experience broaden our understanding, changes in research methods, professional practices, or medical treatment may become necessary.

Practitioners and researchers must always rely on their own experience and knowledge in evaluating and using any information, methods, compounds, or experiments described herein. In using such information or methods they should be mindful of their own safety and the safety of others, including parties for whom they have a professional responsibility.

With respect to any drug or pharmaceutical products identified, readers are advised to check the most current information provided (i) on procedures featured or (ii) by the manufacturer of each product to be administered, to verify the recommended dose or formula, the method and duration of administration, and contraindications. It is the responsibility of practitioners, relying on their own experience and knowledge of their patients, to make diagnoses, to determine dosages and the best treatment for each individual patient, and to take all appropriate safety precautions.

To the fullest extent of the law, neither the Publisher nor the authors, contributors, or editors, assume any liability for any injury and/or damage to persons or property as a matter of products liability, negligence or otherwise, or from any use or operation of any methods, products, instructions, or ideas contained in the material herein.

Library of Congress Cataloging-in-Publication Data

Rosenthal, Ken S.
  Rapid review microbiology and immunology / Ken S. Rosenthal, Michael J. Tan.—3rd ed.
    p. ; cm.—(Rapid review)
  Rev. ed. of: Microbiology and immunology / Ken S. Rosenthal, James S. Tan. 2nd ed. c2007.
  Includes index.
  ISBN 978-0-323-06938-0
  1. Medical microbiology—Outlines, syllabi, etc. 2. Medical microbiology—Examinations, questions, etc. 3. Immunology—Outlines, syllabi, etc. 4. Immunology—Examinations, questions, etc. 5. Physicians—Licenses—United States—Examinations—Study guides. I. Tan, Michael J. II. Rosenthal, Ken S. Microbiology and immunology. III. Title. IV. Title: Microbiology and immunology. V. Series: Rapid review series.
  [DNLM: 1. Viruses—Examination Questions. 2. Bacteria—Examination Questions. 3. Communicable Diseases—immunology—Examination Questions. QW 18.2 R815r 2011]
  QR46.R7535 2011
  616.9'041—dc22

2009045667

Acquisitions Editor: James Merritt
Developmental Editor: Christine Abshire
Publishing Services Manager: Hemamalini Rajendrababu
Project Manager: Gopika Sasidharan
Design Direction: Steve Stave

Printed in the United States of America

Last digit is the print number: 9 8 7 6 5 4 3 2

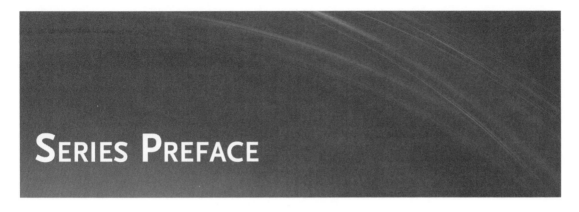

SERIES PREFACE

The First and Second Editions of the *Rapid Review Series* have received high critical acclaim from students studying for the United States Medical Licensing Examination (USMLE) Step 1 and consistently high ratings in *First Aid for the USMLE Step 1*. The new editions will continue to be invaluable resources for time-pressed students. As a result of reader feedback, we have improved upon an already successful formula. We have created a learning system, including a print and electronic package, that is easier to use and more concise than other review products on the market.

SPECIAL FEATURES

Book

- **Outline format:** Concise, high-yield subject matter is presented in a study-friendly format.
- **High-yield margin notes:** Key content that is most likely to appear on the exam is reinforced in the margin notes.
- **Visual elements:** Full-color photographs are utilized to enhance your study and recognition of key pathology images. Abundant two-color schematics and summary tables enhance your study experience.
- **Two-color design:** Colored text and headings make studying more efficient and pleasing.

New! Online Study and Testing Tool

- A minimum of **350 USMLE Step 1–type MCQs:** Clinically oriented, multiple-choice questions that mimic the current USMLE format, including high-yield images and complete rationales for all answer options.
- **Online benefits:** New review and testing tool delivered via the USMLE Consult platform, the most realistic USMLE review product on the market. Online feedback includes results analyzed to the subtopic level (discipline and organ system).
- **Test mode:** Create a test from a random mix of questions or by subject or keyword using the timed **test mode.** USMLE Consult simulates the actual test-taking experience using NBME's FRED interface, including style and level of difficulty of the questions and timing information. Detailed feedback and analysis shows your strengths and weaknesses and allows for more focused study.
- **Practice mode:** Create a test from randomized question sets or by subject or keyword for a dynamic study session. The **practice mode** features unlimited attempts at each question, instant feedback, complete rationales for all answer options, and a detailed progress report.
- **Online access:** Online access allows you to study from an internet-enabled computer wherever and whenever it is convenient. This access is activated through registration on www.studentconsult.com with the pin code printed inside the front cover.

Student Consult

- **Full online access:** You can access the complete text and illustrations of this book on www.studentconsult.com.
- **Save content to your PDA:** Through our unique Pocket Consult platform, you can clip selected text and illustrations and save them to your PDA for study on the fly!
- **Free content:** An interactive community center with a wealth of additional valuable resources is available.

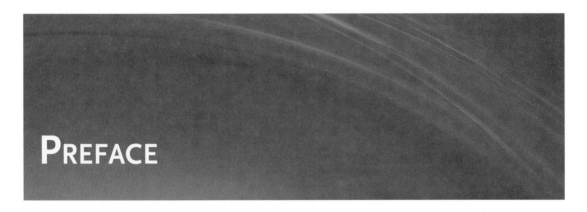

PREFACE

Rapid Review Microbiology and Immunology, Third Edition provides updated, relevant material in an easy-to-read and understandable outline format, with excellent figures and summary tables to help you SEE and REMEMBER the concepts. KEY WORDS and CONCEPTS are highlighted to promote **RAPID** recognition and recall. For **RAPID** study, the relevant facts for all of the microbes are summarized in tables. TRIGGER WORDS for each of the microbes spark **RAPID** word associations on exam questions and in the clinic. Case scenarios and clinical presentations are offered to help you think in terms of the USMLE Step 1 exam. Most importantly, questions are provided online to reinforce your knowledge and help you practice taking the exam. These questions have been carefully written, reviewed, and edited for content to emulate USMLE Step 1 questions. Detailed answers continue the review process.

Rapid Review Microbiology and Immunology can be an important part of your training for the USMLE exam. Success on the exam requires more than a thorough knowledge of the subject. As with any big challenge—a race, match, or championship game—a positive winning attitude as well as mental, physical, and emotional preparedness are necessary. Make sure to go into the exam strong. Good luck on the examination.

ACKNOWLEDGMENT OF REVIEWERS

The publisher expresses sincere thanks to the medical students and faculty who provided many useful comments and suggestions for improving both the text and the questions. Our publishing program will continue to benefit from the combined insight and experience provided by your reviews. For always encouraging us to focus on our target, the USMLE Step 1, we thank the following:

Bhaswati Bhattacharya, MD, MPH, Columbia University, Rosenthal Center for Complementary and Alternative Medicine

Natasha L. Chen, University of Maryland School of Medicine

Patricia C. Daniel, PhD, University of Kansas Medical Center

Kasey Edison, University of Pittsburgh School of Medicine

Charles E. Galaviz, University of Iowa College of Medicine

Georgina Garcia, University of Iowa College of Medicine

Dane A. Hassani, Rush Medical College

Harry C. Kellermier, Jr., MD, Northeastern Ohio Universities College of Medicine

Joan Kho, New York Medical College

Michael W. Lawlor, Loyola University Chicago Stritch School of Medicine

Ronald B. Luftig, PhD, Louisiana State University Health Science Center

Christopher Lupold, Jefferson Medical College

Michael J. Parmely, PhD, University of Kansas Medical Science Center

Mrugeshkumar K. Shah, MD, MPH, Tulane University Medical School, Harvard Medical School/Spaulding Rehabilitation Hospital

John K. Su, MPH, Boston University School of Medicine, School of Public Health

Ryan Walsh, University of Illinois College of Medicine at Peoria

ACKNOWLEDGMENTS

This book is dedicated to our parents, who were excellent parents, teachers, and role models. Joseph and Muriel Rosenthal instilled a love of learning and teaching in their children and students. James Tan, MD, previous co-author of this book, was an excellent infectious disease specialist, physician, colleague, father, and mentor. June Tan is a perpetual source of support who raised three children in a medical family while maintaining her own endeavors. We also want to acknowledge our students and patients from whom we learn and who hold us to very high standards.

This book could not have been written without the expert editing of the first edition by Susan Kelly, Ruth Steyn, and Donna Frasseto. We wish to also thank Jim Merritt, Ed Goljian, Christine Abshire, Hemamalini Rajendrababu, and Gopika Sasidharan for their work on this edition. Finally, we want to thank our families, Judy, Joshua, and Rachel Rosenthal and Jackie Peckham and Jameson Tan who allowed us to disappear and work on this project.

CONTENTS

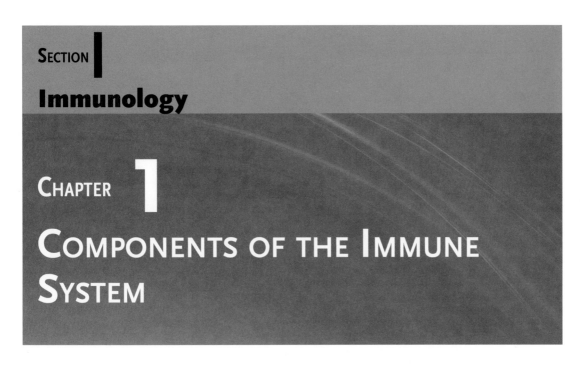

CHAPTER 1

COMPONENTS OF THE IMMUNE SYSTEM

I. **Types and Goals of Host Defense Mechanisms**
  A. **Nonspecific (innate) immunity**
    • Involves antigen-independent mechanisms that provide the first defense against pathogens
    1. Anatomic and physiologic barriers exclude many microbes (Fig. 1-1).
    2. Inflammation and the resulting increase in vascular permeability permit leakage of antibacterial serum proteins (acute phase proteins) and phagocytic cells into damaged or infected sites.
    3. Phagocytosis, initially by neutrophils and later by macrophages, destroys whole microorganisms, especially bacteria.
    4. Complement system can be activated by microbial surfaces (alternate and lectin pathways) and by immune complexes (classical pathway).
  B. **Specific (acquired) immunity**
    • Results from random recombination of immunoglobulin and T cell receptor genes within lymphocytes and selection by **antigen-dependent** activation, proliferation **(clonal expansion)**, and differentiation of these cells to resolve or control infections.
    1. **Defining properties**
      • **Antigenic specificity**
        a. Ability to discriminate subtle molecular differences among molecules
      • **Diversity**
        a. Ability to recognize and respond to a vast number of different antigens
      • **Memory**
        a. Ability to "remember" prior encounter with a specific antigen and mount a more effective secondary response
      • **Self and nonself recognition**
        a. Lack of response **(tolerance)** to self antigens but response to foreign antigens
    2. **Functional branches**
      • **Cell-mediated immune (CMI) response** effected by **T lymphocytes** (see Chapter 2)
      • **Humoral immune response** effected by **antibodies** expressed on the surface of **B lymphocytes** and secreted by B lymphocytes and terminally differentiated B lymphocytes called **plasma cells** (see Chapter 3)
II. **Immune Organs**
  A. **Primary**
    1. Thymus is the site for maturation of T cells
    2. Bone marrow and fetal liver are the sites for maturation of B cells
  B. **Secondary**
    1. Lymph node (see Chapter 4, Fig. 4-1)
      • Site where immune response is initiated
      • Swollen lymph node denotes stimulation of immunity and cell growth.

Margin notes:

Innate immunity: antigen independent; first defense

Innate protections are immediate.

Innate protections may be triggered by microbial structures.

Specific immunity: antigen dependent

Activation, expansion, and movement of specific immunity to an infection takes time.

CMI response: T cells

Humoral response: B cells → plasma cells → antibodies

Thymus: maturation of T cells

Bone marrow, fetal liver: maturation of B cells

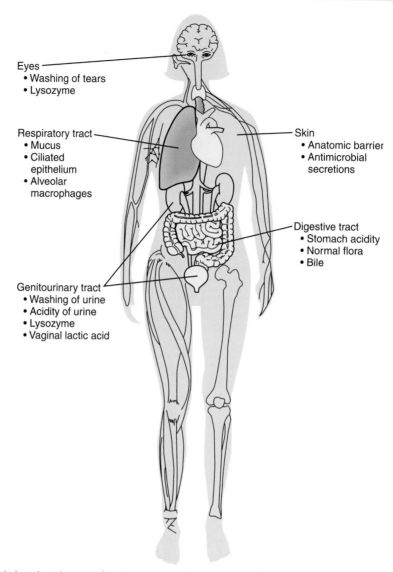

Eyes
• Washing of tears
• Lysozyme

Respiratory tract
• Mucus
• Ciliated epithelium
• Alveolar macrophages

Skin
• Anatomic barrier
• Antimicrobial secretions

Digestive tract
• Stomach acidity
• Normal flora
• Bile

Genitourinary tract
• Washing of urine
• Acidity of urine
• Lysozyme
• Vaginal lactic acid

1-1: Anatomic and physiologic barriers of the human body. These and other elements of innate immunity prevent infection by many microbes.

- Dendritic cells and antigen from the periphery enter through the **afferent lymphatic vessel** into the **medulla** where the **T cells** reside.
- B cells wait in follicles for T cell activation, and antigenically stimulated B cells are in the **germinal centers** within the follicles.

B cells: located in germinal centers

2. Spleen
   - Site of immune responses to antigens in blood
   - Filter for dead erythrocytes and microbial particulates, especially encapsulated bacteria
3. Mucosa-associated lymphoid tissue (MALT)
   - Intestine
     a. Gut-associated lymphoid tissue (GALT)
       - M cell in mucosal epithelium is the door keeper to Peyer patch.
       - Peyer patch is a mini lymph node.
       - Intraepithelial lymphocytes patrol mucosal lining.

M cell: "door keeper" to Peyer patches

   - Tonsils and adenoids
     a. Highly populated by B cells

III. **Immune System Cells**
   A. **Overview**
   1. Immune cells can be distinguished by morphology, cell surface markers, and/or function (Box 1-1, Fig. 1-2, and Tables 1-1 and 1-2).
   2. Development of the various cell lineages from stem cells in the bone marrow requires specific hematopoietic growth factors, cytokines, and/or cell-cell interactions (Fig. 1-3).

BOX 1-1 "MUST-KNOWS" FOR EACH CELL: CARP

Cell surface determinants
Actions: activate, suppress, and kill
Role of cell and type of response
Products: cytokines, antibodies, etc.

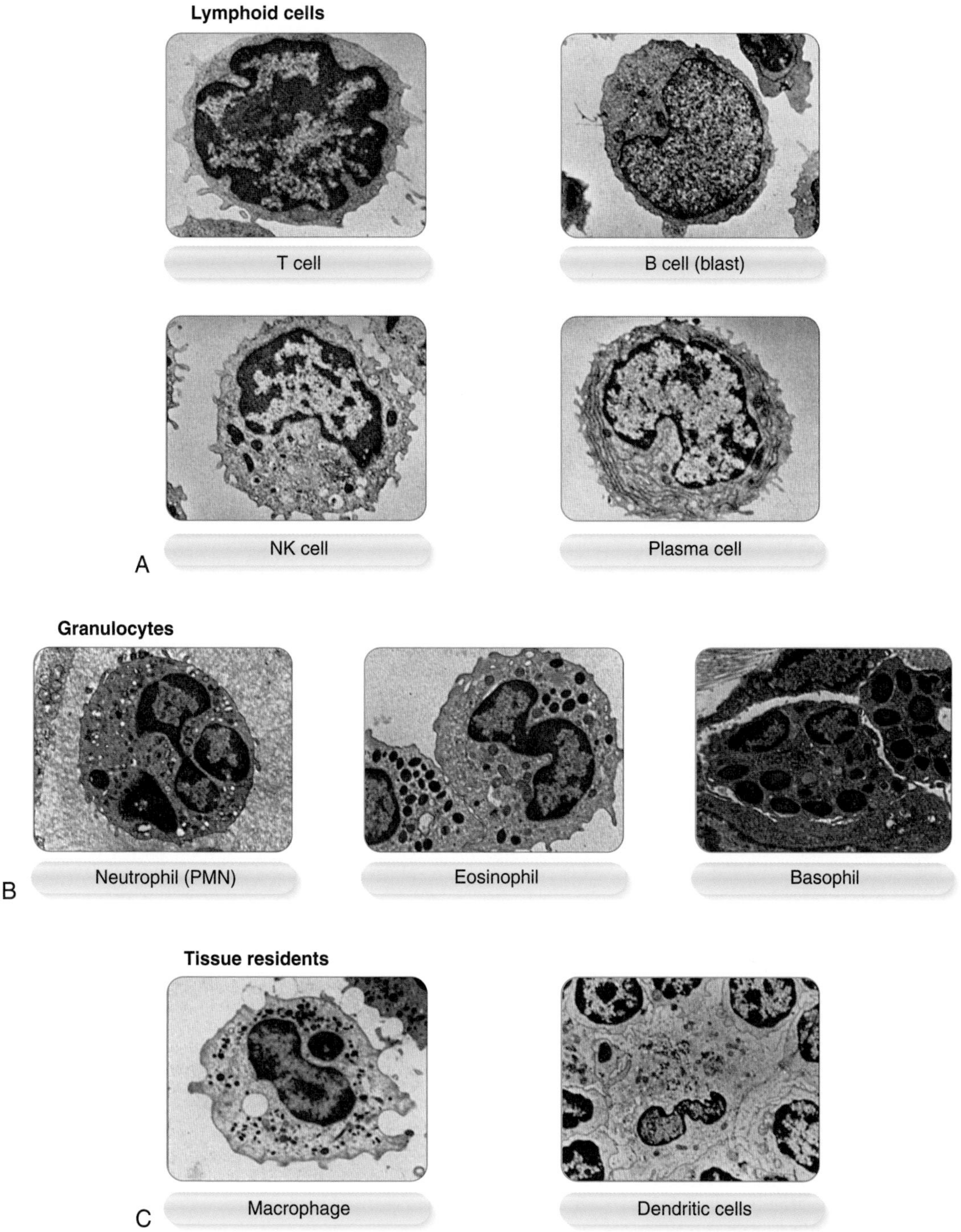

Lymphoid cells
T cell
B cell (blast)
NK cell
Plasma cell
A
Granulocytes
Neutrophil (PMN)
Eosinophil
Basophil
B
Tissue residents
Macrophage
Dendritic cells
C

1-2: Morphology of primary cells involved in the immune response. **A,** T and B lymphocytes are the only cells that possess antigen-binding surface molecules. Antigen-stimulated B cells proliferate and differentiate into plasma cells, the body's antibody-producing factories. Natural killer (NK) cells are large granular lymphocytes that lack the major B and T cell markers. **B,** Granulocytes can be distinguished by their nuclear shapes and cell type–specific granules. **C,** Macrophages and dendritic cells are phagocytic and function in presenting antigen to T cells.

TABLE 1-1 **Major Cells of the Immune System**

CELL TYPE	MORPHOLOGY	SURFACE MARKERS	PRIMARY FUNCTIONS
Granulocytes			
Neutrophils (PMNs)	Multilobed nucleus, small granules, band form (immature)	IgG receptors IgM receptors C3b receptors	Phagocytose and kill bacteria nonspecifically Mediate ADCC of Ab-coated bacteria
Eosinophils	Bilobed nucleus, numerous granules with core of major basic protein	IgE receptors	Involved in allergic reactions Mediate ADCC of parasites
Basophils, mast cells	Irregular nucleus, relatively few large granules	IgE receptors	Release histamine and other mediators of allergic and anaphylactic responses
Myeloid Cells			
Macrophages*	Large, granular mononuclear phagocytes present in tissues	**Class II MHC** IgG receptors IgM receptors C′ receptors Toll-like receptors	Phagocytose and digest bacteria, dead host cells, and cellular debris Mediate ADCC of Ab-coated bacteria Process and present Ag to CD4 T$_H$ cells Secrete cytokines that promote acute phase and T cell responses
Dendritic cells	Granular, mononuclear phagocytes with long processes; found in skin (Langerhans cells), lymph nodes, spleen	High levels of **class II MHC,** B7 coreceptors Toll-like receptors	Process and present Ag to T cells Secrete cytokines that promote and direct T cell response Required to initiate T cell response
Lymphocytes			
B cells	Large nucleus, scant cytoplasm, agranular	**Membrane Ig Class II MHC** C3d receptor (CR2 or CD21)	Process and present Ag to class II MHC-restricted T cells On activation, generate memory B cells and plasma cells
Plasma cells	Small nucleus, abundant cytoplasm		Synthesize and **secrete Ab**
Helper T cells (T$_H$ cells)	Large nucleus, scant cytoplasm	**CD4 TCR complex** CD2, CD3, CD5	Recognize Ag associated with class II MHC molecules On activation, generate memory T$_H$ cells and cytokine-secreting effector cells
Cytotoxic T (T$_C$) cells)	Large nucleus, scant cytoplasm	**CD8 TCR complex** CD2, CD3, CD5	Recognize Ag associated with class I MHC molecules On activation, generate memory T$_C$ cells and effector cells (CTLs) that destroy virus-infected, tumor, and foreign graft cells
Memory B or T cells	Large nucleus, scant cytoplasm	**CD45RO** Usual B or T cell markers	Generated during primary response to an Ag and mediate **more rapid secondary response** on subsequent exposure to same Ag
Natural killer cells	Large granular lymphocytes	IgG receptors KIRs, CD16 **None of usual B or T cell markers**	Kill virus-infected and tumor cells by perforin or Fas-mediated, MHC-independent mechanism Kill Ab-coated cells by ADCC

* Activation of macrophages, by interferon-γ or other cytokines, enhances all their activities and leads to secretion of cytotoxic substances with antiviral, antitumor, and antibacterial effects.
Ab, antibody; ADCC, antibody-dependent cell-mediated cytotoxicity; Ag, antigen; C′, complement; CTL, cytotoxic T lymphocyte; Ig, immunoglobulin; KIR, killer cell immunoglobulin-like receptor; MHC, major histocompatibility complex; TCR, T cell receptor (antigen specific).

B. Antigen-recognizing lymphoid cells

1. B lymphocytes express **surface antibodies** that recognize antigen.
2. T lymphocytes express **T cell receptors (TCRs)** that recognize antigenic peptides only when displayed on a major histocompatibility complex (MHC) molecule (Box 1-2).
   - Helper T (T$_H$) cells
     a. CD4 surface marker
     b. Class II MHC restricted
   - Cytolytic T (T$_C$) cells
     a. CD8 surface marker
     b. Class I MHC restricted
3. Memory cells are generated during clonal expansion of antigen-stimulated lymphocytes.

TABLE 1-2 **Selected CD Markers of Importance**

MARKER	FUNCTION	CELL EXPRESSION
CD1	Class I MHC–like, nonpeptide antigen presentation	DCs, macrophages
CD2 (LFA-3R)	Erythrocyte receptor	T cells
CD3	TCR subunit (γ, δ, ω, ζ, η); activation	T cells
CD4	Class II MHC receptor	T cell subset, monocytes, some DCs
CD8	Class I MHC receptor	T cell subset, some DCs
CD14	LPS-binding protein	Myeloid cells (DCs, monocytes, macrophages)
CD21 (CR2)	C3d complement receptor, EBV receptor, B cell activation	B cells
CD25	IL-2 receptor (α chain), early activation marker, marker for regulatory cells	Activated T cells, regulatory T cells
CD28	Receptor for B-7 costimulation: activation	T cells
CD40	Stimulation of B cells, DCs, and macrophages	B cells, macrophages
CD40 L	Ligand for CD40	T cells
CD80 (B7-1)	Costimulation of T cells on APCs	DC, macrophages, B cells
CD86 (B7-2)	Costimulation of T cells on APCs	DC, macrophages, B cells
CD95 (Fas)	Apoptosis inducer	Many cells
CD152 (CTLA-4)	Receptor for B-7; tolerance	T cells
CD178 (FasL)	Fas ligand: apoptosis inducer	Killer T and NK cells
Adhesion Molecules		
CD11a	LFA-1 (α chain)	
CD29	VLA (β chain)	
VLA-1, VLA-2, VLA-3	α Integrins	T cells
VLA-4	α_4-Integrin homing receptor	T cells, B cells, monocytes
CD50	ICAM-3	Lymphocytes and leukocytes
CD54	ICAM-1	
CD58	LFA-3	

APCs, antigen-presenting cell; CTLA, cytotoxic T lymphocyte–associated protein; DC, dendritic cell; EBV, Epstein-Barr virus; ICAM, intercellular adhesion molecule; IL, interleukin; LFA, leukocyte function–associated antigen; LPS, lipopolysaccharide; MHC, major histocompatibility complex; NK, natural killer; TCR, T cell antigen receptor; VLA, very late activation (antigen).

C. Granulocytes
1. Neutrophils (polymorphonuclear leukocytes)
   - Strongly phagocytic cells important in controlling bacterial infections
   - Normally are **first cells** to arrive at site of infection and have a short life span and rapid turnover (apoptosis)
2. Eosinophils
   - Weakly phagocytic
   - Main role in allergic reactions and destruction of parasites
3. Basophils and mast cells
   - Nonphagocytic granulocytes that possess cell surface receptors for immunoglobulin E (IgE)
   - Mediate **allergic** and **antiparasitic responses** due to release of **histamine** and other mediators following activation

D. Myeloid cells
   - **Monocytes** are released from the bone marrow, circulate in the blood, and enter tissues where they **mature into dendritic cells or macrophages.**
1. Dendritic cells (DCs)
   - Found in various tissues (e.g., Langerhans cells of the skin), peripheral blood, and lymph
   - Have long arm-like processes
   - **Required to initiate** an immune response and very efficient at presenting antigen to both CD4 T$_H$ and CD8 T$_C$ cells
   - Secrete cytokines that direct the nature of the T cell response (e.g., IL-12 for T$_H$1)

Neutrophil: phagocytic; first line of cellular defense

Neutrophils die and make pus.

Eosinophils: allergic reactions; destroys intestinal worms.

Basophils, mast cells: release histamine

DCs initiate, direct and control the T cell response through interactions and cytokines.

Langerhans cells: DCs of skin; process antigens

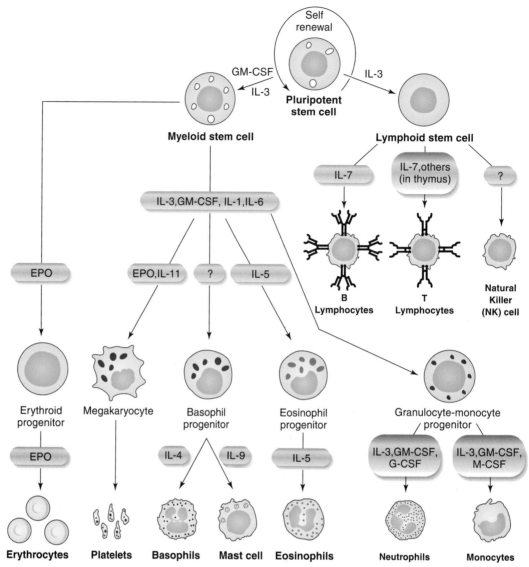

1-3: Overview of hematopoiesis and involvement of key hematopoietic factors. The pluripotent stem cell is the source of all hematopoietic cells, which develop along two main pathways—the lymphoid and the myeloid paths of development. Factors secreted from bone marrow stromal cells maintain a steady-state level of hematopoiesis that balances the normal loss of blood cells. Cytokines produced by activated macrophages and helper T (T_H) cells in response to infection induce increased hematopoietic activity. EPO, erythropoietin; G-CSF, granulocyte colony-stimulating factor; GM-CSF, granulocyte-macrophage colony-stimulating factor; IL, interleukin; M-CSF, macrophage colony-stimulating factor.

BOX 1-2 MAJOR HISTOCOMPATIBILITY COMPLEX

All MHC molecules have **antigen-binding sites** that noncovalently bind short peptides produced by intracellular degradation of proteins. Recognition of MHC-bound peptides derived from foreign proteins triggers immune responses by T cells. **CD8** cytolytic T cells recognize antigens associated with **class I MHC** molecules, which are expressed by **all nucleated cells. CD4** helper T cells recognize antigens associated with **class II MHC** molecules, which are expressed by a limited number of cell types, collectively called **antigen-presenting cells.**

Macrophages:
follow neutrophils
in inflammation;
phagocytose; process
antigen

2. Macrophages
- Help to initiate early innate immune response (Table 1-3)
- Secrete numerous cytokines that promote immune responses (Box 1-3)
- Secrete antibacterial substances, inflammatory mediators, and complement
- Phagocytose and inactivate microbes (see later in this chapter)
- Present antigen associated with class II MHC molecules to CD4 T_H cells

TABLE 1-3 **Macrophages Versus Neutrophils**

PROPERTY	NEUTROPHILS	MACROPHAGES
	First to arrive at local site of infection or tissue damage	Arrive later
Phagocytic activity	Yes	Yes
Bacterial destruction	Very effective	Less effective unless activated
Oxidative burst	Yes	Only when activated
Antigen presentation on class II MHC molecules	No	Yes
Cytokine secretion	No	Yes (IL-1, IL-6, IL-12, TNF-α, etc)
Antibody-dependent cell-mediated cytotoxicity	Yes	Yes
Life span	Short	Long

IL, interleukin; MHC, major histocompatibility complex; TNF-α, tumor necrosis factor-α.

BOX 1-3 KEY CYTOKINES SECRETED BY DENDRITIC CELLS AND MACROPHAGES

In response to infection and inflammation, dendritic cells and macrophages secrete **IL-1, TNF-α, and IL-6,** which activate **acute phase responses.** All three cytokines are endogenous **pyrogens** (induce fever), stimulate liver production of acute phase proteins (e.g., complement components, clotting factors, and C-reactive protein), increase vascular permeability, and promote lymphocyte activation.

Dendritic cells and macrophages also secrete **IL-12** in response to appropriate TLR stimuli, which promotes release of interferon-γ (macrophage-activating factor) by certain T_H cells (discussed in Chapter 2). Activation of macrophages increases their phagocytic, secretory, and antigen-presenting activity.

---

3. Activated ("angry") macrophages: larger and exhibit enhanced antibacterial, inflammatory, and antigen-presenting activity
   - Activation is initiated by phagocytosis of particulate antigens and enhanced by interferon-γ produced by T cells and natural killer cells.

E. Natural killer (NK) cells
- These large granular lymphocytes lack the major B and T cell surface markers.
1. Targets of NK cell killing
   - Specificity of NK cells for virus-infected and tumor cells may depend on reduced expression of class I MHC molecules and alterations in surface carbohydrates on these target cells.
2. Mechanism of NK cell killing
   - Direct cytotoxicity involving contact with target cell and lysis by perforin-mediated mechanism similar to that used by T_C cells
     a. Perforin-mediated lysis by NK cells is **antigen independent** and **not MHC restricted,** whereas T_C cells only attack cells bearing specific antigenic peptides bound to a class I MHC molecule.
   - Fas (on target cell) and Fas ligand (on NK or T cell) killing of target cell through tumor necrosis factor receptor–like apoptosis pathway
   - Antibody-dependent cellular cytotoxicity (ADCC)
     a. Binding of Fc receptors on NK cells to **antibody-coated target cells** initiates killing.
     b. Neutrophils, eosinophils, and macrophages also exhibit ADCC.

IV. Complement System
  A. Overview
   1. The complement system consists of numerous serum and cell surface proteins that form an **enzymatic cascade.**
   2. Cleavage of inactive components converts them into **proteases** that cleave and activate the next component in the cascade.
  B. Complement pathways (Fig. 1-4)
   - The three complement pathways differ initially, but all form **C3 and C5 convertases** and ultimately generate a common **membrane attack complex (MAC).**
   1. **Alternate pathway** (properdin system) most commonly is activated by **microbial surfaces** and **cell surface components** (e.g., lipopolysaccharide and teichoic acid).
     - Generates **early, innate response** that does not require antibody for activation
   2. **Lectin pathway** interacts with mannose on bacterial, viral, and fungal surfaces.

Macrophages eat (phagocytize) and secrete (cytokines) but must be angry to kill.

Asplenic individuals are prone to infections with encapsulated bacteria.

NK cells: large granular lymphocytes; direct cytotoxicity; ADCC

NK cells provide an early, rapid defense against virus-infected and tumor cells.

NK cells and cytotoxic T cells have similar killing mechanisms, but NK killing is turned off by MHC, and cytotoxic T cells are targeted to MHC.

Complement is the earliest antibacterial response.

Complement kills, opens the vasculature (C3a, C4a, C5a), and attracts cell-mediated protections (C3a, C5a).

Activation of alternate and lectin pathways: microbial surfaces, cell surface components (e.g., endotoxin)

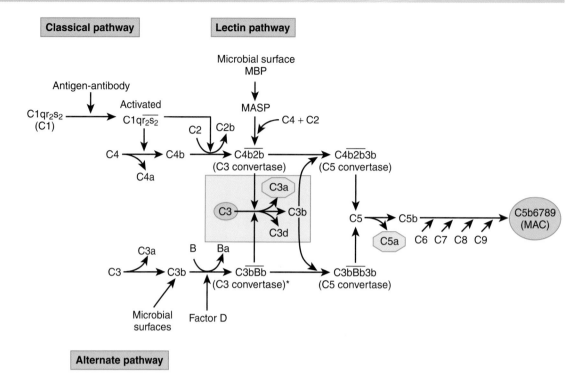

* Stabilized by properdin.

1-4: The classical, lectin and alternate complement pathways. *Thick arrows* indicate enzymatic or activating activity; *thin arrows* indicate reaction steps. The goal of these pathways is activation of C3 and C5 to provide chemoattractants and anaphylotoxins (C3a, C5a) and an opsonin (C3b), which adheres to membranes, and to initiate and anchor the membrane attack complex (MAC). MASP, mannose binding protein associated serine protease; MBP, mannose binding protein. *(From Murray PR, Rosenthal KS, Pfaller MA: Medical Microbiology, 6th ed. Philadelphia, Mosby, 2009.)*

Classical pathway: activated by antigen-antibody complexes

For complement cleavage products: *b* means binding (e.g., C3b); *a* means attract, "anaphylact" (e.g., C3a, C4a, C5a)

MAC: punctures cell membranes

3. **Classical pathway** is activated primarily by **antigen-antibody complexes** containing IgM or IgG.
   * Constitutes a major effector mechanism of humoral immunity
C. **Biologic activities of complement products**
   1. **MAC** acts as a molecular drill to puncture cell membranes.
      * Formation of MAC begins with **cleavage of C5 by C5 convertases** formed in all pathways (see Fig. 1-4).
      * Sequential addition of C6, C7, and C8 to C5b yields **C5b678,** a complex that **inserts stably into cell membranes** but has limited cytotoxic ability.
      * Binding of multiple C9 molecules produces a **highly cytotoxic MAC (C5b6789$_n$)** that forms holes in the cell membrane, killing the cell.
         a. C9 resembles the perforin molecule used by NK and T_C cells to permeabilize target cells.
   2. **Complement cleavage products** promote inflammatory responses, opsonization, and other effects summarized in Table 1-4.
      * Some of these activities depend on the presence of complement receptors on specific target cells.
D. **Regulation of complement**
   * Various regulatory proteins, which bacteria do not produce, protect host cells from complement activity.
   1. **C1 esterase inhibitor** prevents inappropriate activation of the classical pathway.
      * Also inhibits bradykinin pathway
   2. **Inactivators of C3 and C5 convertases** include decay-accelerating factor (DAF), factor H, and factor I.
   3. **Anaphylotoxin inhibitor** blocks anaphylactic activity of C3a and C5a.
E. **Consequences of complement abnormalities**
   1. **C1, C2, or C4 deficiency** (classical pathway); examples include:
      * Immune complex diseases such as **glomerulonephritis, systemic lupus erythematosus (SLE),** and **vasculitis**
      * **Pyogenic staphylococcal and streptococcal** infections

TABLE 1-4 **Major Biologic Activities of Complement Cleavage Products**

ACTIVITY	MEDIATORS	EFFECT
Opsonization of antigen	C3b and C4b	Increased phagocytosis by macrophages and neutrophils
Chemotaxis	C3a and C5a	Attraction of neutrophils and monocytes to inflammatory site
Degranulation	C3a and C5a (anaphylotoxins)	Release of inflammatory mediators from mast cells and basophils
Clearance of immune complexes	C3b	Reduced buildup of potentially harmful antigen-antibody complexes
B cell activation	C3d	Promotion of humoral immune response

2. **C3, factor B, or factor D deficiency** (alternate pathway); examples include:
   - Disseminated pyogenic infections, vasculitis, nephritis
3. C5 through C9 deficiency; examples include:
   - *Neisseria* species infections; some types of SLE
4. C1 esterase inhibitor deficiency (hereditary angioedema)
   - Marked by recurrent, acute attacks of skin and mucosal edema
5. DAF deficiency (paroxysmal nocturnal hemoglobinuria)
   - Complement-mediated intravascular hemolysis

V. **Phagocytic Clearance of Infectious Agents**
   A. **Mechanism of phagocytosis**
      1. Attachment of phagocytic cells to microbes, dead cells, and large particles is enhanced by opsonins (Fig. 1-5A).

Individuals with C1 to C4 deficiencies are prone to pyogenic infections; those with C5 to C9 deficiencies are prone to neisserial infections.

Hereditary angioedema: C1 esterase inhibitor deficiency

Paroxysmal nocturnal hemoglobinuria: deficiency of DAF

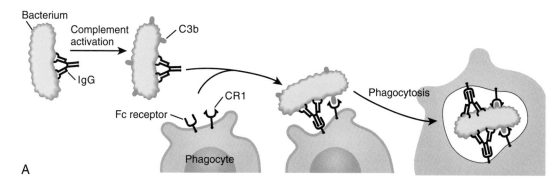

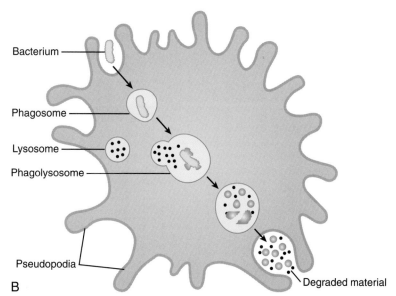

1-5: Phagocytic destruction of bacteria. **A,** Bacteria are opsonized by immunoglobulin M (IgM), IgG, C3b, and C4b, promoting their adherence and uptake by phagocytes. **B,** Hydrolytic enzymes, bactericides, and various reactive toxic compounds kill and degrade internalized bacteria (see Box 1-4). Some of these agents are also released from the cell surface in response to bacterial adherence and kill nearby bacteria.

BOX 1-4 MEDIATORS OF ANTIBACTERIAL ACTIVITY OF NEUTROPHILS AND MACROPHAGES

The killing activity of both neutrophils and macrophages is enhanced by highly reactive compounds whose formation by NADPH oxidase, NADH oxidase, or myeloperoxidase is stimulated by a powerful **oxidative burst** following phagocytosis of bacteria. Macrophages must be activated to produce these oxygen-dependent compounds.

Oxygen-Dependent Compounds	Oxygen-Independent Compounds
Hydrogen peroxide (H_2O_2)	Acids
Superoxide anion	Lysozyme (degrades bacterial peptidoglycan)
Hydroxyl radicals	Defensins (damage membranes)
Hypochlorous acid (HOCl)	Lysosomal proteases
Nitric oxide (NO)	Lactoferrin (chelates iron)

Opsonins: IgG, C3b

- C3b and C4b coated bacteria bind to CR1 receptors on phagocytes.
- IgM and IgG bound to surface antigens on microbes interact with Fc receptors on phagocytes.
2. Internalization and formation of phagolysosome promote destruction of bacteria (Fig. 1-5B).
3. Destructive agents kill internalized bacteria and also are released to kill bacteria in the vicinity of the phagocyte surface (Box 1-4).
   - Neutrophils are always active and ready to kill, but macrophages must be activated (see Table 1-3)

Oxygen-dependent myeloperoxidase system: most potent microbicidal system

   - Oxygen (respiratory) burst and glucose use lead to production of toxic oxygen, nitrogen, and chloride compounds that mediate oxygen-dependent killing.
   - Degradative enzymes and antibacterial peptides released from cytoplasmic granules mediate oxygen-independent killing.

B. Genetic defects in phagocytic activity
   - Defects in phagocyte killing and digestion of pathogens increase the risk for bacterial and yeast infection (Table 1-5).

C. Microbial resistance to phagocytic clearance
   - Many pathogens have mechanisms for avoiding phagocytosis or subsequent destruction, thereby increasing their virulence (see Chapters 6 and 19).

VI. Inflammation: Induced by tissue damage due to trauma, injurious agents, or invasion of microbes; Mediated primarily by innate and immune cells, cytokines, and other small molecules (Table 1-6).

A. Acute inflammation occurs in response to bacteria and physical injury.
   1. Localized response is characterized by increased blood flow, vessel permeability, and phagocyte influx (redness, swelling, and warmth).

Acute inflammation: chemical, vascular, cellular (neutrophil) components

      - Anaphylotoxins C3a and C5a stimulate mast cells to release histamine and serotonin (↑ vascular permeability) and prostaglandins (↑ vasodilation).

Classic signs of local acute inflammation: rubor (redness), calor (heat), tumor (swelling), and dolor (pain)

Inflammatory response and phagocytic killing are sufficient to contain and resolve many infections by extracellular bacteria.

TABLE 1-5 Inherited Phagocytic Disorders

DISEASE	DEFECT	CLINICAL FEATURES
Chédiak-Higashi syndrome	Reduced ability of phagocytes to store materials in lysosomes and/or release their contents	Recurrent pyogenic infections (e.g., *Staphylococcus* and *Streptococcus* species)
Chronic granulomatous disease	Reduced production of H_2O_2 and superoxide anion due to lack of NADPH oxidase (especially in neutrophils)	Increased susceptibility to catalase-producing bacteria (e.g., *Staphylococcus* species) and fungal infections
Job syndrome	Reduced chemotactic response by neutrophils and high immunoglobulin E levels	Recurrent cold staphylococcal abscesses; eczema; often associated with red hair and fair skin
Lazy leukocyte syndrome	Severe impairment of neutrophil chemotaxis and migration	Recurrent low-grade infections
Leukocyte adhesion deficiency	Defect in adhesion proteins reducing leukocyte migration into tissues and adherence to target cells	Recurrent bacterial and fungal infections; poor wound healing; delayed separation of umbilical cord
Myeloperoxidase deficiency	Decreased production of HOCl and other reactive intermediates	Delayed killing of staphylococci and *Candida albicans*

TABLE 1-6 Acute Versus Chronic Inflammation

	ACUTE	CHRONIC
Cells	Infection: neutrophils, macrophages Allergy: eosinophils, mast cells	Macrophages, lymphocytes
Mediators	Complement, kinins, prostaglandins, leukotrienes, acute phase cytokines, chemokines	Cytokines from macrophages and T cells
Lesion	Rash, pus, abscess	Rash, fibrosis, granuloma
Examples	Response to infection, hypersensitivity response	Autoimmunity, response to intracellular bacterial infection

- Endothelial damage activates plasma enzymes, leading to production of bradykinin, a potent vasoactive mediator, and formation of fibrin clot, which helps prevent the spread of infection.
- Initially **neutrophils** and later **macrophages** migrate into the affected tissue and are chemotactically attracted to invading bacteria.
    a. Subsequent destruction of bacteria by these phagocytic cells is often sufficient to control infection.
    b. Dead neutrophils are a major component of pus.
  2. **Systemic acute phase response** accompanies localized response (see Box 1-3).
B. **Chronic inflammation**
  1. Often follows acute inflammation but can be the only inflammatory response in certain **viral infections** and **hypersensitivity reactions**
  2. Infiltration of tissue with macrophages, lymphocytes and plasma cells, or eosinophils characterizes chronic inflammatory diseases.

CHAPTER 2
ROLE OF T CELLS IN IMMUNE RESPONSES

I. T Cell Surface Molecules

A. T cell receptor (TCR) complex

- Comprises an antigen-recognizing heterodimer associated with a multimeric activation unit (CD3) (Box 2-1; Fig. 2-1)
    1. All TCRs expressed by a single T cell are specific for the same antigen.
        - The gene and protein structures of TCRs resemble those of immunoglobulins.
    2. TCRs only recognize antigenic peptides bound to class I or II major histocompatibility complex (MHC) molecules.
        - α,β TCR is present on most T cells.
            a. Slightly different γ,δ TCR is present on different T cells.
        - The CD3 activation unit consists of several subunits (γ, δ, ε, and ζ) that are noncovalently linked to TCR.
            a. Binding of antigen to TCR activates a cascade of phosphorylation events, the first step in intracellular signaling leading to activation of T cells.

B. Accessory molecules

- Promote adhesion of T cells and/or signal transduction leading to T cell activation
    1. CD4 and CD8 coreceptors define two main functional subtypes of T cells.
        - CD4, present on helper T (T_H) cells, binds to class II MHC molecules on the surface of antigen-presenting cells (APCs).
        - CD8, present on cytolytic T (T_C) and suppressor T (T_S) cells, binds to class I MHC molecules on the surface of all nucleated cells.
    2. Adhesion molecules (e.g., CD2, LFA-1) help bind T cells to APCs and target cells or direct T cells to sites of inflammation and lymph nodes.
    3. Coreceptor activating molecules (e.g., CD28 and CTLA-4) transduce signals important in regulating functional responses of T cells.

II. Development and Activation of T Cells

A. Antigen-independent maturation

1. Begins in bone marrow and is completed in the thymus, generates immunocompetent, MHC-restricted, naive T cells
2. Diversity of antigenic specificity of TCRs results from rearrangement of V, D, and J gene segments during maturation (similar to rearrangement of immunoglobulin genes).
    - Each T cell possesses only one functional TCR gene and thus recognizes a single antigen (or a small number of related cross-reacting antigens).
3. Thymic selection eliminates developing thymocytes that react with self-antigens (including self MHC molecules).

TCR: associated with CD3 on T cells

TCRs resemble immunoglobulins but have to be presented with antigen by MHC.

CD4: binds to class II MHC

CD8: binds to class I MHC

BOX 2-1 "MUST-KNOWS" FOR EACH OF THE IMMUNE CELL RECEPTORS: CLAP

Cell it is on
Ligand it binds
Action it causes
Purpose in immunity

B. Antigen-dependent activation

1. Leads to proliferation and differentiation of naive T cells (clonal expansion) into effector cells and memory T cells (Fig. 2-2)
2. Effective stimulation requires primary and coactivating signals (fail-safe mechanism) that trigger intracellular signal transduction cascades, ultimately resulting in new gene expression (Fig. 2-3).
   - Signal 1 (primary): **specificity**—dependent on antigen and MHC
     a. Antigen-specific binding of TCR to antigenic peptide:MHC molecule on APC or target cell
     b. Binding of CD4 or CD8 coreceptor to MHC molecule on APC or target cell

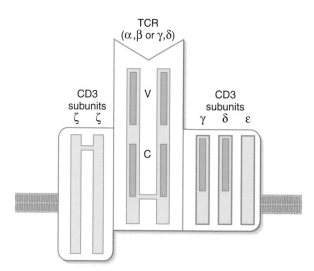

2-1: T cell receptor (TCR) complex. The TCR consists of α and β subunits (most common) or γ and δ subunits, which recognize antigen in association with major histocompatibility complex molecules. Differences in the variable (V) regions of the TCR subunits account for the diversity of antigenic specificity among T cells. Activation of T cells requires the closely associated CD3, a complex of four different types of subunits. C, constant region; V, variable region.

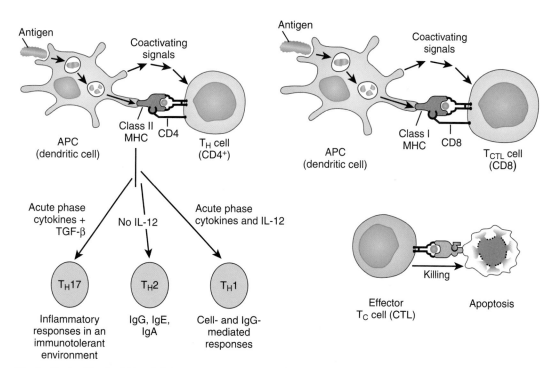

2-2: Overview of T cell activation. The dendritic cell (DC) initiates an interaction with CD4 or CD8 T cell through an MHC-peptide interaction with the T cell receptor. The DC provides an 11–amino acid peptide on the class II MHC, B7 coreceptor, and cytokines to activate CD4 T cells. Activation of CD8 T cell is through the class I MHC and 8– to 9–amino acid peptide plus the B7 coreceptor and cytokines. Presentation of antigen to CD4 T cells and cross presentation to CD8 T cells is shown in the diagram. The cytokines produced by the DC determine the type of T helper cell. Activated CD8 T cells can interact with and lyse target cells through T cell receptor recognition of peptide in class I MHC molecules on target cell. APC, antigen-presenting cell; CTL, cytotoxic T lymphocyte; Ig, immunoglobulin.

ACTIVATION OF CD4 T CELL

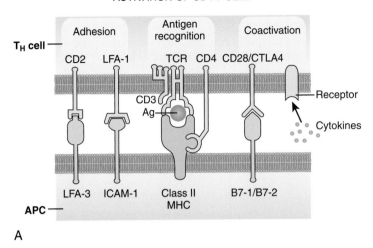

A

T CELL ACTIVATION OF B CELL OR APC

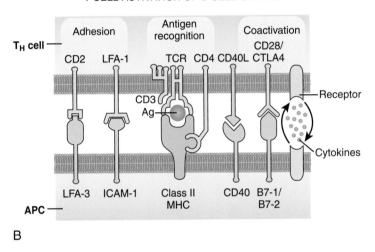

B

CTL RECOGNITION OF TARGET CELL

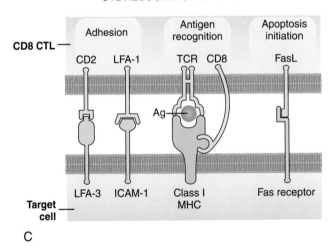

C

2-3: Cell-cell interactions that initiate and deliver T cell responses. **A,** Dendritic cells initiate specific immune responses by presenting antigenic peptides on class II MHC molecules to CD4 T cells with binding of coreceptors and release of cytokines. **B,** CD4 T cells activate B cells, macrophages, and dendritic cells (antigen-presenting cells [APCs]) by adding the CD40 ligand (CD40L) binding to CD40 and cytokines. **C,** CD8 cytotoxic lymphocytes (CTLs) recognize targets through T cell receptor and CD8 binding to antigenic peptides on class I major histocompatibility (MHC) molecules.

- Signal 2 (coactivating): **permission**—independent of antigen and MHC
    a. Lack of signal 2 results in tolerance due to anergy or apoptosis.
    b. Interaction between coreceptor activating molecules on T cell and APC or target cell (e.g., CD28-B7 interaction)
3. Signal 3 (determines nature of response): **direction**—cytokine from dendritic cell (DC) or APC
    - Determines the cytokine response and function of the T cell (T_H1, T_H2, T_H17, regulatory T [Treg] cell)
4. Adhesion molecules: selectin (E-, L-, P-), ICAM (-1, -2, -3, LFA-3 CD2), and integrin (VLA, LFA-1, CR3)
    - Strengthens cell-cell interactions; binds cells to epithelium in immune organs or facilitates migration and homing of cells.

C. **Antigen processing and presentation by class I and II MHC molecules (Fig. 2-4)**
    - Different pathways are used for degradation of intracellular and internalized extracellular protein trash. Peptides resulting from digestion of nonhost (foreign) protein trash are recognized by the T cell surveillance squad, which mounts an appropriate defense (Box 2-2).

Antigen specificity (TCR-MHC) + permission (CD28-B7) + direction (cytokine) = T cell activation

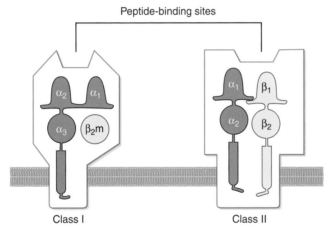

2-4: Structures of class I and II major histocompatibility complex (MHC) molecules. Class I molecules comprise a large α chain and a much smaller β_2-microglobulin molecule (β_2m), which is encoded by a gene located outside of the MHC. The class I peptide binding site is a pocket-like cleft (like pita bread) that holds peptides of 8 to 10 residues. Class II molecules comprise α and β chains of about equal size. The class II peptide binding site is an open-ended cleft (like a hotdog roll) that holds peptides with 12 or more residues. Noncovalent interactions hold the subunits together in both class I and II molecules.

BOX 2-2   CELLULAR TRASH AND T CELL POLICEMEN

Extracellular, or **exogenous,** trash (e.g., dead cells, intact microbes, and soluble proteins) is picked up by **APCs,** the body's garbage trucks. Once internalized, extracellular trash is degraded within **lysosomes** (garbage disposal), and the resulting peptides bind to **class II MHC** molecules, which then move to the cell surface. As the APCs circulate through lymph nodes, **CD4 T_H cell** police officers view the displayed peptide trash. The presence of foreign peptides activates the CD4 T cells to move, producing and secreting cytokines that alert other immune system cells to the presence of intruders within the lymph node and at the site of infection. **Cross-presented** antigens (to activate CD8 T cells) from dead cells containing from dead cells containing viral, tumor, or intracellular bacterial antigens leak out into the cytoplasm and are processed for presentation on class I MHC molecules, as described for endogenous proteins. DCs use this process to initiate the CD8 T cell response.

Intracellular (endogenous) proteins are marked as trash by attachment of multiple **ubiquitin** molecules and then degraded in large, multifunctional protease complexes called **proteasomes.** These cytosolic garbage disposals, present in all cells, generate peptides that pass through **TAP** transporters into the rough endoplasmic reticulum, where they bind to **class I MHC** molecules, which act like garbage cans. Once an MHC garbage can is filled with a peptide, it moves to the cell surface. **CD8 T_c** cells, like neighborhood policemen searching for contraband, continually check the class I garbage cans for **nonself** peptides derived from viral intruders, foreign grafts, and tumor cells. Such antigenic peptides alert CD8 T cells to attack and kill the offending cells.

Both normal self proteins and foreign proteins are processed and presented in the endogenous and exogenous pathways. However, **patrolling T cells normally recognize only foreign peptide–MHC complexes** and ignore the large number of self peptide–MHC complexes on cells.

1. Endogenous antigen (class I MHC) pathway generates and presents antigenic peptides derived from intracellular viral, foreign graft, and tumor cell proteins (Fig. 2-5A).
   - Recognition of displayed antigenic peptides directs CD8 T cell activation and killing.
2. Exogenous antigen (class II MHC) pathway generates and presents antigenic peptides derived from internalized microbes and extracellular proteins (Fig. 2-5B).
   - Recognition of displayed antigenic peptides triggers CD4 T cell activation.
3. Cross-presentation pathway in DCs allows extracellular proteins (e.g., virus, tumor) to activate CD8 T cells (Fig. 2-5C).

III. **T Cell Effector Mechanisms**

A. **Cytokine production by CD4 T cells**
   1. Overview
      - DCs activate the naive T cells and determine the type of T cell.
      - CD4 T cells differentiate into subsets of effector cells defined by the cytokines they secrete (Fig. 2-6; Table 2-1).
   2. T_H0 cells: presumed precursor of T_H1 and T_H2 subsets

Class II MHC presents phagocytized protein trash to CD4 T cells.

Class I MHC presents intercellular protein trash to CD8 T cells.

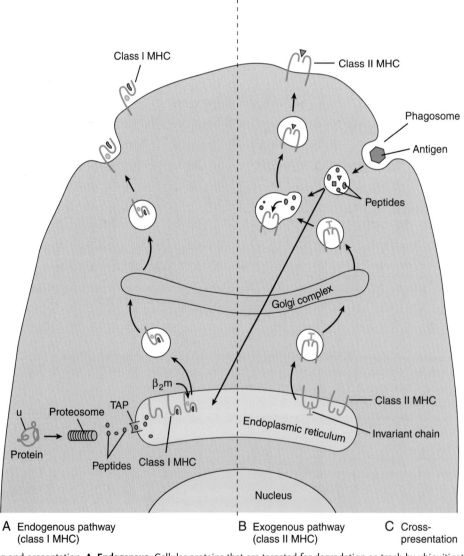

A Endogenous pathway (class I MHC)   **B** Exogenous pathway (class II MHC)   **C** Cross-presentation

2-5: Antigen processing and presentation. **A, Endogenous.** Cellular proteins that are targeted for degradation as trash by ubiquitination (u) are digested in the proteosome. Peptides of 8 or 9 amino acids pass through the transporter associated with processing (TAP) into the endoplasmic reticulum (ER). The peptide binds to a groove in the heavy chain of class I MHC molecules, the complex acquires β_2-microglobulin and is shuttled through the Golgi apparatus to the cell surface where the class I MHC molecule presents the peptide to CD8 T cells. **B, Exogenous.** Phagocytized proteins are degraded in endosomes, which fuse with vesicles that carry class II MHC molecules from the ER. The class II molecules acquire an invariant chain in the ER to prevent acquisition of a peptide in the ER. The class II molecules then acquire an 11– to 13–amino acid peptide, which is delivered to the cell surface for presentation to CD4 cells. **C, Cross-presentation.** Proteins phagocytized by antigen presenting cells (e.g., from viruses or tumor cells) are released into the cytoplasm and pass through the TAP to the ER, where they can fill class I MHC molecules to be presented to and activate CD8 T cells. (*From Murray PR, Rosenthal KS, Pfaller MA: Medical Microbiology, 6th ed. Philadelphia, Mosby, 2009, Fig. 11-8.*)

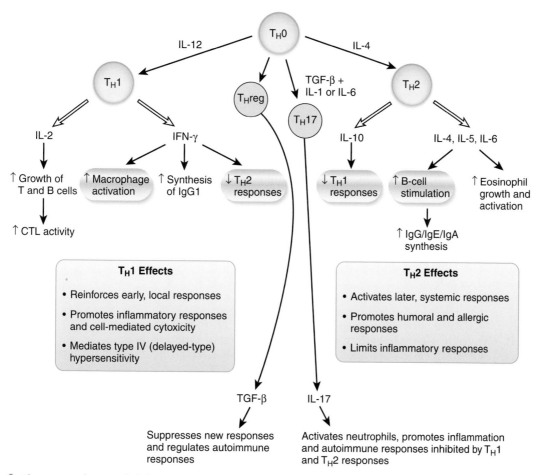

2-6: Characteristic features of T helper cell responses. CD4 T_H cells form subsets defined by the cytokines they produce. The T_H1 and T_H2 subsets and the responses they elicit are the best characterized. T_H17 responses are initiated by an acute phase response in a TGF-β tissue environment. Note that the responses control each other. CTL, cytotoxic T lymphocyte; IFN-γ, interferon-γ; Ig, immunoglobulin.

TABLE 2-1 **Cytokine: STAT (Source, Trigger, Action, Target)**

RESPONSE	CYTOKINE	SOURCE	TRIGGER	ACTION	TARGET
Acute phase	IL-1 TNF-α IL-6 IL-12	MP, DC	TLR stimulation by microbes	Fever, acute phase liver, sepsis, etc. Activate T_H1	Many cell types NK, CD4T
T_H1	IL-2 IFN-γ Lymphotoxin	CD4T CD4T, CD8T, NK CD4T	DC: MHC:Ag-TCR B7-CD28 IL-12	Lymphocyte growth MP activation IgG class switch cytotoxicity	B, T, NK cells MP, DC, B cell, T cell Target cell
T_H2	IL-4 IL-5 IL-10	CD4 T	DC: MHC:Ag-TCR B7-CD28	IgG, IgE, IgA class switch, inhibit T_H1 Inhibit T_H1 Stimulate B cell	B cell, T cell B cell T cell, MP, etc. B cell
T_H17	IL-17	CD4T	DC: MHC:Ag-TCR B7-CD28 IL6 + TGF-β, IL23	Neutrophil activation, autoimmune responses	Neutrophils and other cells
Treg	TGF-β, IL-10	CD4T and other cells	Unknown	Prevent naive T cell activation	T cell and other

Ag, antigen; DC, dendritic cell; IFN-γ, interferon-γ; IL, interleukin; MHC, major histocompatibility complex; MP, macrophage; NK, natural killer; TCR, T cell receptor; TGF-β, transforming growth factor-β; TLR, toll-like receptor; TNF-α, tumor necrosis factor-α; Treg, regulatory T cell.

3. T_H1 cells: characteristic responses mediated by interferon-γ (IFN-γ), lymphotoxin (LT) (tumor necrosis factor-β [TNF-β]), and interleukin-2 (IL-2)
   - IL-12 stimulates development and maintenance of T_H1 responses.
   - Promote cell-mediated and IgG antibody responses
   - Reinforce local, innate defense by activating macrophages and stimulating lymphocyte proliferation
   - Mediate type IV (delayed-type) hypersensitivity (see Chapter 4)
   - Important for intracellular infections (viral, tuberculosis), fungi, and tumors
4. T_H2 cells: characteristic responses mediated by IL-4, IL-5, IL-6, and IL-10
   - Activate humoral (antibody) responses
   - Promote allergic responses (type I hypersensitivity)
   - Stimulate antiparasitic eosinophil response (immunoglobulin E [IgE])
5. T_H17 cells: characteristic responses mediated by IL-17
   - Acute phase cytokines IL-6 and IL-1 in the presence of transforming growth factor-β (TGF-β) stimulate T_H17 response.
   - Important for anti-bacterial and anti-fungal infections responses
   - Activates neutrophils
   - Involved in autoimmune responses.
6. Treg cells
   - Produce TGF-β and IL-10
   - Suppress naive and inappropriate T cell responses
   - Can be overridden by appropriate dendritic cell and cytokine action

B. Cytotoxic T lymphocyte (CTL)-mediated killing of target cells
1. CD8 T_C cells are activated in lymph node by DCs, which cross-present phagocytosed or internal antigen on class I MHC molecules.
   - CD8 T_C cells kill virus-infected cells, tumor cells, and transplanted cells expressing antigen on class I MHC molecules.
   - Multiple interactions create an immune synapse between the CTL and target cell.
2. Cytotoxic substances released from granules in the CTL attack the target cell.
   - Perforin pokes holes in the membrane (similar to complement component C9).
   - Granzymes (serine esterases) and other toxic molecules that enter target cell through holes promote apoptosis.
3. Fas ligand on CTLs binds to Fas receptor on the target cell, stimulating apoptosis of target cell.

IV. MHC and the Immune Response to Transplanted Tissue (Box 2-3)
   A. Clinical classification of allograft rejection
   1. Hyperacute reaction is a rapid response (within hours) mediated by preexisting antibodies to transplanted alloantigens leading to complement-dependent damage to the graft.
      - Preexisting antibodies can arise owing to exposure to alloantigens during previous blood transfusions, transplantation, or multiple pregnancies.
   2. Acute reaction, mediated primarily by T cells, begins about 10 days after transplantation.
      - Massive infiltration of host cells, especially CTLs, destroys graft cells bearing alloantigens.

BOX 2-3   MAJOR HISTOCOMPATIBILITY COMPLEX AND ALLOANTIGENS

MHC molecules, also known as **human leukocyte antigens (HLAs)** in humans, are encoded by several highly polymorphic genes clustered together on chromosome 6. The α chain of **class I MHC** molecules is encoded by three separate genes—**HLA-A, HLA-B,** and **HLA-C.** (The gene for the $β_2$-microglobulin subunit of class I molecules is located outside the MHC complex.) **Class II MHC** molecules are encoded by the **HLA-DP, HLA-DQ,** and **HLA-DR** loci, each containing an α chain and β chain gene. Genes encoding TNF, some complement proteins, and several other proteins are also located within the MHC complex.

An individual inherits two sets of alleles **(haplotypes),** one from each parent. Each nucleated cell expresses both the maternal and the paternal alleles of all class I genes. Each APC also expresses all alleles of the class II genes. All nucleated cells thus express several HLA antigens on their surface. Given the numerous alleles of each HLA gene (>100), individuals can vary widely in their HLA haplotypes. The diversity of HLA molecules allows binding of diverse antigenic peptides for antigen presentation and activation of protective immune responses. **HLA differences trigger host rejection of transplanted tissue,** including allografts between individuals of the same species. Although red blood cells do not express HLA antigens, the ABO blood group glycoproteins function as alloantigens that can trigger antibody-mediated transfusion reactions.

3. Chronic reaction is marked by fibrosis and vascular injury developing months to years after transplantation.
   - Both cell-mediated mechanisms (e.g., chronic type IV hypersensitivity) and antibody-dependent mechanisms (e.g., complement-mediated cell damage) contribute to chronic reaction.

B. Graft-versus-host disease (GVHD)

1. Represents cell-mediated response mounted by lymphocytes in the graft against allogeneic host cells
2. Occurs when a graft containing many lymphocytes (e.g., bone marrow transplant) is transplanted into a host with a compromised immune system due to disease or treatment with immunosuppressive agents.

GVH reaction: jaundice, diarrhea, dermatitis

GVHD develops most commonly after allogeneic bone marrow transplantation.

C. Determination of tissue compatibility

1. HLA typing with anti-HLA antibodies tests for the presence of specific HLA antigens on host and potential donor cells.
2. Mixed lymphocyte reaction is a laboratory test of the reaction of host T cells to donor cells or for GVHD.

V. Cytokines

- Cytokines are low-molecular-weight proteins that induce characteristic cellular responses when they bind to specific receptors on their target cells.

A. Cytokine functions and sources (Table 2-2)

- The diverse functions of cytokines can be grouped into several broad classes, but many cytokines exert more than one class of effect.

TABLE 2-2 **Selected Cytokines**

CYTOKINE	MAJOR SOURCES	MAJOR EFFECTS AND TARGET CELLS
IL-1	Macrophage, dendritic cell, B cell	Acts on various nonimmune cells to initiate acute phase responses, fever Coactivates T_H cells
IL-2	T_H1 cell	Promotes growth and activation of T and B cells
IL-3	T_H cell	Stimulates hematopoiesis in bone marrow
IL-4	T_H2 cell, mast cell	Promotes growth and differentiation of B cells Enhances IgG and IgE synthesis Stimulates T_H2 response
IL-5	T_H2 cell	Promotes growth and differentiation of B cells Enhances IgA synthesis Stimulates growth and activation of eosinophils
IL-6	T_H2 cell, macrophage, dendritic cell	Promotes formation of plasma cells from B cells and antibody production Induces synthesis of acute phase proteins by liver cells
IL-10	T_H2 cell	Reduces T_H1 response by inhibiting IL-12 production by macrophages Reduces class II MHC expression by APCs
IL-12	Macrophage, dendritic cell, B cell	Stimulates formation of T_H1 cells Acts with IL-2 to promote formation of CTLs, activates NK cells
IL-17	T_H17 cell	Promotes neutrophil activation and inflammatory responses
IL-23	Dendritic cell	Promotes T_H17 responses
IFN-γ	T_H1 cell, NK cell	Enhances macrophage activity Inhibits T_H2 response Mediates aspects of type IV hypersensitivity
TNF-α	Macrophage and other cells	Has effects similar to IL-1 Promotes cachexia associated with chronic inflammation Is cytotoxic for tumor cells
TNF-β (lymphotoxin)	T_H1 cell, T_C cell	Enhances phagocytic activity of macrophages and neutrophils Is cytotoxic for tumor cells
TGF-β	Macrophage, Treg cell, B cell	Generally limits inflammatory response, enhances IgA synthesis
CXC-type chemokines (e.g., IL-8)	Macrophage, neutrophil, endothelium, fibroblast	Attracts neutrophils and promotes their migration into tissues
CC-type chemokines (e.g., MIP, RANTES)	Macrophage, neutrophil, endothelium, T cell	Attracts macrophages, eosinophils, basophils, and lymphocytes

APC, antigen-presenting cell; CTL, cytotoxic T lymphocyte; IFN, interferon; Ig, immunoglobulin; IL, interleukin; MHC, major histocompatibility complex; TGF, transforming growth factor; TNF, tumor necrosis factor.

1. Acute phase, innate, and inflammatory responses
   - Include IL-1, TNF-α, IL-6, IL-8, and chemokines
   - Secreted primarily by macrophages, DCs, and other nonlymphocytes
2. T_H17 antibacterial and inflammatory responses
   - Activated by IL-6, IL-1, TGF-β, and mediated by IL-17, IL-23
3. T_H1-related local cell-mediated and antibody immune responses
   - Activated by IL-12, TNF-α (secreted by DC and macrophage) and mediated by TNF-β, IFN-γ, IL-2
4. T_H2 humoral
   - IL-4, IL-5, IL-6, and IL-10
5. Treg immunosuppressive responses
   - TGF-β and IL-10 immunosuppressive cytokines
6. Stimulators of inducible hematopoiesis in response to infection
   - Include IL-3, IL-5, IL-6, and colony-stimulating factors
   - Produced by activated T_H cells, macrophages, and mesenchymal bone marrow cells

B. **Cytokine-related disorders**
   - Both the overexpression and underexpression of cytokines or their receptors can be pathogenic.
   1. Overproduction of IL-1, IL-6, and TNF causes a drop in blood pressure, shock, fever, and widespread blood clotting.
      - Endotoxin stimulation of dendritic cells and macrophages following infection by some gram-negative bacteria → bacterial septic shock
   2. Massive release of cytokines can affect many systems.
      - Superantigen stimulation of T cells by TSST-1 (a bacterial exotoxin) → toxic shock syndrome
   3. Inappropriate cytokine production dysregulates the immune system.
      - IL-6 secretion by cardiac myxoma (benign tumor) and other tumor cells leads to fever, weight loss, and increased antibody production.
      - Overproduction of IL-2 and the IL-2 receptor by T cells infected with the HTLV-1 retrovirus stimulates cell growth and contributes to development of adult T cell leukemia.

Cytokine storm can be due to excessive IL-1, TNF, and other cytokines adn lead to sepsis, and systemic failures.

Cardiac myxoma: IL-6 responsible for fever, weight loss, ↑ antibody synthesis

TAX protein product of the virus stimulates IL-2.

CHAPTER 3

IMMUNOGLOBULINS AND THEIR PRODUCTION BY B CELLS

I. Immunoglobulin Structure and Functions
- Immunoglobulins, synthesized by B cells, are antigen-binding glycoproteins (antibodies) that function in the recognition of and defense against antigens (Table 3-1).

A. Chain structure of immunoglobulins (Fig. 3-1A)
1. Each monomeric antibody molecule comprises two identical heavy (H) chains and two identical light (L) chains (κ or λ).
2. Antigenic specificity is determined by the amino acid sequence of the variable domains near the amino-terminal end of each chain.
   - Light chains contain one variable domain (V_L) and one constant domain (C_L).
     a. Sequence differences in the constant-region domain define two types of light chains: κ and λ.
   - Heavy chains contain one variable domain (V_H) and three or four constant domains (C_H1, C_H2, etc.).
     a. Sequence differences in the constant-region domains define five major types of heavy chains: μ, γ, δ, α, and ε.
     b. Each type of heavy chain can be expressed as a membrane-bound or membrane-soluble (secreted) form.

B. Functional regions of antibody molecules
1. Papain digestion cleaves the antibody molecule into two Fab fragments and one Fc fragment (Fig. 3-1B).
   - Pepsin digestion cleaves the antibody molecule into one $F(ab')_2$ and one Fc fragment.
2. The Fab portion contains variable region (V_L/V_H) domains, which bind antigen.
3. The Fc portion mediates antigen clearance by binding to complement and to Fc receptors on immune system cells (Table 3-2).
4. Membrane-spanning region is a heavy-chain carboxyl-terminal domain present only in immunoglobulins expressed on the surface of B cells.

C. Properties of immunoglobulin isotypes
- The five major immunoglobulin classes, or isotypes, exhibit different functions and roles in immunity (Table 3-3; Fig. 3-2).
1. IgM
   - Pentameric secreted IgM
     a. First secreted antibody produced during initial exposure to an antigen (primary response)
     b. Too large to spread into tissue from serum
     c. Held in multimeric form by J chain and disulfide bonds
     d. Effective antibacterial, complement-binding antibody
     e. Major component of rheumatoid factor (an autoantibody against the Fc portion of IgG)
     f. Most potent activator of the complement system
   - Monomeric IgM: present in membrane form on surface of B cells
2. IgD
   - Present almost exclusively in membrane form on B cells
   - Functions as antigen receptor in activation of B cells

Heavy chains define the specificity of the immunoglobulin.

Papain cleaves immunoglobulin G (IgG) into two monovalent Fab and one Fc fragment.

Pepsin cleaves IgG into one divalent $F(ab')_2$ and one Fc fragment.

Fab interacts with antigen, and Fc interacts with complement and immune cells.

Fc is sometimes referred to as: fragment, crystallizable.

IgM: first immunoglobulin produced after antigen exposure (e.g., bacteria)

IgM has capacity for binding 10 antigenic epitopes.

TABLE 3-1 **Antigen and Antibody Terminology**

TERM	DEFINITION
Adjuvant	Substance that **enhances immune response** to an antigen when administered with it; used to improve response to vaccines
Affinity	Binding strength of a **single variable region** of an antibody for a corresponding epitope on the larger antigen structure
Antigen	Substance that **binds to antibodies and T cell receptors.** Although most antigens are also immunogens, some small molecules are antigenic but not immunogenic.
Avidity	Combined binding strength of the **multiple interactions** between a multivalent antibody molecule and all the corresponding epitopes on an antigen
Epitope (antigenic determinant)	Region on an antigen molecule to which a **single antibody molecule or T cell receptor binds.** An antigen usually has multiple epitopes and thus can react with antibodies of different specificities.
Fab fragment	Portion of antibody molecule, produced by papain digestion, that contains a **single antigen-binding site.** All antibodies have two or more Fab regions and thus are **bivalent** or **multivalent.**
Fc fragment	Portion of antibody molecule, produced by papain digestion, that **fixes complement** and **binds to Fc receptors**; varies among immunoglobulin isotypes
Hinge region	**Flexible portion** of antibody heavy chains located **between the Fab and Fc regions** and containing intrachain disulfide bonds; present in **IgG, IgA, and IgD**
Immunogen	Substance capable of eliciting a specific immune response
Monoclonal antibody	Homogeneous antibody that **recognizes only one epitope**; produced by a **single clone** of plasma cells
Polyclonal antibody	Mixture of antibodies that **recognize different epitopes** on an antigen; produced by **multiple clones** of plasma cells in response to an antigen containing different epitopes. Natural antiserum to a microbial antigen is polyclonal.
Thymus-dependent antigens	Antigens that **require helper T cells** to induce antibody production (humoral response); most **protein antigens**
Thymus-independent antigens	Antigens possessing many repetitive structures (e.g., flagellin, polysaccharide, and **LPS**) that can induce antibody production (humoral response) **without helper T cells**

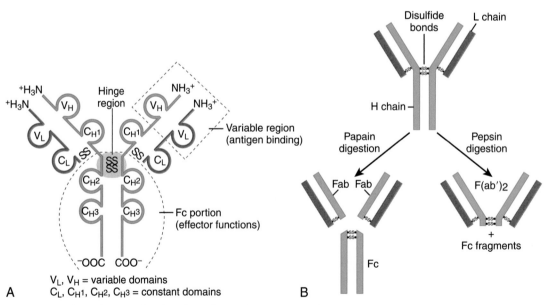

3-1: Structure of IgG, the most abundant class of antibody in serum. **A,** Chain and domain structure of IgG. Variable domains of light and heavy chains (V_L and V_H) contribute to the antigen-binding sites. Only the heavy chain constant domains C_H2 and C_H3 contribute to effector functions. **B,** Products of papain digestion of IgG. Fab fragments have one antigen-binding site **(monovalent),** whereas $F(ab')_2$ fragments have two antigen-binding sites **(bivalent).** Fc fragments interact with C1 complement and cellular Fc receptors.

TABLE 3-2 **Functions Mediated by Interactions with Antibody Fc Region**

FUNCTION	FC REGION INTERACTS WITH
Opsonization	Fc receptors on macrophages and neutrophils
Killing by means of ADCC	Fc receptors on neutrophils, macrophages, NK cells, eosinophils
Degranulation leading to allergic and antiparasitic responses	Fc receptors for IgE on mast cells
Activation of cells	Fc receptors on lymphocytes
Transmucosal movement	Fc receptors for dimeric IgA on epithelial cells
Activation of classical complement pathway leading to cell lysis (especially of bacteria), opsonization, and inflammatory response	Initial component of pathway (C1)

ADCC, antibody-dependent cellular cytotoxicity; NK, natural killer.

TABLE 3-3 **Immunoglobulin Isotypes**

	IgG	IgM	IgA	IgD	IgE
Property					
Heavy chain class	γ	μ	α	δ	ε
Subclasses	$\gamma_1, \gamma_2, \gamma_3, \gamma_4$	—	α_1, α_2	—	—
Molecular weight of secreted antibody (kDa)*	154	900	160-320	185	190
Maximal valence*	2	10	4	2	2
Percentage of total immunoglobulin in serum	75-85	5-10	5-15	<1	<1
Half-life in serum (days)	23	5	6	2-3	2-3
Activity[†]					
Site of action	Serum, tissue	Serum	Secretions	B cell surface	Mast cells
Primary effect	Antigen clearance from host **(secondary response)**	Antigen clearance from host **(primary response)**	Prevention of antigen crossing membranes	Activation of B cells	Type I hypersensitivity (anaphylaxis)
Complement activation	+	++	−	−	−
Opsonization	++	−	+	−	−
ADCC	+	−	−	−	+
Mast cell degranulation	−	−	−	−	++
Crosses placenta	+	−	−	−	−
Crosses mucous membranes	−	−	++	−	−

ADCC, antibody-dependent cellular cytotoxicity.
*IgG, IgD, and IgE always exist as monomers. IgM always exists as a pentamer. IgA exists as a monomer (160 kDa) or dimer.
[†]Relative activity levels: ++, high; +, moderate; −, none.

3. IgG
   - Major isotype of circulating (serum) antibody; longest half-life
   - Only isotype to cross placenta
   - Fixes complement; acts as opsonin; stimulates chemotaxis
   - Occurs as several subtypes, which have slightly different structures and vary slightly in their functional activity
      a. IgG1 is the most abundant subtype.
4. IgA
   - Predominant antibody isotype in external secretions (e.g., saliva, mucus, breast milk)
   - Found mostly as monomer in serum and as dimer in secretions (secretory IgA) held together by J chain
   - Acquires secretory component as it moves across epithelial cells (Fig. 3-3)
   - Prevents adherence of microbes to mucous membranes
5. IgE
   - Mediator of type I (immediate) hypersensitivity and promotes antiparasitic responses
   - Binds tightly to Fc receptor on mast cells

IgG is the most abundant immunoglobulin.

IgG: only immunoglobulin to cross the placenta

IgA: only immunoglobulin with a secretory component

IgE: mediator for type I hypersensitivity reactions

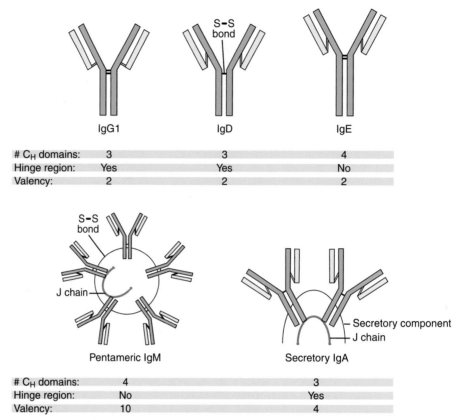

# C$_H$ domains:	3	3	4
Hinge region:	Yes	Yes	No
Valency:	2	2	2

# C$_H$ domains:	4	3
Hinge region:	No	Yes
Valency:	10	4

3-2: Comparative structures of the major immunoglobulin isotypes in humans. Variations occur in the number of antigen-binding sites (valency), heavy chain constant domains (C$_H$), and interchain disulfide (S-S) bonds and in the presence of a hinge region. Serum IgM always exists as a pentamer held together by disulfide bonds and a J chain. Serum IgA exists primarily as a monomer. Secretory IgA (shown here) is a dimer stabilized by a J chain and secretory component.

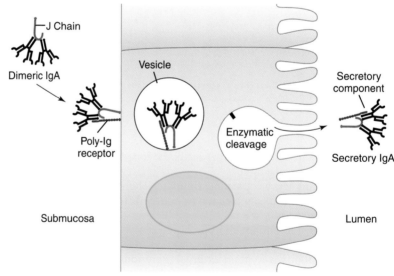

3-3: Formation of secretory IgA. Poly-Ig receptor on epithelial cells specifically binds Fc portion of dimeric IgA molecules. As it traverses an epithelial cell, dimeric IgA acquires a secretory component, which is released by cleavage of the receptor.

Everyone has the same (*iso*) types (IgG, IgM, IgD, IgE, IgA) of immunoglobulin. "All'o" us have our own personal immunoglobulins. Just as in the world, there are many "idiot types" of immunoglobulin in each of us for all the different variable regions.

D. Antigenic determinants on antibodies

1. **Immunoglobulins,** like other proteins, can induce an **immune response.**
2. Three major groups of immunoglobulin epitopes—**isotypic, allotypic,** and **idiotypic**—differ in their location within antibody molecules and/or distribution among individuals (Table 3-4).

TABLE 3-4 Antigenic Determinants on Antibodies

EPITOPE CLASS	LOCATION	COMMENT
Isotype	Constant region	These epitopes, which **define each class of Ig heavy chains**, are **identical in all members of a species**. The five human isotypes are IgA, IgD, IgE, IgG, and IgM. (*Iso* = same.)
Allotype	Constant region	These epitopes **vary among individuals**. IgG exhibits the most allotypic differences. (*Allo* = different.)
Idiotype	Variable region	These epitopes **differ among antibodies because of different antigen-binding specificities**. Monoclonal antibodies have the same idiotype. (There are many "idiot" types.)

II. Development and Activation of B Cells
A. Antigen-independent maturation of B cells
- Naive, immunocompetent B cells are generated in the bone marrow from hematopoietic precursors (see Fig. 1-3).
  1. Germline Ig DNA consists of multiple coding segments separated by noncoding regions.
     - Light chain germline DNA contains many V, 5 J, and 1 C segments in humans.
     - Heavy chain germline DNA contains many V, many D, 6 J, and multiple C segments in humans.
  2. Random recombination of gene segments forms V_LJ (light chain) or V_HDJ (heavy chain) units, which encode the variable region of each chain and determine the antigenic specificity of mature B cells (Fig. 3-4).
  3. Splicing of primary RNA transcripts formed by mature B cells yields messenger RNAs (mRNAs) with a single variable region and single constant region.

All the antibodies produced by an individual B cell have the same antigenic specificity.

Light chain gene has VJC segments.

Heavy chain gene has VDJC segments.

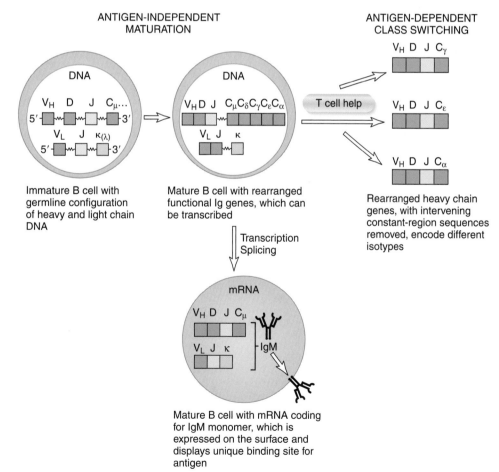

ANTIGEN-INDEPENDENT MATURATION

Immature B cell with germline configuration of heavy and light chain DNA

Mature B cell with rearranged functional Ig genes, which can be transcribed

Transcription Splicing

Mature B cell with mRNA coding for IgM monomer, which is expressed on the surface and displays unique binding site for antigen

T cell help

ANTIGEN-DEPENDENT CLASS SWITCHING

Rearranged heavy chain genes, with intervening constant-region sequences removed, encode different isotypes

3-4: Immunogenetics of B cell development. Germline immunoglobulin DNA within B cell precursors undergoes random genetic recombination during antigen-independent maturation in the bone marrow. Germline DNA contains multiple V, D, and J segments, although only one of each type is shown. After transcription of the rearranged genes, splicing of the messenger RNA (mRNA) joins the V_LJ or V_HDJ unit to a constant segment (κ or $C\mu$), with removal of the remaining intervening sequences. During differentiation of mature B cells triggered by antigen stimulation and cytokine from T_H cells, recombination attaches different heavy chain genes, resulting in expression of different isotypes (class switching).

BOX 3-1 GEARING UP FOR ANTIBODY SECRETION
A **mature, naive B cell** is an antibody factory waiting to get turned on for production of secreted antibody. Membrane antibodies are "tester" molecules looking for antigen to occupy them. B cells expressing membrane antibody that best "fits" the antigen will be the ones that are turned on to grow **(clonal expansion)** and differentiate into **antibody-secreting plasma cells.** During clonal expansion and differentiation, the affinity of the antibody mixture for antigen may increase **(affinity maturation),** and the biologic activities of the antibody molecule can change as the result of **class switching.** B cells require T_H cells and cytokines to respond to most antigens.

IgM and IgD come from the same mRNA.

IgM and IgD are the only immunoglobulins that are expressed on the same cell.

TI antigens are repetitive structures, like bacterial surface molecules.

IgG, IgE, and IgA production require T cell help.

- Exception: Alternative splicing of heavy chain primary transcripts in unstimulated B cells yields mRNAs encoding membrane IgM, IgM, or membrane IgD.

B. Stimulation by T-independent (TI) antigens
1. Restricted to IgM response
2. Repetitive, polymeric antigens (e.g., lipopolysaccharide, dextran, capsular polysaccharides, and flagellin) activate B cells in the absence of T_H cells.
3. B cell response to TI antigens does *not* exhibit isotype switching, affinity maturation, or production of memory cells.

C. Stimulation by T-dependent (TD) antigens (Box 3-1)
- Activation, proliferation, and differentiation of naive B cells in response to most protein antigens is driven by direct interaction with CD4 T_H cells and the action of various cytokines.
1. Three types of signals are required for response to TD antigens.
  - Antigen-triggered signal: antigen binds to immunoglobulin and triggers tyrosine kinase activation cascade.
    a. Coreceptors (e.g., CD21 [C3d receptor] and CD19) intensify initial signal triggered by cross-linkage of membrane immunoglobulin molecules by antigen.
    b. Increased expression of class II major histocompatibility complex (MHC) molecules is induced.
    c. Antigen is endocytosed and degraded, and peptides are displayed on B cell surface associated with class II MHC molecules.
  - Costimulatory signal.
    a. Binding of CD40L on T_H cell to CD40 on B cell promotes increased expression of cytokine receptors on B cell.
  - Cytokine signals
    a. Binding of cytokines secreted primarily by activated T_H cells stimulates subsequent proliferation and differentiation of B cells.
    b. Plasma cells are terminally differentiated B cells (do not divide) that secrete antibody.
    c. Memory B cells, which express membrane-bound antibody of any isotype, respond faster than naive B cells to second exposure to antigen.

Direct B cell–T_H cell interaction and cytokines secreted by T_H cells are required for B cells to respond to most antigens.

Memory response is faster than primary response.

Antibody diversity is generated during random recombination of VDJ regions, nucleotide insertion during recombination, and somatic mutation.

Somatic mutation during B cell proliferation and clonal selection of the producing cells improves the antibody product, and isotype switching changes its biologic properties.

Isotype switching: IgM-producing plasma cell now produces IgG or other immunoglobulins.

T cell help induces generation of memory B cells and antibody-secreting plasma cells.

T_H1 responses include IgG. T_H2 responses include IgG, IgE, and IgA.

2. Affinity maturation (clonal expansion) results from selective expansion of B cell clones that make the best antibody.
  - The immunoglobulins produced by these cells have increased average binding strength improving the antibody mixture to the antigen.
    a. Somatic mutation occurs randomly within the variable region of heavy and light chain genes during the course of the B cell response.
  - As a result, some B cells begin to produce higher-affinity immunoglobulin.
    a. B cells bearing higher-affinity membrane immunoglobulin proliferate and differentiate most rapidly because they interact preferentially with antigen (clonal selection).
3. Class (isotype) switching occurs as the immune response progresses.
  - IgM-producing plasma cells are generated first after antigen stimulation.
  - With T cell help, heavy chain DNA in later-differentiating B cells undergoes further rearrangement, resulting in expression of antibody with the same antigenic specificity but different heavy chains (see Fig. 3-4).
    a. Interferon-γ (T_H1 response) promotes switching to IgG1.
    b. Interleukin (IL)-4, and IL-5 (T_H2 response) promote switching to IgE, IgA, and other IgG subclasses.

III. Antibody Effector Mechanisms
A. Neutralization of viruses and toxins
- Occurs when these agents become coated with antibody, which interferes with their binding to their receptors and prevents the infectious or toxic process from proceeding

B. Opsonization (IgG)
- Promotes ingestion and killing by phagocytic cells (see Chapter 1, Fig. 1-5)

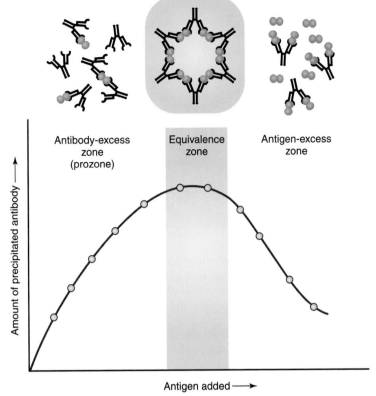

3-5: Precipitin curve. If increasing amounts of an antigen are added to a constant amount of its specific antibodies, maximal precipitation occurs when the relative antigen and antibody concentrations favor formation of large insoluble complexes (equivalence zone). Minimal precipitation occurs on either side of the equivalence zone.

    C. Complement activation (IgG and IgM)
- Induces inflammatory response and cytolytic destruction of extracellular microbes

    D. Antibody-mediated agglutination (IgM) of bacteria
- May aid in their clearance

    E. Antibody-dependent cellular cytotoxicity
- Leads to the destruction of microbes and virus-infected cells coated with **IgG** antibody

    F. Binding of secretory IgA to microbes at mucosal surfaces
- Prevents adherence and colonization

    G. Hypersensitivity reactions
- Can be triggered by antibody or antigen-antibody complexes (see Chapter 4)

IV. Antigen-Antibody Reactions
- Antigen-antibody reactions provide the basis for **qualitative** and **quantitative tests** for both **antigen (Ag)** and **antibody (Ab)** (see Chapter 5).

    A. Precipitation-based assays
1. **Precipitin** reaction
   - At appropriate concentrations of antibody and antigen **(zone of equivalence)**, each antibody molecule binds more than one antigen molecule, leading to formation of large complexes that precipitate from the solution (Fig. 3-5).

    B. Agglutination-based assays
1. Interaction between antibody and particulate antigens (e.g., bacteria and erythrocytes) results in visible clumping (agglutination).
2. IgM antibodies are good agglutinins, whereas smaller IgG antibodies often do not cause agglutination.

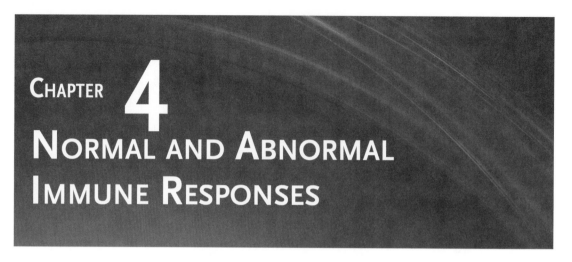

CHAPTER 4

NORMAL AND ABNORMAL IMMUNE RESPONSES

I. Cascade of Events in Typical Immune Responses (Box 4-1)

  A. Localized antigen-nonspecific responses at site of antigen exposure

  1. Fast: activation of alternate or lectin complement pathway leading to inflammatory response, opsonization, and bacterial killing
  2. Fast: interferon-mediated protection against viral infection and natural killer (NK) cell killing of virus-infected cells
  3. Soon after: migration of phagocytes (neutrophils, macrophages, dendritic cells [DCs]) to site of antigen and phagocytosis
  4. Early: pathogen-associated molecular patterns (PAMPs) on microbial structures (e.g., lipopolysaccharide and peptidoglycan) stimulate toll-like receptors (TLRs) and other receptors on DCs and macrophages that make cytokines
  5. Early: acute phase response induced by interleukin-1 (IL-1), IL-6, and tumor necrosis factor (TNF) secreted from macrophages and DCs
  6. Early: DC maturation
      - TLR stimulation promotes maturation and mobilization of DCs to lymph nodes
      - IL-12 from DCs and macrophages activates NK cells and promotes helper T cell subset 1 (T_H1) responses.

  B. Primary antigen-specific responses

  - Lymphocytes interact with antigen-presenting cells (APCs) in lymph nodes (Fig. 4-1), the spleen, and mucosal-associated lymphoid tissue, which includes tonsils, adenoids, appendix, and Peyer patches; cytokines define the nature of the response (Table 4-1).
  1. Initial activation of naive CD4 T_H cells triggered by binding to antigenic peptides associated with class II major histocompatibility complex (MHC) molecules on DCs, but not other APCs
  2. Activation of naive B cells (T dependent) expressing membrane immunoglobulin M (IgM) triggered by binding of antigen and interaction with T_H cells
  3. Proliferation of activated CD4 T_H cells and differentiation into cytokine-secreting T_H1 and T_H2 subsets
  4. Initial activation and proliferation of naive CD8 cytotoxic T (T_C) cells triggered by binding of antigenic peptides associated with class I MHC molecules on DCs for recognition of infected cells, tumor cells, and grafts

Acute phase (proinflammatory) cytokines are IL-1, IL-6, and TNF-α.

IL-12 production signals need for local cellular and antibody protections (T_H1).

Primary antibody response: slow onset, initially IgM, low titer. Presence of IgM is good indication of a primary response.

Secondary antibody response: fast onset, primarily IgG, high titer

BOX 4-1 "MUST-KNOWS" FOR THE NATURE OF THE RESPONSE: TICTOC
Trigger
Inducer
Cells
Time course
Outcome
Cytokines

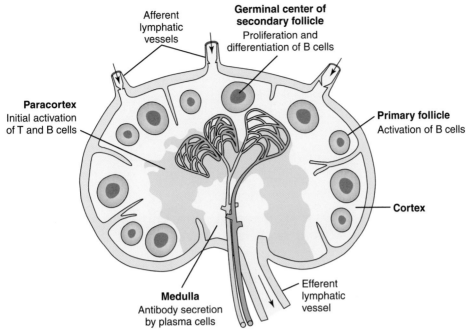

4-1: Antigen-dependent lymphocyte activity in peripheral lymph node. Antigen carried in the lymph becomes associated with dendritic cells (DCs) to be presented to lymphocytes. The paracortex contains mainly T cells, many of which are associated with interdigitating antigen-presenting cells (DCs). After initial activation, T cells migrate to the cortex, where they interact with B cells in primary follicles, which develop into secondary follicles, with active B cell proliferation and differentiation occurring in the germinal centers. Lymphocytes leave the node through the efferent lymphatic vessel.

TABLE 4-1 **Cytokine Responses**

TYPE OF RESPONSE	ACUTE PHASE	T_H1	T_H17	T_H2	TREG/SUP
Inducer	PAMP	IL-12	TGF-β	IL-6	IL-10
		IL-6	IL-6		TGF-β
			IL-23		
Mediator	IL-1	IL-2	IL-17	IL-4	IL-10
	TNF-α	Lymphotoxin		IL-5	TGF-β
	IL-6	IFN-γ		IL-10	
	IFN-α; IFN-β				
	IL-12*				

*IL-12 is not always part of an acute phase response.
IFN, interferon; IL, interleukin; PAMP, pathogen-associated molecular pattern; TGF, transforming growth factor; T_H, helper T cell; TNF, tumor necrosis factor; Treg/sup, regulatory or suppressive T cell.

5. Cytokine-induced proliferation of activated B cells and differentiation into memory cells and antibody-secreting plasma cells
   - Class switching (gene recombination) and affinity maturation (somatic mutation) occur.
   - T_H1 cytokines stimulate B cells to make IgG1 (human).
   - T_H2 cytokines stimulate production of other IgG subclasses, IgE, or IgA.
6. Swelling of lymph nodes because of lymphoid proliferation
7. Exit of activated lymphocytes from lymph node or other peripheral lymphoid tissue and mobilization to site of infection
8. Activation of macrophages and DCs by interferon-γ (IFN-γ; T_H1 cytokine), leading to enhancement of their antigen-presenting, antibacterial, antiviral, and antitumor activities

C. **Secondary immune response**
   1. Rechallenge with an antigen produces a secondary specific response that is faster and stronger (anamnestic response) than primary response to the same antigen because DCs and any APCs can present antigen to T cells and because of the presence of memory B and T cells (Fig. 4-2).
   2. Persistence of memory B cells accounts for the phenomenon called "original antigenic sin" (Box 4-2).

Acute inflammation produces painful swelling of lymph nodes.

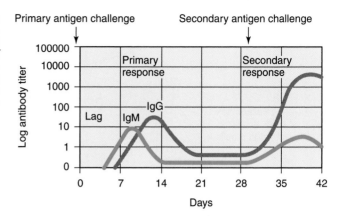

4-2: Time course of primary and secondary humoral (antibody) immune responses. After initial challenge with a particular antigen, secreted antibody is detectable only after a lag period of several days and initially consists of IgM. The secondary immune response (anamnestic response) after rechallenge with the same antigen reaches a higher titer, lasts longer, and consists predominantly of IgG.

BOX 4-2 ORIGINAL ANTIGENIC SIN

Once generated during a primary response, antigen-specific memory B cells stop dividing (G$_o$ phase of cell cycle) and may have a life span of years. When these quiescent cells later encounter the same epitope on a closely related antigen X, they sometimes are preferentially activated, producing antibody that binds to antigen X and prevents activation of naive B cells specific for other epitopes on antigen X, thereby **inhibiting a new primary antibody response to X.** This phenomenon is often observed with strains of type A influenza virus and may contribute to **influenza epidemics.**

II. Hypersensitivity Reactions

- Hypersensitivity reactions are important in the immune response to certain antigens, but they also cause pathologic changes associated with many autoimmune diseases and infections, especially viral infections (Table 4-2).

A. Type I (immediate) hypersensitivity

- IgE-mediated atopic (allergic) and anaphylactic reactions in previously exposed (sensitized) individuals (Fig. 4-3)
1. Initiation: cross-linkage by antigen (allergen) of IgE bound to Fc receptors on mast cells and basophils after reexposure of sensitized host to allergen
2. Effector mechanism: degranulation of mast cells and basophils releasing numerous vasoactive and other mediators, such as histamine and SRS-A (slow-reacting substance of anaphylaxis)
3. Clinical manifestations
   - Acute generalized anaphylaxis: shock, vascular collapse, respiratory collapse
   - Chronic, recurrent localized reactions: asthma, allergic rhinitis (hay fever), and wheal and flare (hives)
4. Desensitization therapy: repeated injections of increasing doses of allergen induce production of IgG, which binds the allergen and prevents its binding to IgE on sensitized cells.

B. Type II hypersensitivity

- Antibody-dependent cytotoxicity
1. Initiation: binding of antibody to cell surface antigens
2. Effector mechanisms
   - Complement activated by cell surface antigen-antibody complex → cell lysis by membrane attack complex
   - Antibody-dependent cellular cytotoxicity (ADCC) triggered by binding of antibody to Fc receptors on macrophages and NK cells → cell destruction
   - C3a and C5a attract neutrophils and promote inflammation.
3. Clinical manifestations
   - **Hemolytic transfusion reactions:** antibodies to red blood cell (RBC) antigens
   - **Drug-induced thrombocytopenia and hemolytic anemia:** antibodies to drugs absorbed on platelets and RBCs
   - **Hemolytic disease of the newborn (erythroblastosis fetalis):** maternal antibody to antigens on fetal RBCs, especially **Rh antigens** (Box 4-3)
   - **Autoimmune diseases:** see section V

C. Type III hypersensitivity

- Immune complex–induced tissue-damaging inflammation (Fig. 4-4)
1. Initiation: formation of large amounts of circulating antigen-antibody (immune) complexes and their deposition in various tissues or on vessel walls

Type I: Soluble mediators, preformed actors—fast reactions of less than 30 minutes

Type II : soluble mediators, cellular actors—slower reactions of less than 8 hours

Type III: soluble mediators, cellular actors—slower reactions of less than 8 hours

Type IV: cellular mediators, cellular actors—slow reactions of more than 1 day

Type I hypersensitivity: IgE; mast cell degranulation; rapid local (allergic) or systemic (anaphylactic) effects

Type II hypersensitivity: complement fixation on cells; acute inflammation

TABLE 4-2 **Hypersensitivity Reactions**

ONSET TIME	KEY FEATURES	BENEFICIAL EFFECTS	PATHOLOGIC EFFECTS
Type I Reaction			
<30 min	IgE-dependent release of various mediators	Antiparasitic responses and toxin neutralization	Localized allergies (e.g., **hay fever, asthma**) Systemic anaphylaxis
Type II Reaction*			
<8 hr	Antibody- and antibody (with complement)–mediated cytotoxicity	Opsonization and direct lysis of extracellular bacteria and other susceptible microbes	Hemolytic anemias (e.g., **transfusion reactions, Rh disease,** Hapten [penicillin]), modified red blood cells Organ-specific tissue damage in some autoimmune diseases (e.g., **Goodpasture syndrome**) Autoantibody activation of receptors (e.g., **Graves disease, myasthenia gravis**)
Type III Reaction*			
<8 hr	Deposition of soluble antigen-antibody complexes, which activate complement	Acute inflammatory reaction at site of extracellular microbes and their clearance	Arthus reaction (localized) **Serum sickness** and drug reactions (generalized) (e.g., **hypersensitivity pneumonitis** [farmer's lung], **glomerulonephritis** [*Streptococcus pyogenes* sequelae]) Systemic autoimmune diseases (e.g., **systemic lupus erythematosus**)
Type IV Reaction			
24-72 hr (acute); >1 wk (chronic)	Delayed release of T_H1 cytokines; activation of macrophages and cytotoxic lymphocytes	Protection against infection by fungi, intracellular bacteria, and viruses	Acute: contact dermatitis, tuberculosis skin test Chronic: granuloma formation, **graft rejection**

*Antibody (with complement)–initiated autoimmune diseases like rheumatoid arthritis, systemic lupus erythematosus, and possibly multiple sclerosis develop into T cell–mediated chronic diseases.
T_H1, helper T cell subset 1.

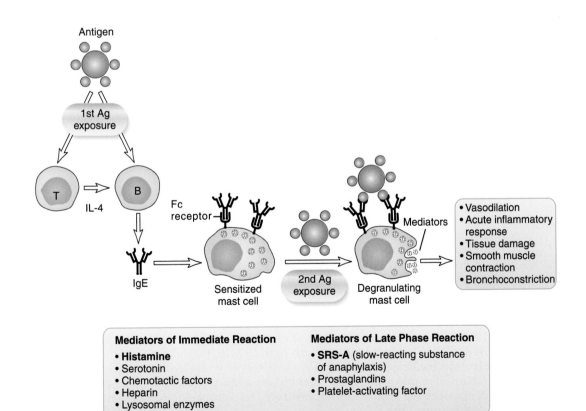

Mediators of Immediate Reaction
- **Histamine**
- Serotonin
- Chemotactic factors
- Heparin
- Lysosomal enzymes

Mediators of Late Phase Reaction
- **SRS-A** (slow-reacting substance of anaphylaxis)
- Prostaglandins
- Platelet-activating factor

4-3: Type I hypersensitivity. IgE produced in response to initial allergen exposure binds to Fc receptors on mast cells and basophils. Rechallenge with the same allergen leads to release of histamine and other mediators, which produce various symptoms of localized atopic reaction or generalized anaphylaxis. Ag, antigen; IL-4, interleukin-4.

BOX 4-3 HEMOLYTIC DISEASE OF THE NEWBORN

An **Rh-negative** woman normally becomes **sensitized** to Rh antigens during birth of her first Rh-positive child. During a subsequent pregnancy with an Rh-positive infant, the sensitized mother produces **anti-Rh IgG antibody,** which crosses the placenta, leading to **destruction of fetal RBCs** by type II hypersensitivity reaction. Hemolysis causes hemoglobinemia, jaundice, and accumulation of indirect bilirubin, which can result in respiratory and brain damage to the fetus.

Anti-Rh antibody **(RhoGAM)** administered to the mother soon after delivery of her first Rh-positive child prevents sensitization by neutralizing fetal Rh antigens that enter the mother's circulation during removal of the placenta. A Rhogam-treated mother will not mount an anti-Rh immune response in subsequent pregnancies.

Direct Coombs test detects maternal anti-Rh antibody on fetal RBCs. **Indirect Coombs test** detects anti-Rh antibody in maternal serum.

4-4: Type III hypersensitivity. Circulating immune complexes formed in the presence of excess soluble antigen are deposited in the kidney and elsewhere in the body. Activation of complement and other damaging responses occur at the site of deposition.

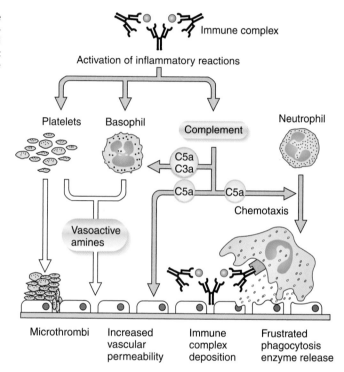

Production of C3a and C5a during Types II and III hypersensitivity *attract* and *activate* inflammatory neutrophils.

Type III hypersensitivity: deposition of immune complexes; complement activation; acute inflammation

Large amount of hepatitis B surface antigen (HBsAg) and antibody during hepatitis B infection can cause immune complexes and type III hypersensitivity.

Type IV hypersensitivity: cytokines from CD4 T_H1 cells; activated macrophages; skin reactions (acute); granulomatous and rejection reactions (chronic)

2. Effector mechanism: activation of the complement cascade by immune complexes leading to acute inflammatory reactions
3. Clinical manifestations
   - Arthus reaction: local skin reaction (redness and swelling) induced by intradermally injected antigen or insect bite
     a. Intrapulmonary Arthus-type reaction can be induced by inhalation of bacterial spores or fungi (e.g., farmer's lung).
   - Serum sickness: generalized reaction developing 1 or 2 weeks after a second administration of immunoglobulin of another species (e.g., in passive immunization with horse serum)
     a. Penicillin and other drugs can cause similar reaction marked by fever, urticaria, lymphadenopathy, and arthralgia.
   - Vasculitis, nephritis, arthritis, and skin lesions associated with some infectious and autoimmune diseases

D. **Type IV (delayed-type) hypersensitivity**
   - Delayed inflammatory response and cell-mediated cytotoxicity
   1. Initiation: antigen-stimulated release of cytokines (e.g., IL-2, IFN-γ, tumor necrosis factor-β [TNF-β]) from sensitized (activated) CD4 T_H1 cells
   2. Effector mechanisms
      - Primary inflammatory response: recruitment and activation of macrophages, which kill microbes and release various substances responsible for local inflammation and tissue damage
      - Secondary cytolytic response: activation of CD8 T_C cells and subsequent killing of target cells bearing antigen associated with class I MHC molecules
   3. Clinical manifestations (Table 4-3)

TABLE 4-3 **Clinical Manifestations of Delayed-Type Hypersensitivity Reactions**

TYPE	ANTIGEN	CLINICAL AND HISTOLOGIC FEATURES
Acute Reaction (1-3 days)		
Contact dermatitis	Epidermal (e.g., poison ivy, chemicals, cosmetics)	Eczema with edema Raised epidermis, many macrophages
Tuberculin reaction	Dermal (e.g., purified protein derivative, other mycobacterial and fungal antigens)	Local induration and swelling ± fever T cells, fewer macrophages
Chronic (>1 wk)		
Graft rejection	Persistent exposure to alloantigens	Thrombosis and necrosis of graft T cells, many macrophages
Granuloma formation	Persistent exposure to infectious or noninfectious agents	Skin induration Nodule composed of epithelioid cells (activated macrophages), giant cells, and helper T cells; fibrosis ± caseous necrosis

III. Antimicrobial and Antitumor Host Defenses
- Table 4-4 summarizes the contribution of the various immune effector components in host responses to different types of pathogens.
- Several anatomic and physiologic barriers inhibit entry of microbes into tissues (see Chapter 1, Fig. 1-1).

A. Antibacterial responses (Fig. 4-5)
1. Initial innate (nonspecific) events
   - Complement-mediated lysis, opsonization, and phagocytic destruction often can control infection by extracellular bacteria.
   - PAMP stimulation of TLRs on DCs and macrophages stimulates cytokine production to stimulate acute, innate, and immune responses (Box 4-4).
     a. Neutrophils are the initial antibacterial phagocytic response.
     b. Activation of macrophages is necessary for killing of phagocytized bacteria.
        - Activation stimulates enzymes, nitrous oxide (NO), and reactive oxygen species (ROS) production.
2. Antigen-specific events
   - T_H1 response (IFN-γ) is important in activating macrophages to control extracellular and intracellular bacteria (e.g., mycobacteria and *Listeria monocytogenes*) and wall-off infection (e.g., *Mycobacterium tuberculosis*).
   - T_H2 response stimulates and promotes class switch in B cells, thus promoting antibody production.
   - Secreted antibody (B cell response) is most important against extracellular bacteria and toxins.
     a. Antibody promotes opsonization and complement-mediated lysis of bacteria.
     b. Antibody is important for binding and neutralizing toxins.

B. Antiviral responses (Fig. 4-6)
1. Initial innate (nonspecific) events
   - IFN-α and IFN-β secreted by infected cells protect surrounding noninfected cells from infection (local response) and trigger systemic immune responses (Box 4-5).

Increase in number of banded (immature) versus segmented neutrophils in complete blood count, referred to as a left shift, usually accompanies bacterial infection.

Neutrophils always eat and kill bacteria; macrophages eat but must be activated to kill bacteria.

Antibody is the primary antigen-specific protection.

Antibody blocks toxin action and opsonizes and initiates complement reactions to bacteria.

TABLE 4-4 **Role of Various Immune Effectors in Antimicrobial Responses**

EFFECTOR	EXTRACELLULAR BACTERIA	INTRACELLULAR BACTERIA	VIRUSES	FUNGI	PARASITES
Neutrophils	++	−	−	+	+
Macrophages	+	++	+	+	−
Complement	++	−	−	−	−
Natural killer cells	−	−	+	−	−
CD4 T_H1 cells	+	++	++	+	+
CD8 cytotoxic lymphocytes	−	+	++	−	−
Secreted antibody	++	+	+	+	++ (IgE)*

*IgE-mediated degranulation of mast cells is especially important in response to worm (helminthic) infections.
Relative contribution: ++, major role; +, important secondary role; −, minimal or no role. T_H1 cells, helper T cells subtype 1.

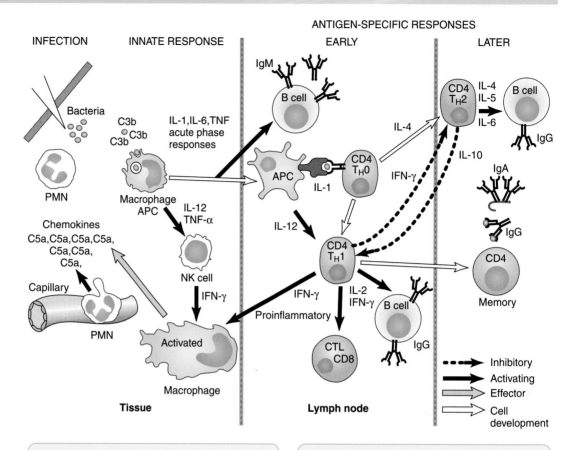

ANTIGEN-SPECIFIC RESPONSES

INFECTION   INNATE RESPONSE   EARLY   LATER

Complement (C′)
- Activation by bacterial surfaces or Ab-Ag complexes
- Chemotaxis and anaphylaxis (C3a, C5a)
- Opsonization of bacteria (C3b)

Neutrophils
- O_2-dependent and O_2-independent killing of extracellular bacteria

Macrophages
- O_2-dependent and O_2-independent killing of extracellular bacteria
- Production of IL-1, IL-6, IL-12, and TNF-α
- Activation of acute phase responses
- Antigen presentation to CD4 T_H cells

T cells
- T_H1 cell cytokines important in cellular response to intracellular bacteria
- T_H2 cell cytokines important in antibody response to all bacteria

Secreted antibody
- Binding of Ab to bacterial surface antigens blocks adherence of bacteria to host tissues
- Opsonization of bacteria
- Activation of complement (classical pathway)
- Clearance of bacteria
- Neutralization of bacterial toxins and toxic enzymes

4-5: *Top,* Overview of time course of antibacterial responses. The response begins with complement activation, which promotes recruitment and activation of polymorphonuclear lymphocytes (PMNs; neutrophils) and macrophages. After reaching lymph nodes, antigen-presenting cells (APCs) and antigen induce early specific responses (helper T cell subset 1 [T_H1] cytokines, activated macrophages, and secreted IgM and IgG). Later, T_H2 cytokines promote mature antibody response (IgG, IgA, and IgE). Much later, memory cells will develop. *Bottom,* Summary of major components in antibacterial responses. Ab, antibody; Ag, antigen; IFN, interferon; IL, interleukin; NK, natural killer; TNF, tumor necrosis factor.

BOX 4-4 TOLL-LIKE RECEPTORS ACTIVATE ANTIMICROBIAL RESPONSES

Microbial structures bind to specific TLRs on dendritic cells, macrophages, and other cells to activate antimicrobial responses. There are at least 10 TLRs to sense bacteria, viruses, fungi, and parasites. Microbial structures that trigger TLR responses include lipopolysaccharide, lipoteichoic acid, flagellin, viral and bacterial DNA and RNA, and fungal cell wall mannans. Activation of TLRs initiates a cascade of events that lead to production of mRNA for activation of cells and production of interferons, cytokines, and chemokines.

INNATE RESPONSES   ANTIGEN-SPECIFIC RESPONSES

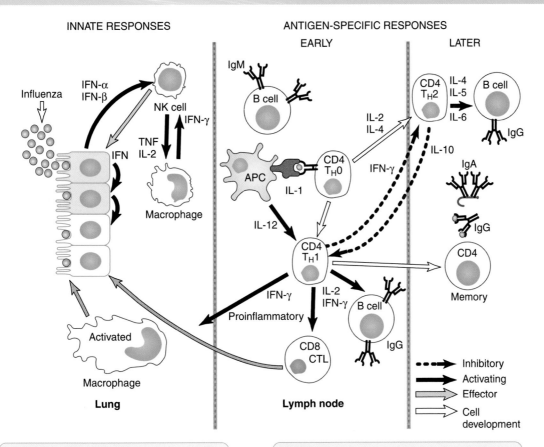

Interferons (IFN-α and IFN-β)
- Protection of noninfected cells by blocking viral replication
- Activation of NK cells

NK cells
- Direct killing of virus-infected cells
- Activation of macrophages via secreted IFN-γ

Macrophages
- Presentation of viral antigens to CD4 T_H cells
- Phagocytosis of opsonized virions
- Filtration of virions from blood in liver

T cells
- Cytolytic T_H1 response more important than T_H2 response in resolving nonlytic and enveloped viral infections
- Destruction of virus-infected cells by CTLs

Secreted antibody
- Resolution of lytic viral infections
- Neutralization of extracellular virions by Ab binding to viral attachment proteins
- Inhibition of viremic spread to target tissues
- Protection of mucosal surfaces from infection by secretory IgA
- Opsonization of virions
- Destruction of virus-infected cells by ADCC

4-6: *Top,* Overview of time course of antiviral responses. The response begins with production of IFN-α and IFN-β by virus-infected cells (*gray shading*) and involvement of natural killer (NK) cells. Subsequent specific responses resemble those induced in bacterial infections, except that CD8 cytotoxic T lymphocytes (CTLs) are important effectors in defense against viruses. *Bottom,* Summary of major components in antiviral responses. Ab, antibody; ADCC, antibody-dependent cellular cytotoxicity; APC, antigen-presenting cell; IFN, interferon; T_H, helper T cell; TNF, tumor necrosis factor.

BOX 4-5 INTERFERONS AND ANTIVIRAL RESPONSE

Viral infection, particularly by **RNA viruses,** stimulates some cells (e.g., leukocytes, epithelial cells, and fibroblasts) to synthesize and secrete **IFN-α** and **IFN-β**. These secreted molecules act on neighboring noninfected cells to induce an **antiviral state.** Protein kinase R (PKR) and 2,5'-adenosine polymerase are produced, but subsequent infection of the cells activates these enzymes that degrade viral mRNA and inhibit viral protein synthesis, thus aborting the infection process. IFN-α and IFN-β also activate **NK cells,** which can destroy virus-infected cells. **IFN-γ**, produced primarily by CD4 T_H1 cells, activates macrophages and promotes antigen-specific cytolytic responses.

By quickly limiting the number of infected host cells that churn out new virions and by activating NK cells, interferons set the stage for final elimination of virus-infected cells by cell-mediated processes and of free virions by antibody-dependent processes.

IFN-α, IFN-β, and NK cells may be sufficient to stop virus infection.

IFN-α and IFN-β cause the flu-like symptoms associated with prodrome of many viral diseases.

Double-stranded RNA is the best inducer of IFN-α and IFN-β activation of the antiviral state.

Antibody cleans up free virus, and cell-mediated immunity kills virus factories to resolve infection.

Vaccine-induced antibody prevents viremic spread of virus to disease target organ.

Passive immunization is common treatment for individuals exposed to tetanus toxin, botulinum toxin, rabies virus, or hepatitis A or B virus.

Vaccine-induced cell-mediated immune responses are not dependable before 12 months of age. Thus, attenuated measles-mumps-rubella (MMR) and varicella-zoster virus (VZV) vaccines commonly are administered at 15 months.

Killed vaccines are safer than live attenuated vaccines for immunodeficient individuals.

Live vaccines induce both cellular and antibody responses and better memory.

      a. Double-stranded RNA produced during replication of RNA viruses is the best inducer of IFN-α and IFN-β and the antiviral response.
- IFN-α activates NK cells to kill infected cells.

2. Later specific events
- Antibody neutralizes cell-free virus particles (virions; antibody), and cell-mediated immunity kills virus-infected cells, especially those not killed by virus replication.
- T_H1 response is essential for control of enveloped and nonlytic viruses, which can replicate and spread within the host without killing infected cells.
   a. T_H1 cytokines promote antibody (IgG) production, which neutralizes virus and activation of cell-mediated responses, including CD8 cytotoxic T lymphocytes (CTLs), which kill infected cells.
- T_H2 response stimulates antibody production.
   a. Overactive T_H2 response during early phase of viral infection can exacerbate disease by inhibiting development of protective inflammatory and cytolytic T_H1 responses.
- Secreted antibody (B cell response) directed against viral surface antigens is essential in controlling infection by lytic viruses, which kill infected cells, and in preventing spread of virus by viremia.

C. **Antiparasite and antifungal responses**
1. IgE-mediated degranulation of mast cells is critical to the control of parasitic worm infections.
2. Macrophages and delayed-type hypersensitivity (T_H1 response) are essential for controlling most fungal infections and for intracellular parasites.

D. **Antitumor responses**
- Tumor-cell antigens elicit T cell responses and, to a lesser extent, an antibody response.
1. CTL-mediated destruction of tumor cells is a major antitumor effector response.
2. Antibody response plays a small or no role but may promote ADCC of tumor cells by NK cells and macrophages.
- Antibodies to tumor antigens, such as carcinoembryonic antigen, are monitors of tumor progression.
3. NK cells and activated macrophages exhibit nonspecific antitumor activity.
- Reduced levels of class I MHC molecules on tumor cells may act as a signal for direct perforin-mediated killing by NK cells.
- TNF secreted by activated macrophages contributes to their antitumor effect.

IV. **Vaccines and Immunization (see Chapters 8 and 20)**
  A. **Passive immunization**
1. Administration of preformed antibodies, which provide rapid, temporary (2 or 3 months) protection against current infection or symptoms
2. Use of human gammaglobulin, rather than animal-derived serum, avoids possible induction of serum sickness.

  B. **Active immunization**
1. Administration of agents that induce slowly developing but long-lasting immune protection against subsequent exposure to an infectious agent
2. Attenuated vaccines are live, weakened forms of an infectious agent; used primarily against viruses.
- Elicit both **cell-mediated** and **antibody responses** and long-term memory without need for multiple boosters
3. Inactivated vaccines include **killed microbes** and **purified** macromolecules.
- Elicit mainly **antibody response** and require **periodic boosters** to maintain immunity
   a. Aggregation of antigens into particles increases their immunogenicity, such as hepatitis B and human papillomavirus–like particles.
- Bacterial polysaccharide capsular antigens elicit a relatively weak T-independent response, but when conjugated to a protein, they will elicit a strong T-dependent response with memory.
4. DNA vaccines are plasmids encoding a viral antigen (not yet licensed).
- Uptake of plasmids by macrophages or DCs leads to expression of antigen and its presentation to T cells, inducing cell-mediated and antibody responses.

V. **Autoimmune Responses**
  A. **Causes of autoimmune disorders**
1. Inherited absence of tolerance to certain self antigens
2. Cross-reactivity of antimicrobial antibody with host tissue (e.g., antibody to group A streptococci)

3. Polyclonal activation induced by tumors or infection (e.g., multiple myeloma, Epstein-Barr virus infection)

B. **Mechanisms of autoimmune pathology (Table 4-5)**
1. Autoantibodies to cell surface proteins or circulating molecules blocking normal function or stimulating abnormal activity (also can be considered a *type II hypersensitivity reaction*)
   - Examples: Graves disease, myasthenia gravis
2. Hypersensitivity-type reactions
   - Type II reaction
     a. Autoantibodies to cell surface antigens mediate antibody plus complement lysis and ADCC of host cells.
     b. Examples: autoimmune hemolytic anemia, Goodpasture syndrome
   - Type III reaction
     a. Immune complexes between autoantibodies and self antigens mediate inflammatory reaction.
     b. Examples: rheumatoid arthritis, systemic lupus erythematosus (SLE)
   - Type IV reaction
     a. T_H17 cells, T_{DTH} cells, and CTLs sensitized against self antigens mediate inflammation and cell destruction.
     b. Examples: multiple sclerosis, type 1 (insulin-dependent) diabetes mellitus

TABLE 4-5 **Autoimmune Diseases**

DISEASE	PROBABLE PATHOLOGIC MECHANISMS	CLINICAL FEATURES
Organ-Specific Diseases		
Autoimmune hemolytic anemia	Type II reaction against RBC (phagocytosis of RBCs)	Anemia, positive direct Coombs test
Goodpasture syndrome	Type II reaction against capillary basement membranes in kidneys and lungs	Lung hemorrhages; nephritis with proteinuria, hematuria, renal failure
Graves disease	Stimulation of receptor for thyroid-stimulating hormone by autoantibody (type II)	Hyperthyroidism, diffuse goiter, ophthalmic symptoms (exophthalmos)
Hashimoto disease	Type II and IV reactions (damage to thyroid tissue); inhibition of iodine uptake by autoantibody to thyroid peroxidase and thyroglobulin	Thyroiditis, goiter, hypothyroidism
Type 1 diabetes mellitus (insulin dependent)	Type II and IV reactions against pancreatic β cells	No insulin production; insulitis
Myasthenia gravis	Blocking of neural stimulation of muscle by autoantibody against acetylcholine receptor	Muscle weakness, fatigue
Pernicious anemia	Inhibition of vitamin B_{12} uptake by autoantibody to intrinsic factor (type II); type IV reaction against gastric parietal cells	Abnormal erythropoiesis caused by deficiency of vitamin B_{12}
Poststreptococcal rheumatic fever	Type II and III reactions induced by cross-reaction of antistreptococcal antibodies with host tissues	Heart valve lesions, myocarditis, arthritis, chorea
Poststreptococcal glomerulonephritis	Type III reactions induced by streptococcal antigen C3 complexes	Kidney damage and dysfunction
Thrombocytopenic purpura	Type II reaction (lysis of platelets)	Bleeding disorders due to platelet deficiency
Systemic Diseases		
Multiple sclerosis	Type IV reaction against central nervous system leading to demyelination and inflammatory lesions	Periodic episodes of weakness, incoordination, speech disturbances, paresthesia
Rheumatoid arthritis	Type III and Th17 responses reaction against connective tissue and IgG	Chronic inflammation of joints marked by granulation tissue, subcutaneous nodules, and vasculitis
Systemic lupus erythematosus	Type III reaction involving autoantibodies against DNA, histones, RBCs, clotting factors, and other tissue antigens	Vasculitis, erythematous rash, arthritis, nephritis

RBC, red blood cell.

3. Cytokine responses
- Tissue damage produces self antigen, which combines with cytokines to create a cycle of T cell and macrophage activation to cause continued release of TNF-α and other acute phase cytokines that induce tissue destruction and inflammation.

C. **Association between HLA alleles and autoimmunity**
- Individuals who express particular MHC antigens are at significantly higher risk for certain autoimmune diseases than the general population.
1. **HLA-B27:** juvenile rheumatoid arthritis, ankylosing spondylitis, Reiter syndrome
2. **HLA-DR2:** Goodpasture syndrome, multiple sclerosis
3. **HLA-DR3:** type 1 diabetes mellitus, myasthenia gravis, SLE
4. **HLA-DR4:** rheumatoid arthritis, type 1 diabetes mellitus

VI. **Transplantation**
A. **Pregnancy**
1. The most common tissue graft is the fetus, and this requires that the mother have natural immunosuppression.
2. Trophoblasts express different HLA molecules (inhibit NK cells), decay antibody-accelerating factor (DAF; inhibits complement), inhibitors of T cells, and other immunosuppressive factors.
3. Cell-mediated immunity (CMI) autoimmunity wanes (rheumatoid arthritis), but antibody-mediated processes get worse (SLE).
4. Failures of immunotolerance to fetus
- Hemolytic disease of the newborn due to Rh incompatibility (see Box 4-3)
- Passive transfer of antibodies: Graves disease, myasthenia gravis, fetal alloimmune thrombocytopenia (anti–HPA-1 on platelets), fetal alloimmune neutropenia (anti–HNA-1 on neutrophils)

B. **Blood transfusion**
1. ABO antigens: tolerance initiated to self antigens; therefore, reactivity to others
2. Rh antigens

C. **Solid organ**
1. Hyperacute rejection (minutes to hours): due to preexisting antidonor antibodies (e.g., ABO)
2. Acute (days to weeks): T cells reacting to HLA mismatch
3. Chronic (months): due to minor HLA mismatch
4. Graft versus host (e.g., bone marrow transplantation): T cells from graft react to host, release cytokines, kill cells, dysfunctional immune response

D. **Treatments**
1. Calcineurin inhibitors: cyclosporine, tacrolimus
2. Antimetabolites: azathioprine
3. Steroids: prednisone
4. Immune therapy: anti–T cell reagents to kill T cells or promote tolerance

VII. **Immunodeficiency Diseases**
A. **Overview**
1. Neonates are naturally immunodeficient and susceptible to viral and intracellular microbial infections that cannot be controlled by maternal antibody due to inability to mount effective T cell responses.
2. Primary immunodeficiency results from congenital defects in some component of the immune system.
3. Secondary (acquired) immunodeficiency is associated with HIV infection, certain noninfectious diseases (e.g., nephrotic syndrome), cancer chemotherapy, and use of immunosuppressive drugs.

B. **Phagocyte disorders** (see Chapter 1, Table 1-5)
C. **Complement abnormalities** (see Chapter 1, section IV. E)
D. **Lymphocyte deficiencies** (Table 4-6)
1. Humoral deficiencies: decreased production of some or all antibody isotypes due to B cell defects or impaired T_H cell function
2. Cell-mediated deficiencies: compromised delayed-type hypersensitivity response, T_C-mediated cytotoxicity, or both
- Associated with numerous opportunistic infections (Box 4-6)
3. Combined immunodeficiencies: most severe with marked reduction in both cell-mediated and antibody responses

---

Blood transfusions: type O is the universal donor but picky about transfusions. O has antibodies to A and B; A has antibodies to B; B has antibodies to A.

Antibody deficiencies → increased susceptibility to bacterial infections, especially by encapsulated bacteria

T cell deficiencies → increased susceptibility to opportunistic infections by viruses, intracellular bacteria, and fungi

Inherited deficiency of adenine deaminase (ADA) causes one form of severe combined immunodeficiency disease (SCID). ADA-SCID has been treated successfully with gene therapy.

TABLE 4-6 **Primary Lymphocyte Immunodeficiencies**

DISEASE	IMMUNOLOGIC DEFECTS*	OTHER FEATURES
B Cell Deficiencies		
Bruton agammaglobulinemia	Defect in maturation of B cells: ↓ B cell count; ↓ Ig of all isotypes	Recurrent pyogenic infections (e.g., *Streptococcus pneumoniae*); small lymph nodes with poorly developed germinal centers; X-linked recessive
Common variable hypogammaglobulinemia	Defect in differentiation of B cells to plasma cells: ↓ Ig of all isotypes	Recurrent pyogenic infections (e.g., *Streptococcus* species, pneumoniae, giardiasis); often associated with blood or autoimmune disorders
Selective IgA deficiency	Failure of B cells expressing membrane IgA to differentiate into plasma cells: ↓ IgA and secretory IgA but normal levels of other isotypes	Recurrent respiratory and gastrointestinal infections (giardiasis); most common congenital B cell defect
T Cell Deficiencies		
Chronic mucocutaneous candidiasis	Absence of T cell response to *Candida* species despite normal T cell count and function	Recurrent candidal skin and mucous membrane infections; often associated with endocrine dysfunction
DiGeorge syndrome	Thymic aplasia due to defect in development of third and fourth pharyngeal arches: ↓ T cell count; ↓ or normal Ig levels	Recurrent viral, fungal, and protozoan infections due to absent thymus; tetany resulting from hypocalcemia due to absent parathyroid glands
Hyper-IgM syndrome	Decreased B cell activation and class switching due to T cell defect: ↑ IgM; ↓ IgG and IgA	Poor response to thymus-dependent antigens; recurrent infections, especially by *Pneumocystis jiroveci;* often associated with autoimmune blood disorders
Combined B and T Cell Deficiencies		
Ataxia-telangiectasia	↓ T cell count and function; ↓ IgA, IgE, and IgG2	Cerebellar dysfunction (ataxia), dilation of small vessels (telangiectasia); recurrent bacterial infections of respiratory tract; autosomal recessive
Severe combined immunodeficiency (SCID)	Various defects that interrupt early lymphocyte development: ↓ T and B cell counts; ↓ Ig of all isotypes	Recurrent infections of all types; short life span; may be X-linked (X-SCID) or autosomal recessive (e.g., adenine deaminase deficiency)
Wiskott-Aldrich syndrome	Poor response to polysaccharide antigens and depressed T cell function: ↓ IgM; ↑ IgA and IgE	Eczema, thrombocytopenia, and recurrent infections with encapsulated pyogenic bacteria; X-linked recessive

* ↓, Below normal; ↑, above normal. Immunoglobulin (Ig) entries refer to serum antibody levels of indicated isotype.

BOX 4-6 MAJOR OPPORTUNISTIC INFECTIONS

Some microbes rarely cause disease in individuals with a normal immune system, but they may do so in those with compromised immunity. Diseases caused by such **opportunistic organisms** include the following:

Fungal and Parasitic Disease

Pneumocystis species pneumonia

Chronic cryptosporidiosis

Toxoplasmal cerebral abscess

Extraintestinal strongyloidiasis

Isosporiasis

Esophageal and bronchial candidiasis

Cryptococcosis

Histoplasmosis

Bacterial and Viral Disease

Atypical mycobacterial infection

Cytomegalovirus infection

Herpes simplex ulceration

Disseminated herpesvirus infection

Progressive multifocal leukoencephalopathy

CHAPTER 5

LABORATORY TESTS FOR DIAGNOSIS

I. Laboratory Assays for Detecting Nucleic Acids (Table 5-1)

- Detection of RNA or DNA is rapid and sensitive and can detect microbes that are too virulent or not readily grown in the laboratory.
- Methods depend on hybridization of a probe (primer) sequence with a complementary sequence in the sample.
- Probes are either radioactive or chemically labeled to allow detection on hybridization with sample.

A. Southern blotting for DNA and Northern blotting for RNA detect electrophoretically separated genome sequences.

B. In situ hybridization detects viral DNA or RNA within infected cells.

C. Polymerase chain reaction (PCR) (DNA), reverse transcriptase (RT)-PCR (RNA), and related technologies permit detection, identification, and amplification of specific nucleic acid sequences.

1. PCR: heat-stable DNA polymerase amplifies DNA between sequence specific primers (Fig. 5-1)
2. RT-PCR: RT makes a complementary DNA copy of RNA, which is then amplified by PCR using sequence specific primers.
   - Detects RNA virus genomes, such as HIV
   - Detects messenger RNA for cytokine genes activated in an immune response

PCR is a rapid, sensitive, and specific means for detecting microbes and distinguishing microbial strains.

PCR of cerebrospinal fluid (CSF) replaced immunofluorescence of a brain biopsy for confirmation of herpes simplex virus (HSV) encephalitis.

RT-PCR is the method of choice for detecting most RNA viruses.

Viral load of human immunodeficiency virus (HIV) is determined by quantitative RT-PCR of patient serum.

TABLE 5-1 Common Diagnostic Procedures Used in Microbiology

METHOD	APPLICATIONS	SPECIFIC EXAMPLES
Genomic		
PCR	Rapid detection and identification of bacteria, DNA viruses, or fungi	Analysis of CSF for HSV encephalitis
RT-PCR	Rapid detection and identification of RNA viruses, mRNA expression	Detection of arboviruses, influenza strains
Quantitative RT-PCR	Quantity of virus Extent of mRNA expression	Viral load of HIV Extent of activation of immune cells
Serology		
ELISA	Quantitation of antibody Quantitation of antigen	Diagnosis of HBV and EBV infection Diagnosis of rotavirus, HBV, HIV, and other infections Pregnancy test
Immunofluorescence	Detection of virus infection	Cytomegalovirus infection of tissue culture cells
Ouchterlony	Presence of antibody or antigen in serum	Analysis of serum for *Histoplasma* or *Blastomyces* species infection
Western blot	Specificity of antibody	Confirmation test for HIV seropositivity
Flow cytometry	Quantitation of immune cell populations	CD4:CD8 T cell ratio for an AIDS patient

AIDS, acquired immunodeficiency syndrome; CSF, cerebrospinal fluid; ELISA, enzyme-linked immunosorbent assay; HBV, hepatitis B virus; HIV, human immunodeficiency virus; HSV, herpes simplex virus; mRNA, messenger RNA; RT, reverse transcriptase; PCR, polymerase chain reaction.

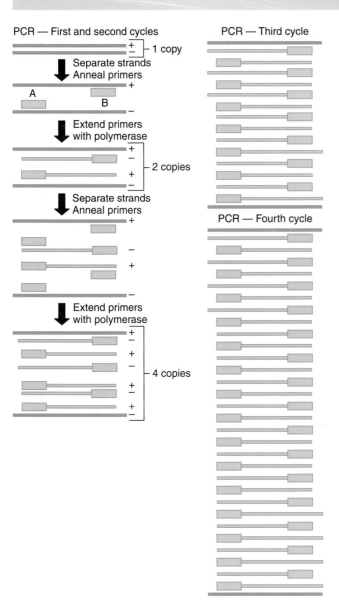

PCR — First and second cycles

1 copy

Separate strands
Anneal primers

A

B

Extend primers
with polymerase

2 copies

Separate strands
Anneal primers

Extend primers
with polymerase

4 copies

PCR — Third cycle

PCR — Fourth cycle

5-1: Polymerase chain reaction (PCR). After heating and melting a DNA sample, specific DNA primer sequences find, bind, and define the sample to be amplified. After cooling, a heat-stable DNA polymerase amplifies the DNA. The cycle is repeated 20 to 30 times, amplifying the sequence $2^{20\text{-}30}$ times. *(Modified from Blair GE, Blair Zajdel ME: Biochem Educ 20:87-90, 1992. In Murray PR, Rosenthal KS, Pfaller MA: Medical Microbiology, 6th ed. Philadelphia, Mosby, 2009, Fig. 16-4.)*

3. Quantitative PCR (qPCR; real-time PCR): rate of production of DNA during PCR reaction determines concentration of DNA in sample.
   - qPCR after reverse transcription of HIV genome can be used to quantitate the serum concentration of virus (genome load of infection).
4. Other DNA and RNA detection methods include branched-chain DNA assay and antibody capture solution hybridization assay.

II. Immunologic Assays (see Table 5-1)
- Assays can be used to detect immune responses to infection, or specific antibody can be used to detect soluble and cell-associated antigen.

A. Antibody-antigen binding (see also Chapter 3, section IV)
1. Precipitin reactions: Ouchterlony immunodiffusion distinguishes identical, similar, and different antigens based on the precipitin line formed by antigen-antibody precipitation (Fig. 5-2)
   - Used for testing serum for antibody in the diagnosis of *Histoplasma* and *Blastomyces* species fungi
2. Agglutination reactions include hemagglutination, passive agglutination, Coombs test, and ABO blood typing (Table 5-2).
3. Antibody-antigen binding is detected by a probe such as a fluorescent marker, radiolabel, or enzyme (e.g., horseradish peroxidase, alkaline phosphatase, and β-galactosidase) that produces a colored product on addition of substrate.

IgG anti-Rh antibodies, which are nonagglutinating, are detected by the Coombs test. This test employs antihuman antibody to cause agglutination of red blood cells (RBCs).

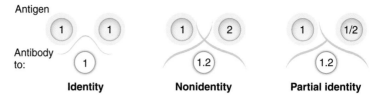

Identity **Nonidentity** **Partial identity**

5-2: Ouchterlony test. In this double-immunodiffusion method, antigen and antibody diffuse from wells in a gel and form a precipitin line (Ag-Ab precipitate) within the zone of equivalence. *Identity:* If two antigens share a common epitope specific for the antibody, a single continuous V-shaped precipitin line forms. In this example, both antigens contain epitope 1. *Nonidentity:* If two antigens have no common epitope, two distinct precipitin lines that cross are produced. In this example, one antigen contains epitope 1, and the other contains epitope 2. *Partial identity:* If two antigens share one epitope but not another, a continuous line with a spur forms. In this example, the right antigen contains epitopes 1 and 2, whereas the left antigen contains only one of these epitopes.

TABLE 5-2 **ABO Blood Types**

RECIPIENT BLOOD TYPE	ANTIGENS ON RED BLOOD CELLS	ANTIBODIES IN SERUM	COMPATIBLE DONOR BLOOD TYPES
A	A	Anti-B-IgM	A and O
B	B	Anti-A-IgM	B and O
AB	A and B	Neither	All (universal recipient)
O	Neither	Anti-A and anti-B; IgM and IgG (most people)	Only O (universal donor)

B. Immunofluorescence (IF) and enzyme immunoassay (EIA) detect proteins expressed on the surface or inside of cells (Fig. 5-3).

C. Direct versus indirect assays

1. For **direct assays,** antibody is covalently linked to the probe.
2. For **indirect assays,** the probe is linked to a secondary antibody that binds to the primary antiviral antibody after it interacts with viral antigen.

D. Enzyme-linked immunosorbent assay (ELISA) and radioimmunoassay (RIA) can be used to detect and quantitate antigen or antibody.

1. ELISA (Fig. 5-4)
   - For analysis of antigen: antibody is attached to plate and captures antigen, and an enzyme-linked antibody is used to detect and quantitate the antigen.
   - For analysis of antibody: antigen is attached to plate, antibody binds, and an enzyme-linked anti-antibody is used to detect and quantitate the antigen.
2. RIA: direct or competitive methods are used to detect and quantitate antigen.
   - Quantitative precipitation of radioactive antigen or antibody by the sample
   - Sample competes for radioactive material in a predetermined reaction with antibody.

ELISA can detect antigen or antibody depending on the adhered molecule used to capture the sample.

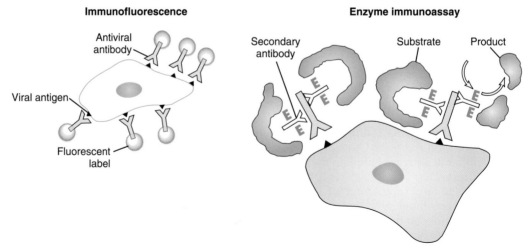

5-3: Immunofluorescence and enzyme immunoassay (EIA) for antigen localization. A biopsy specimen or tissue culture cells are incubated with an antigen-specific fluorescent conjugated antibody (e.g., fluorescein isothiocyanate; direct immunofluorescence) or an antigen-specific or patient serum and a second fluorescent-labeled anti-immunoglobulin antibody (indirect immunofluorescence) and then viewed under the fluorescent microscope. For EIA, antigen is detected with an enzyme-conjugated antibody (e.g., horseradish peroxidase), which converts a substrate into a chromophore visible under the light microscope.

ANTIBODY DETECTION   ANTIGEN CAPTURE AND DETECTION

5-4: Enzyme-linked immunosorbent assay quantitates antigen or antibody similar to enzyme immunoassay. For antigen, a capture antibody immobilized to the bottom of a well specifically captures antigen from a sample. Enzyme-conjugated antibody specific for the captured antigen is added, and quantitation of antigen is indicated by the amount of color (absorption) produced by conversion of substrate. *(From Murray PR, Rosenthal KS, Pfaller MA: Medical Microbiology, 6th ed. Philadelphia, Mosby, 2009, Fig. 17-5.)*

E. **Western blot can determine true-positive ELISA reactions by showing the specific proteins recognized by patient sera.**
   1. **Western Blot analysis** uses antibody to identify proteins that were blotted onto special paper membranes after molecular size separation by sodium dodecyl sulfate polyacrylamide gel electrophoresis (Fig. 5-5).
   2. True-positive reactions in ELISA can be confirmed by serum recognition of multiple proteins in the Western blot (confirmation test for HIV).
F. **Antibody inhibitory tests: hemagglutination inhibition, virus or toxin neutralization**
   1. Stock antibody is used to distinguish specific virus strain or toxin, such as strain of influenza.
   2. Stock virus or toxin is used to determine titer of antibody to a specific virus strain or toxin.

Western blot

5-5: Western blot analysis. Proteins separated by size are blotted onto a special filter paper and then reacted with antigen-specific or patient antibody (primary antibody) and then an enzyme conjugated antibody and enzyme substrate. A band is seen where antibody identifies a protein. 1° Ab, primary antibody; 2° Ab, secondary antibody; NC, nitrocellulose; SDS-PAGE, sodium dodecyl sulfate polyacrylamide gel electrophoresis. (From Murray PR, Rosenthal KS, Pfaller MA: Medical Microbiology, 6th ed. Philadelphia, Mosby, 2009, Fig. 17-6.)

BOX 5-1 CLINICAL USES OF SEROLOGY

Determination of the types and relative amounts of antibody and the identity of infectious agents in serum provides a history of a patient's infection. The **antibody titer** is the **reciprocal of the greatest dilution of antiserum** detectable by one or more antibody assays (e.g., passive agglutination, ELISA, and RIA). Serologic testing for antibody isotypes can detect certain immunodeficiency diseases (e.g., **Bruton agammaglobulinemia** and **selective IgA deficiency**).

The time course of an infection can be tracked by determining whether production of specific antibody in response to infection (**seroconversion**) has begun. Seroconversion, indicated by a **fourfold or greater increase in the specific antibody titer,** occurs 2 or 3 weeks after primary infection by many microbes. However, **HIV** and other pathogens exhibit a longer and more variable lag period between infection and seroconversion.

Pathogens, particularly viruses that are difficult to isolate and culture may be identified by assays for their antigens or for antibodies they induce. Viruses commonly identified by serology include **rubella virus, hepatitis viruses, Epstein-Barr virus,** and **HIV.**

III. Serology (History of the Infection) (Box 5-1)

　　A. Serologic testing can determine the type and titer of antiviral antibodies in serum and the identity of viral antigens.
　　　　1. Titer is defined as the lowest dilution that still gives a positive test result in a standardized assay.
　　　　2. A fourfold difference in antibody titer is required to indicate a significant response to antigen (seroconversion). (A fourfold difference means two tubes in a dilution scheme.)
　　　　3. A fourfold increase in antibody titer between acute and convalescent sera is necessary to indicate specific response.
　　　　4. Detection of specific immunoglobulin M (IgM) indicates recent exposure to antigen.

IV. Flow Cytometry
　　　　• Laser is used to rapidly evaluate size, granularity, and fluorescence properties of large numbers of cells (Fig. 5-6).
　　　　• A **fluorescence-activated cell sorter (FACS)** is a flow cytometer that can analyze and separate cells based on their properties as they flow through the instrument.
　　A. Light scatter measurements can distinguish lymphocytes, macrophages, and granulocytes.
　　　　1. Forward scatter determines size of cell.
　　　　2. Side scatter determines granularity.
　　B. DNA-binding fluorescent dyes can be used to evaluate cell cycle.
　　　　1. Cells in G_0, G_1 phase have fluorescence equivalent to 2N (N = normal chromosome number).
　　　　2. Cells in G_2 phase or mitosis have twice the fluorescence of G_0, G_1 phase cells.
　　　　3. Cells in S phase have intermediary fluorescence.
　　C. Immunofluorescence measurements indicate the phenotype of the cell.
　　　　1. Multiple antibodies marked with different fluorescent colors can be analyzed simultaneously.
　　　　2. Cells can be identified and quantitated by analysis of multiple cell surface markers (e.g., helper T cell expresses CD3, CD4).
　　　　3. Analysis can be presented as a histogram or a two-dimensional dot plot (see Fig. 5-6B to D).

Flow cytometry determination of CD4 T cell levels is often sufficient for a diagnosis of acquired immunodeficiency syndrome (AIDS).

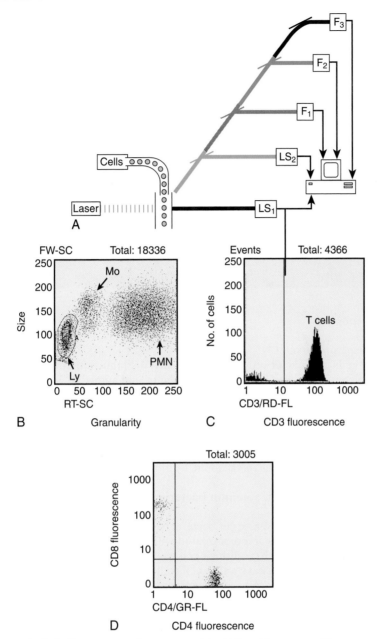

5-6: Flow cytometry. **A,** Individual cell parameters such as size, granularity (GR), and the presence of fluorescent markers (e.g., fluorescent antibodies or DNA stains) are detected at rates greater than 5000 per second as the cells pass through a laser beam. Computer analysis allows "gating" of the data to focus on subsets of cells for further analysis. Panels **B** to **D** depict T cell analysis of a normal individual. **B,** Laser light scatter depicts size and granularity of cells to distinguish type of cell. **C,** Only the lymphocyte (Ly) population is analyzed for CD3 expression. **D,** Only the T cells (CD3 expressing) are analyzed for CD4 or CD8 expression. F1, F2,F3, fluorescence detectors; LS1, LS2, light scatter detectors; FW-SC, forward light scatter: size; RT-SC, right angle light scatter: granularity; CD3/RD-FL, red fluorescence for CD3 antigen; CD4/GR-FL, green fluorescence for CD4 antigen. *(Data provided by Dr. Tom Alexander, Akron, Ohio.)*

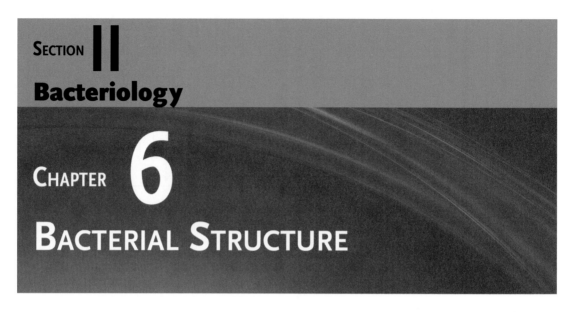

I. Bacterial Morphology

A. Overview

1. Bacteria are prokaryotes
   - Their cells lack nuclei and organelles, which distinguish them from the "true" cells of eukaryotes (i.e., algae, fungi, protozoa, plants, and animals).
2. The differences between eukaryotic and prokaryotic cells, summarized in Table 6-1, are the basis for antimicrobial drugs.

B. Size of bacterial cells

1. Bacterial cells range from 0.2 μm (e.g., *Mycoplasma* species) to 3 μm (e.g., *Bacillus anthracis*) in diameter.
2. The ubiquitous *Escherichia coli* is about 1 μm in diameter. By comparison, erythrocytes are 8 μm in diameter.

C. Shape and arrangement of common bacteria (Fig. 6-1)

D. Gram staining

1. Distinguishes two major classes of bacteria (see Chapter 8)
2. Bacteria that have been starved or treated with antibiotics exhibit variable staining.
3. **Gram-positive bacteria** have a thick cell wall and stain purple.
4. **Gram-negative bacteria** have a thin cell wall and stain red.
5. **Gram-resistant bacteria** (e.g., *Mycobacterium* and *Mycoplasma* species) stain poorly or not at all with Gram stain.

II. Bacterial Ultrastructure

- Gram-positive and gram-negative bacteria have similar internal structures but structurally dissimilar cell envelopes (Fig. 6-2; Table 6-2).

Gram staining:
- Purple = P = gram POSITIVE
- Red = NOT P = gram NEGATIVE

TABLE 6-1 **Prokaryotic Versus Eukaryotic Cells**

CHARACTERISTIC	PROKARYOTIC CELLS	EUKARYOTIC CELLS
Size (approximate) (μm)	0.5–3	>5
Cell wall	Complex structure composed of proteins, peptidoglycan, and lipids	Only in fungal and plant cells; composition differs from that of bacterial cell wall
Plasma (cytoplasmic) membrane	Contains no sterols (except in *Mycoplasma* species)	Contains sterols
Nuclear membrane	Absent	Present
Genome	Single, circular DNA molecule in nucleoid	Multiple, linear DNA molecules in nucleus
Organelles*	Absent	Present
Ribosomes	70S (50S + 30S subunits)	80S (60S + 40S subunits)
Cell division	Via binary fission	Via mitosis and meiosis

*Include mitochondria, Golgi complex, and endoplasmic reticulum.

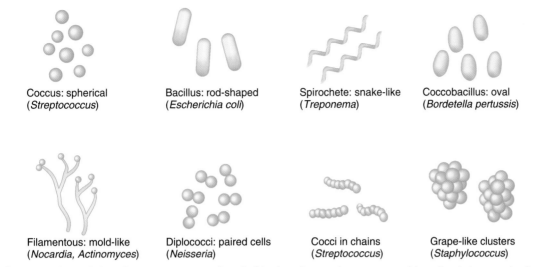

6-1: Bacterial morphologic features. Bacteria are described by their shape and arrangement of the cells relative to each other. Common species in each category are indicated in parentheses.

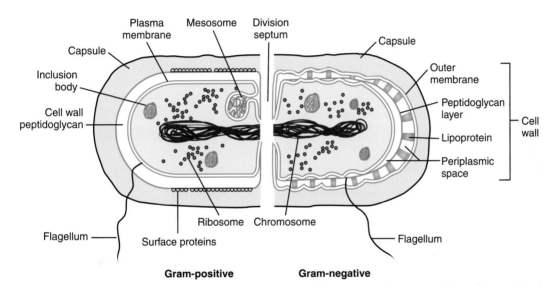

6-2: Gram-positive and gram-negative bacteria. Internal structures and the plasma membrane are similar in all bacteria, but the cell wall is more complex in gram-negative than in gram-positive bacteria. Motile bacteria possess a flagellum. Pili, which are shorter and thinner than flagella, are present on some gram-positive and gram-negative species.

TABLE 6-2 Comparison of Gram-Positive and Gram-Negative Bacteria

CHARACTERISTIC	GRAM-POSITIVE BACTERIA	GRAM-NEGATIVE BACTERIA
Structural		
Outer membrane	Absent	Present
Peptidoglycan layer	Thick	Thin
Lipopolysaccharide	Absent	Present
Teichoic acids	Present in many species	Absent
Capsule, pili, flagella	Present in some species	Present in some species
Functional		
Lysozyme sensitivity	Very sensitive	Largely resistant
Antibiotic permeability	Very permeable to most	Impermeable to many
Sporulation	Some species	None
Exotoxin production	Some species	Some species

A. Internal bacterial structures

1. Nucleoid is the central region of bacterium that contains DNA.
   - There is no nuclear membrane.
2. Bacterial cells contain a single chromosome composed of a circular DNA molecule.
   - Unlike eukaryotic chromosomes, bacterial chromosomes lack histones.
3. Because bacteria lack a nuclear membrane, transcription and translation are coupled (i.e., ribosome-mediated protein synthesis can begin while a messenger RNA [mRNA] is being produced and is still attached to the DNA).
4. Bacterial ribosomes differ in size, components, and shape from eukaryotic ribosomes and thus are a major target of antibiotic action.
5. Plasmids, which are small, circular fragments of extrachromosomal DNA, may be present and often carry antibiotic resistance genes.

B. Cell envelope (Table 6-3)

- Bacterial cell envelope = cytoplasmic membrane + cell wall

1. Cytoplasmic (cell, plasma) membrane
   - Is structurally similar to eukaryotic membranes but lacks sterols, except in some mycoplasmas
   - Membrane contains enzymes and other proteins that carry out energy production (e.g., electron transport chain, F_1 adenosine triphosphatase), transport of nutrients (e.g., permeases), and synthesis of structural components.
2. Cell wall of gram-positive bacteria (Fig. 6-3A)
   - Thick peptidoglycan layer forms a mesh-like exoskeleton essential for bacterial structure.
     a. Peptidoglycan is relatively porous, especially to antibiotics.
   - Teichoic and lipoteichoic acids associated with peptidoglycan are antigenic (strain differences) and may promote adhesion to host tissue.
     a. Weak, endotoxin-like activity is mediated by lipoteichoic acids, which are shed into the culture medium and host tissue.

Ribosome: major antimicrobial target; 30S subunit targeted by tetracycline and aminoglycosides; 50S subunit by chloramphenicol and macrolides, ketolides, and azalides.

Flagellin, lipopolysaccharide (LPS), lipoteichoic acid (LTA), and peptidoglycan are pathogen-associated molecular patterns (PAMPs) that stimulate toll-like receptors (TLRs).

TABLE 6-3 Bacterial Cell Envelope and Associated Structures

STRUCTURE	PRIMARY FUNCTIONS	CHEMICAL CONSTITUENTS
Cytoplasmic (Plasma)		
Membrane	Energy production, metabolite transport, synthesis of cell wall and capsule, support	Phospholipid bilayer, transport proteins, enzymes
Gram-Positive Cell Wall		
Peptidoglycan	Osmotic stability, structural integrity, cell shape; permeable to antibiotics	Thick meshwork of peptide cross-linked polysaccharide chains [(NAG-NAM)$_n$]
Teichoic and lipoteichoic acids	Adhesion to host cells, weak endotoxin activity, antigenic	Polymers of substituted ribitol or glycerol phosphate
Proteins	Adhesion to host cells, antiphagocytic, antigenic	Examples: streptococcal M and R proteins
Gram-Negative Cell Wall		
Peptidoglycan	See above	Thinner version of that found in gram-positive bacteria; linked to lipoproteins that are anchored in outer membrane
Periplasmic space	Transport of nutrients, degradation of macromolecules	Between cytoplasmic and outer membranes; carrier proteins and hydrolytic enzymes (virulence factors)
Outer membrane	Structural support, uptake of metabolites, permeability barrier, protection, antigenic	Phospholipid bilayer, porins, transport and other proteins, lipopolysaccharide
Lipopolysaccharide	Endotoxin activity (lipid A), anticomplement activity (O antigen)	Three parts: lipid A (anchored in outer membrane), core polysaccharide, O antigen (in most)
Porin channel	Allow small and hydrophilic molecules to pass outer membrane	Porin proteins
Other Structures		
Capsule	Antiphagocytic	Layers of polysaccharides or polypeptides
Pili (fimbriae)	Adhesion to host cells, mating	Repeating protein subunits (pilin, adhesin)
Flagella	Motility, antigenic	Flagellin protein

Gram-positive (+) cell wall

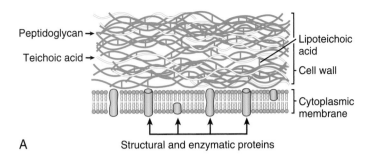

A

Structural and enzymatic proteins

Gram-negative (−) cell wall

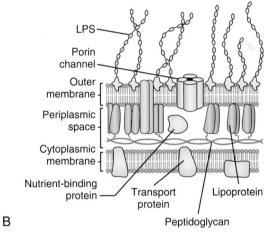

B

6-3: Structure of the cell wall of gram-positive and gram-negative bacteria. **A,** Gram-positive bacteria have a thick peptidoglycan layer that contains teichoic and lipoteichoic acids. **B,** Gram-negative bacteria have a thin peptidoglycan layer that is connected by lipoproteins to an outer membrane. Porin channels and other proteins in the outer membrane allow entry of small hydrophilic molecules. Lipopolysaccharide (LPS; endotoxin) is anchored in the outer membrane and extends into the extracellular environment.

b. Antibody to teichoic acid may indicate recent gram-positive bacterial infection
c. Teichoic acids distinguish different strains.
3. Cell wall of gram-negative bacteria (Fig. 6-3B)
   • Thin peptidoglycan layer is adjacent to cytoplasmic membrane.
   • Outer membrane maintains bacterial structure, acts as a permeability barrier, and provides protection against adverse environmental conditions (e.g., the digestive system of hosts).
   a. Anchors LPS to bacterial surface
   b. Is disrupted by polymyxin antibiotics or EDTA, which removes stabilizing Mg^{2+} and Ca^{2+} ions
   • Periplasmic space, located between the outer membrane and the cytoplasmic membrane, contains degradative enzymes (e.g., β-lactamase) and nutrient-binding and transport proteins.
   • Lipoproteins covalently linked to the peptidoglycan layer are inserted into the outer membrane, connecting the two structures.
   • Porin channels made up of porin proteins allow small, hydrophilic molecules (including some antimicrobials) to pass through the outer membrane and limit entry of large or hydrophobic molecules.
4. Cell wall of **Mycobacterium** species
   • Structure of peptidoglycan in mycobacteria differs slightly from that in other bacteria.
   • **Wax-like** lipid coat containing **mycolic acid** surrounds the peptidoglycan-like layer.
   a. This coat is responsible for **virulence** and **antiphagocytic** activity of mycobacteria.
   b. **Corynebacterium** and **Nocardia** species also produce mycolic acid.
   • Mycobacteria and other mycolic acid–producing bacteria can be identified with **acid-fast** stains.

Gram-negative bacteria have thin peptidoglycan.

Outer membrane has unique structure and composition, with LPS facing outside.

Porin channels allow passage of small and hydrophilic molecules but block others.

Antibiotic's ability to permeate porin channels determines sensitivity and resistance.

An acid-fast stained bacillus in sputum is a mycobacterium.

Teichoic acids are present only in gram-positive bacteria; LPS (endotoxin) is present only in gram-negative bacteria. Mycoplasma lack cell walls, and chlamydia have an outer membrane with LPS but no peptidoglycan.

The polysaccharide capsule surrounding some bacteria is poorly antigenic and antiphagocytic. Bacteria with a prominent, virulence-promoting capsule include *Streptococcus pneumoniae*, *Klebsiella pneumoniae*, *Neisseria meningitidis*, and *Haemophilus influenzae* (type b).

When encapsulated bacteria are mixed with specific anticapsular antisera, the capsule swells, indicating a positive quellung (Neufeld) reaction.

Capsular polysaccharides are used in vaccines against *S. pneumoniae* (Pneumovax), *H. influenzae* type b (Hib), and some meningococcal serotypes.

Capsule is a major virulence factor, is antiphagocytic, and extends the bacteria's time in the bloodstream.

Pili are the major virulence factor providing adherence to especially in urinary tract infections.

Lysozyme in tears and mucus degrades peptidoglycan. Outer membrane protects against lysozyme; therefore, only gram-positive bacteria are sensitive.

C. Other external structures (see Fig. 6-2; Table 6-3)
1. Bacterial capsule
   - Loose layers of polysaccharide or protein that surround the cell wall of some bacteria (Box 6-1)
2. Pili (fimbriae)
   - Short, hair-like appendages composed of protein subunits (pilins) and anchored in plasma membrane of some bacteria
   - Common (somatic) pili
     a. Promote adherence of bacteria to host cells, especially mucosal cells
     b. Are a virulence factor for *Neisseria gonorrhoeae*
   - F pili (sex pili)
     a. Promote transfer of DNA from one bacterium to another through conjugation
     b. Are encoded by a plasmid (F factor)
3. Flagella
   - Long, rope-like appendages that are polymers of the protein flagellin and are anchored to basal bodies in the plasma membrane of some bacteria
   - Confer motility on bacteria and propel them toward food or other chemoattractants (chemotaxis)
   - Express antigenic determinants that distinguish strains of organisms

III. Peptidoglycan
- Peptidoglycan, a rigid mesh-like polymer, is responsible for the structural integrity and shape of the bacterial cell.

A. Structural parts of peptidoglycan (mucopeptide, murein)
- The basic structure consists of polysaccharide (glycan) chains with tetrapeptide or longer side chains that are cross-linked through peptide bonds (Fig. 6-4).
1. Glycan chains are linear polymers of a repeating disaccharide composed of *N*-acetylglucosamine (NAG) and *N*-acetylmuramic acid (NAM).
   - Lysozyme, present in human tears and mucous secretions, cleaves glycan chains.
2. Tetrapeptide side chains contain both L amino acids and D amino acids; the latter are unusual in biologic systems.
   - In a given species, all peptide side chains are identical, but their sequences may vary among species.

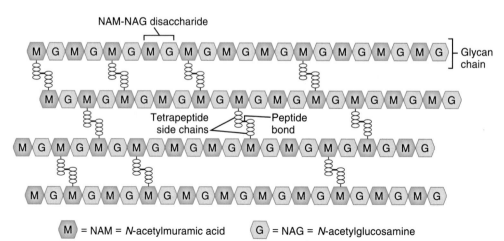

6-4: General structure of the peptidoglycan component of the cell wall. Glycan chains of alternating NAM and NAG residues are connected by peptide bonds between the side chains extending from NAM residues. Side chains are commonly tetrapeptides but are longer in some species. The thickness of the peptidoglycan layer increases as more chains are cross-linked.

3. Peptide bond between a tetrapeptide attached to one glycan chain and that on another chain cross-links the two chains.

B. Biosynthesis of peptidoglycan

1. Peptidoglycan is constantly being synthesized and degraded.
2. Synthesis involves four basic events.
   - Assembly of NAM and NAG precursors and addition of peptide side chain to NAM in the cytoplasm
   - Formation of NAG-NAM disaccharide on inner surface of the cytoplasmic membrane with the aid of bactoprenol, a long carrier molecule embedded in the inner leaflet of the membrane
     a. Bactoprenol with attached NAG-NAM unit then moves to outer leaflet.
   - Transfer of NAG-NAM unit to growing glycan chain extends the chain and frees bactoprenol carrier for reuse
   - Cross-linking of peptide side chains on adjacent glycan chains is catalyzed by transpeptidase (penicillin-binding protein [PBP]) enzymes associated with the outer surface of the membrane (Fig. 6-5)

C. Antibiotics that inhibit peptidoglycan synthesis

   - Degradation of peptidoglycan continues even when synthesis is inhibited, leading to **cell lysis** (death).
1. **Vancomycin** and **teicoplanin** are glycopeptide antibiotics that inhibit elongation of peptidoglycan chains.
2. β-Lactam antibiotics (e.g., penicillins and cephalosporins) inhibit cross-linking reaction.
3. **Bacitracin** interferes with recycling of bactoprenol carrier.

IV. Lipopolysaccharide

   - LPS is the major component of the outer membrane of gram-negative bacteria and is shed into the culture medium or host tissues.

A. Structural parts of LPS (Fig. 6-6)

1. Lipid A, a phosphorylated, fatty acid–modified disaccharide, is anchored in the outer membrane by its fatty acid portion.
   - Endotoxin activity of LPS is mediated by lipid A (see Chapter 7).
2. Core polysaccharide, located adjacent to the outer membrane, is a branched polysaccharide of 9 to 12 sugars attached to lipid A.
   - Core structure is identical for all members of a species but varies among species.
3. O antigen, the outermost part of LPS, is a long, linear polysaccharide composed of 50 to 100 repeating sugar units.
   - Differences in O antigen define serotypes (strains) of a bacterial species.
   - *Neisseria* species lack O antigen, producing a variant form of LPS called *lipooligosaccharide* (LOS), which is readily shed.

> Cross-linking of peptidoglycan is the target for β-lactam antibiotics, vancomycin, and bacitracin.

> Lipid A is endotoxin.

> *Neisseria* species shed LOS, which mediates endotoxin action.

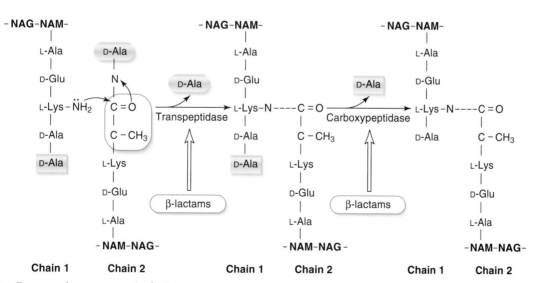

6-5: Transpeptidation reaction, the final step in peptidoglycan synthesis. Free —NH$_2$ on lysine or other diamino-amino acid on chain 1 forms a peptide bond (*dashed line*) with penultimate D-alanine on chain 2, leading to release of the terminal D-alanine from the chain, requiring no new energy. Penicillins and other β-lactam antibiotics bind to and inhibit the enzymes catalyzing these reactions. *Dashed line* represents cross-linking peptide bond.

6-6: General structure of bacterial lipopolysaccharide (LPS). Lipid A and the core polysaccharide are present in all gram-negative bacteria, but some lack the O-antigen component (LOS). Covalent bonds and divalent cation bridges between phosphates of lipid A molecules link LPS into large aggregates, which help stabilize the outer membrane. In addition to contributing to structural integrity of the outer membrane, lipid A mediates the endotoxin activity of LPS.

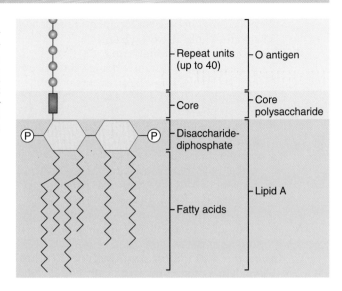

BOX 6-2 ASSEMBLY OF CELL WALL AND CAPSULE CONSTITUENTS

Bacteria use a **membrane-carrier system** for assembling peptidoglycan, LPS, teichoic acids, and capsular polysaccharides. Activated precursors are made inside the cell, where the necessary enzymes and energy are available. With the aid of **bactoprenol,** a membrane-embedded carrier molecule, these prefabricated units are assembled into larger structures on the inner surface of the plasma membrane and then transferred to the outer surface.

B. Synthesis of LPS (Box 6-2)

1. The lipid A and core portions are enzymatically synthesized on the inner surface of the cytoplasmic membrane and then are joined together.
2. Each O antigen repeat unit is assembled on a bactoprenol molecule and then is transferred to a growing O antigen chain (similar to peptidoglycan synthesis).
3. The completed O antigen is transferred to the core lipid A structure, and the entire LPS molecule is translocated to the outer surface of the outer membrane.

CHAPTER 7

BACTERIAL GROWTH, GENETICS, AND VIRULENCE

I. Proliferation of Bacterial Cells

A. Bacterial growth curve
- When placed in a new medium, bacteria exhibit a typical pattern of growth and multiplication marked by four phases (Fig. 7-1).

B. Growth requirements
1. Overview
   - Different bacteria require different nutrients for growth in the body and in culture.
   - Characteristic nutrient requirements and metabolic products can be used to identify bacteria.
2. **Oxygen** requirement
   - Obligate aerobes require oxygen for growth.
   - Anaerobes do *not* require oxygen for growth.
     a. Obligate anaerobes, which are damaged by oxygen, include normal colonizers of the gastrointestinal tract, respiratory tract, and/or skin.
     b. Aerotolerant anaerobes can survive in the presence of small amounts of oxygen but grow best in its absence.
   - Facultative anaerobes can grow under aerobic or anaerobic conditions.
3. Nutrient requirements
   - Undemanding eaters can be cultured on simple media (e.g., *E. coli*, *Salmonella* species, and other gram-negative enteric bacteria).
   - Demanding eaters require complex media containing numerous growth factors (e.g., *Haemophilus* and *Neisseria* species).
4. Temperature requirements
   - Most pathogenic bacteria of medical importance grow optimally at 35°C to 37°C, near normal body temperatures.

Mycobacterium tuberculosis, Neisseria, Nocardia species, and *Pseudomonas aeruginosa* are obligate aerobes.

Bacteroides, Actinomyces, Treponema, and *Propionibacterium* species are obligate anaerobes.

Some *Clostridium* species are aerotolerant anaerobes.

Facultative anaerobes include *Escherichia coli* and *Staphylococcus aureus.*

Aminoglycoside antibiotics (e.g., streptomycin and gentamicin) are ineffective against anaerobic bacteria.

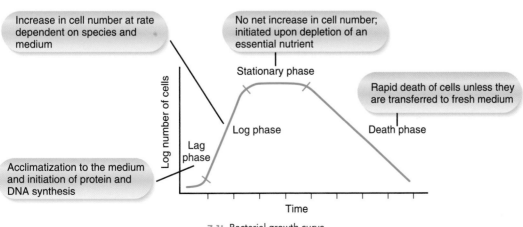

Increase in cell number at rate dependent on species and medium

No net increase in cell number; initiated upon depletion of an essential nutrient

Stationary phase

Rapid death of cells unless they are transferred to fresh medium

Log number of cells

Log phase

Death phase

Lag phase

Acclimatization to the medium and initiation of protein and DNA synthesis

Time

7-1: Bacterial growth curve.

C. Cell division

- Bacteria divide by binary fission, a simpler process than mitotic division of eukaryotic cells.
  1. Chromosome duplication is initiated at a specific sequence (replication origin) in the DNA.
     - If nutrients are available, synthesis of new chromosome begins before previous chromosome synthesis is completed. Once duplication is initiated, the process is completed even when culture conditions (e.g., starvation) are detrimental to the cell.
  2. Synthesis of new membrane and cell wall in the center of the cell forms a septum that eventually divides the cytoplasm into two daughter cells, each containing a complete chromosome.

D. Bacterial spores (endospores)

- Spores, formed by some gram-positive bacteria, represent a dormant state that is resistant to heat, drying, and chemicals.
  1. Spore formation, a variant type of cell division, is induced by depletion of essential nutrients needed for normal growth.
     - Antibiotics and toxins are often produced during sporogenesis, before release of the spore from the bacterial cell.
  2. Germination of spores into vegetative cells is initiated by damage to the spore coat by trauma, water, or aging and requires specific nutrients.
     - Once germination has begun and the spore coat is disrupted, spores are susceptible to the same agents as vegetative cells.

II. Bacterial Genetics

- Important definitions are given in Table 7-1.

A. Bacterial chromosome

1. Single, double-stranded, circular molecule of DNA, containing about 5 million base pairs (or 5000 kilobase pairs)
   - Mycoplasmas have a chromosome about one fourth this size, the smallest bacterial chromosome.
2. Operons provide coordinated control of protein-coding (structural) genes. A bacterial chromosome contains many operons.
   - The enzymes in many bacterial metabolic pathways are encoded by polycistronic operons, which contain multiple structural genes.
   - All the genes in a polycistronic operon are transcribed as a unit, producing a single messenger RNA (mRNA) that is translated into multiple proteins.
   - Transcription of the *lac* operon and many other operons is controlled by presence or absence of metabolites to meet the needs of the cell (Fig. 7-2).

B. Other genetic elements

1. Plasmids
   - Extrachromosomal genetic elements that can replicate independently of the bacterial chromosome
     a. Some plasmids (e.g., *E. coli* F factor) are episomes, which can integrate into the host chromosome.
     b. Drug resistance genes and toxin genes are carried by some plasmids. Plasmids containing a resistance gene are used in gene cloning.

Bacteria initiate new DNA synthesis before cell division (they are born pregnant).

Some gram-positive bacteria can sporulate; gram-negative bacteria *cannot* sporulate.

The most important spore formers are members of *Bacillus* and *Clostridium* genera.

Spores are resistant to boiling and many chemicals (including common disinfectants) and can survive in soil for long times.

Spores are inactivated by autoclaving for 15 minutes and by aldehyde-containing disinfectants.

Transformation: uptake of a segment of naked DNA and its incorporation into the bacterial chromosome

Transduction: uptake of DNA packaged in phage particles and its incorporation into the bacterial chromosome

Conjugation: direct transfer of DNA from a donor (male) cell to a recipient (female) cell through sex (F) pilus, which is encoded by F plasmid in donor cell

Transposition: movement of a transposon (nonreplicable DNA segment) from one DNA site to another, resulting in inactivation of the recipient gene into which it inserts

---

TABLE 7-1 **Bacterial Genetics Terminology**

TERM	DEFINITION
Allele	A particular example of a gene. Each variant of a given gene is a different allele of that gene. Genes that are represented by **multiple alleles** in a population are said to be **polymorphic**.
Cistron	Region of DNA that **codes for a single protein**; a complementation unit
Operator	Nucleotide sequence, located between the promoter and first structural gene of an operon, that **binds a repressor protein**
Operon	Bacterial **transcription unit** comprising a promoter, operator, and one or more structural genes
Plasmid	Small **extrachromosomal DNA** molecule capable of **autonomous replication** in bacteria
Promoter	Nucleotide sequence in an operon that is **recognized by RNA polymerase**
Replicon	Replication unit, consisting of a replication **origin**, a replication terminus, and the intervening coding sequence

Glucose present, lactose absent, low cAMP

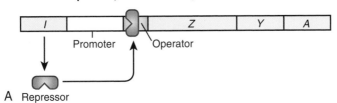

Glucose and lactose present, low cAMP

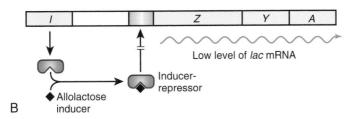

Lactose present, glucose absent, high cAMP

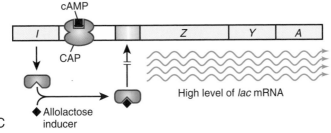

7-2: Regulation of the lactose (*lac*) operon in *Escherichia coli*. The three structural genes in the *lac* operon (Z, Y, and A) encode enzymes that metabolize lactose. Transcription yields a single polycistronic messenger RNA (mRNA), which is translated into the three proteins. **A,** Transcription is directly inhibited by binding of the *lac* repressor (encoded by the *I* gene) to the operator. **B,** In the presence of lactose, the inducer allolactose forms. This molecule binds to the *lac* repressor, forming a complex that cannot bind to the operator, thereby derepressing the operon. **C,** Transcription is stimulated by binding of the activator cAMP-CAP to the promoter. In the absence of glucose, the cAMP level increases, permitting formation of cAMP-CAP. Thus, the *lac* operon is fully "turned on" only when lactose is present and glucose is absent. cAMP, cyclic adenosine monophosphate; CAP, cAMP-binding protein.

    2. Bacteriophages
- Viruses that infect bacteria
  - a. Lytic phages replicate independently of the host chromosome and kill the bacterial host cell.
  - b. Lysogenic phages (e.g., *E. coli* λ phage) can integrate their genome into the host cell chromosome without killing the host.
    - Toxin genes are carried by some lysogenic bacteriophages (e.g., corynephage β carries the gene for diphtheria toxin).
    - A lysogenic bacteriophage becomes lytic and "jumps ship" under certain conditions (e.g., an unhealthy or starving host).

    Lytic phages kill their host; lysogenic phages live in their host but can "jump ship" if the bacteria are sick.

    3. Transposons
- DNA sequences (**"jumping genes"**) that can move from one position to another in a bacterial chromosome or between different molecules of DNA. These elements lack a replication origin.
  - a. **Simple** transposons (insertion sequences) encode only the proteins needed to move.
  - b. **Complex** transposons carry other genes (e.g., **antibiotic-resistance** genes).
    - **Pathogenicity islands** are large transposons that contain all the genes needed for a pathogenic mechanism. They may contain several operons.
    - Pathogenicity islands are coordinately controlled by environmental (temperature), metabolic, and other triggers.

    Salmonella species cellular entry biodevices are encoded within pathogenicity islands turned on by acidic pH and temperature.

C. Mechanisms of genetic transfer
- Although bacteria replicate by binary fission, an asexual process, they have several mechanisms for transferring genetic information, as illustrated in Figure 7-3.

TRANSFORMATION

Donor cell → Cell lysis; release of DNA fragments → DNA enters recipient cell and integrates into DNA

TRANSDUCTION

Phage-infected donor cell

Transducing phage containing donor genomic DNA → Cell lysis; release of phages → Phage infects recipient cell; donor DNA integrates into recipient DNA

CONJUGATION

Genomic DNA

Plasmid DNA

Free plasmid moves from donor to recipient cell via sex (F) pilus

Genomic DNA

Sex pilus

Integrated plasmid (episome) promotes transfer of genomic DNA, which integrates into recipient DNA

TRANSPOSITION

Transposon with inverted repeats

Donor site

gene A gene B′   gene B′ gene C

Recipient site

7-3: Bacterial gene transfer mechanisms. *Shading* indicates recipient cell or DNA.

D. Recombination
1. Homologous recombination occurs between closely related DNA sequences and generally results in substitution of one sequence for another.
   - Basis for periodic shifts in antigens of *Salmonella flagella* and *Neisseria gonorrhoeae* pilus
2. Nonhomologous recombination occurs between dissimilar DNA sequences and generally results in insertions or deletions.
   - Basis for integration of phages into host chromosome and movement of transposons

III. Mechanisms of Bacterial Virulence (Box 7-1)
   - Common routes of bacterial entry are listed in Table 7-2.
   - Disease results from tissue destruction, compromised organ function, or host defense responses that produce systemic symptoms (e.g., fever, nasal congestion, headache, lethargy, and loss of appetite).

   A. Adherence
   - Refers to adherence to epithelial or endothelial cell linings of the bladder, intestine, oropharynx, blood vessels, and other structures that prevent bacteria from being washed away and allows them to colonize these sites

Pili promote adherence.

BOX 7-1 "MUST-KNOWS" FOR BACTERIAL VIRULENCE MECHANISMS: EAT RICE

Enzyme-mediated tissue damage (e.g., hyaluronidase, hemolysin, streptokinase)
Adherence (pili, other adhesins)
Toxin-induced localized and systemic effects (exotoxins, endotoxin)
Resistance to antibiotics
Invasion and growth in normally sterile sites
Circulation via the blood or other means of spreading from primary infection site
Evasion of host immune response by capsule, catalase, intracellular growth, and other mechanisms

TABLE 7-2 **Bacterial Entry into the Body***

ENTRY ROUTE	EXAMPLES
Ingestion	*Bacillus cereus*
	Brucella species
	Campylobacter species
	Clostridium botulinum
	Escherichia coli (enterotoxigenic)
	Listeria species
	Salmonella species
	Shigella species
	Vibrio species
Inhalation	*Bordetella* species
	Chlamydia pneumoniae
	Chlamydia psittaci
	Legionella species
	Mycobacterium species
	Mycoplasma pneumoniae
	Nocardia species
Trauma/needlestick	*Clostridium tetani*
	Pseudomonas species
	Staphylococcus aureus
Arthropod or animal bite	*Borrelia* species
	Coxiella species
	Ehrlichia species
	Francisella species
	Rickettsia species
	Yersinia pestis
Sexual transmission	*Chlamydia trachomatis*
	Neisseria gonorrhoeae
	Treponema pallidum
Transplacental	*Treponema pallidum*

*Most common routes of entry

1. Common pili (fimbriae) are the major structures involved in adherence of enteric bacteria and *N. gonorrhoeae*.
   • Bacteria that lack pili may possess other cell surface adhesins (e.g., lectin protein, lipoteichoic acid, and slime).
2. Adhesin molecules, whether present on pili or elsewhere, interact with receptors on host cells.

B. Invasion
   • Refers to bacteria breaking through tissue barriers and colonizing tissues (Box 7-2)
1. Some enteric bacteria have mechanisms for invading various portions of the gastrointestinal tract.
2. Invasion of normally sterile sites even by normal microbial flora can cause diseases such as bacteremia, meningitis, encephalitis, and pneumonia.

Sterile sites: blood, cerebrospinal fluid, brain, organ parenchyma, lower lung airways, joint spaces, bone

---

BOX 7-2 NORMAL MICROBIAL FLORA

Nonsterile sites in the body (e.g., lumen of the gastrointestinal and urogenital tracts, mouth, saliva, pharynx, and skin) harbor certain organisms that constitute the normal microbial flora. Some dominant members of the **normal flora** and their usual locations include the following:

Skin: *Staphylococcus epidermidis, Propionibacterium acnes*
Upper respiratory tract: *Staphylococcus aureus, Streptococcus pneumoniae, Haemophilus influenzae*
Colon: *Escherichia coli, Bacteroides fragilis*

These and other species composing the normal flora may cause disease when they gain access to organ parenchyma or other sterile sites from which they normally are excluded. Antibiotic elimination of the normal flora can allow excessive growth of competing, drug-resistant organisms (e.g., *Clostridium difficile* in the intestine) that usually are *not* present or are only a minor component of the flora.

Bacterial tissue damage can be caused by metabolic byproducts, degradative enzymes, inhibitors of cell processes, growth on top of cells, and intracellular growth.

3. Colonization of a tissue can cause its destruction or dysfunction or can be a source of spread in the body or release of toxins, including endotoxins.

C. Tissue damage
- Caused in part by bacterial products.
1. Tissue-damaging metabolites (e.g., acids, gases, and other byproducts) may be formed during bacterial growth.
2. Degradative enzymes and cytolytic exotoxins are released by many bacteria.
   - *Clostridium perfringens:* lecithinase (α toxin)
   - Streptococci: hemolysin, streptokinase, hyaluronidase
   - Staphylococci: hyaluronidase, fibrinolysin, lipases, enterotoxins
3. Exotoxins that disrupt normal cellular metabolism (see section G).
4. Intracellular growth can disrupt cell function (e.g., mycobacteria).
5. Bacterial growth on top of tissue can damage and disrupt tissue function (e.g., coagulase-negative staphylococci or viridans streptococci subacute endocarditis)

D. Circulation through the blood (bacteremia)
1. Primary mechanism for spreading bacteria throughout the body
2. Tissue damage promotes bacterial spread, especially if blood vessels are damaged.

E. Pathogen-associated molecular patterns (PAMPs)
Bacteria in blood release cell wall molecules and activate inflammatory processes, including fever.

Cell wall components are PAMPS that activate TLRs to promote acute phase responses.
1. PAMPs are repetitive microbial structures that bind to toll-like receptors (TLRs) and other pathogen pattern receptors on various cells, activate macrophages and dendritic cells, and promote acute phase cytokine release.
2. Examples of PAMPs: peptidoglycan, lipopolysaccharide (LPS), lipoteichoic acid, teichoic acid, flagellin, and CpG oligodeoxynucleotides

F. Endotoxin
All gram-negative bacteria make endotoxin, the lipid A portion of LPS.

Endotoxin causes fever, shock, disseminated intravascular coagulation, and possibly death.
1. The lipid A component of LPS
2. Is present in the cell wall of all gram-negative bacteria
3. Is released during early stages of infection with gram-negative bacteria
4. Initiates complement and clotting pathways
5. LPS is a strong PAMP and binds to TLRs on various cells to induce release of mediators that cause sepsis (Fig. 7-4; Box 7-3).

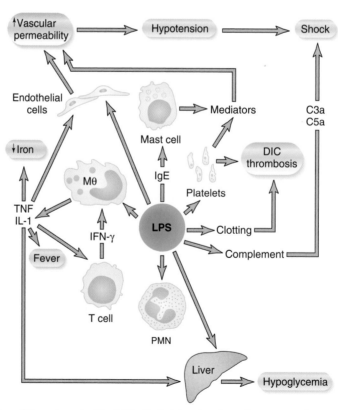

7-4: The many activities of lipopolysaccharide (LPS). Bacterial endotoxin activates many immune mechanisms and the clotting cascade. DIC, disseminated intravascular coagulation; IFN-γ, interferon-γ; IgE, immunoglobulin E; IL-1, interleukin-1; Mθ, macrophage; PMN, polymorphonuclear leukocyte (neutrophil); TNF, tumor necrosis factor.

- Activation of macrophage and dendritic cells through TLRs
- Induction of endogenous pyrogens (e.g., IL-1, TNF, IL-6, prostaglandins) → *fever*
- Increase in capillary permeability → *hypotension and shock*
- Initiation of complement cascade → *shock*
- Initiation of blood coagulation cascades → *disseminated intravascular coagulation*
  Fever + hypotension + shock + multisystem organ failure = possible death

G. Exotoxins
- Secreted by certain gram-positive and gram-negative bacteria (Table 7-3)
1. Cytolytic exotoxins are tissue-degrading enzymes.
2. A-B toxins are composed of one or more B subunits, which bind to the cell surface, and an A subunit, which enters the cell and acts on it (Table 7-4).
3. Superantigen exotoxins activate T cells in the absence of antigen by cross-linking the T cell receptor and class II major histocompatibility complex on antigen-presenting cells.
   - Cause inappropriate release of cytokines (e.g., interleukin-1 [IL-1], IL-6, tumor necrosis factor-α, and other cytokines), with possible life-threatening autoimmune responses and death of T cells
   - Toxic shock syndrome toxin (TSST) of *S. aureus*, staphylococcal enterotoxins, and erythrogenic toxin of *Streptococcus pyogenes* are prime examples.

H. Antibiotic resistance
1. It can spread through a bacterial population by transfer of antibiotic-resistance genes (see Fig. 7-3), or antibiotic may eliminate competing, nonresistant organisms.

I. Escape of host attempts at elimination
- Evasion of host defenses permits bacteria to remain in the host longer, thereby causing more damage.
1. Encapsulation with polysaccharide (slime) layer (Box 7-4)
   - Capsules are poorly antigenic, deter phagocytosis because they are slippery and tear away, and protect against degradation in phagolysosomes of macrophages and neutrophils.
   - Virulence of some encapsulated bacteria (e.g., *S. pneumoniae* and *N. meningitidis*) is lost in mutants lacking a capsule.
2. Biofilms are sticky webs of polysaccharide that can protect the bacteria from host defenses and antimicrobials.
   - Sufficient bacteria must be present to make a biofilm (quorum sensing).
   - *P. aeruginosa* and other bacteria make biofilms. Dental plaque is a biofilm.
3. Intracellular growth *without* inactivation (especially in macrophages)
   - Organisms that can grow and multiply within host cells escape immune detection.
     a. Inhibition of phagolysosome fusion (*M. tuberculosis*), protective outer layers (*M. tuberculosis*), and resistance to lysosomal enzymes allow replication within cells.
     b. Obligate intracellular bacteria: *Rickettsia, Chlamydia, Coxiella* species
   - Chronic stimulation of immune response may result in granuloma formation
     a. Facultative intracellular bacteria: *Mycobacterium, Salmonella, Listeria, Brucella, Francisella, Yersinia, Legionella* species

The B subunit of A-B toxins Binds to the receptor and the A subunit Acts on the cell.

Superantigens and sepsis induce a cytokine storm that dysregulates the immune response, causing hypotension and shock.

The capsule produced by certain gram-positive and gram-negative bacteria is a significant virulence factor that helps bacteria avoid immune detection, phagocytosis, and intracellular killing.

Patients lacking a spleen are more susceptible to encapsulated bacteria.

P. aeruginosa and *Streptococcus mutans* (dental plaque) make biofilms when a quorum of bacteria are present.

TABLE 7-3 **Endotoxin Versus Exotoxins**

PROPERTY	ENDOTOXIN	EXOTOXINS
Produced by	Gram-negative bacteria	Certain gram-positive and gram-negative bacteria
Location of genes	Bacterial chromosome	Bacterial chromosome, plasmid, bacteriophage
Composition	Lipid A part of lipopolysaccharide in cell wall	Polypeptide (secreted)
Stability	Heat stable	Heat labile (usually)
Major biologic actions	Induces tumor necrosis factor-α, interleukin (IL-1), IL-6; initiates complement and clotting pathways	Inhibit protein synthesis, block neuro-transmitter release, increase cyclic adenosine monophosphate level, etc.
Clinical effects	Fever, hypotension, shock, disseminated intravascular coagulation	Various, depending on type (see Table 7-4)
Used as vaccine	No: poorly antigenic	Yes (inactivated **toxoids**): highly antigenic

TABLE 7-4 **A-B Type Bacterial Exotoxins**

TOXIN	ORGANISM	MODE OF ACTION	GENERAL EFFECTS
Increased Production of Cyclic Adenosine Monophosphate			
Anthrax toxin (edema factor)	*Bacillus anthracis*	Has adenylate cyclase activity	Localized edema; cell death
Cholera toxin	*Vibrio cholerae*	Turns on stimulatory G protein	Secretory diarrhea with ion loss
Enterotoxins, heat labile	*Escherichia coli*	Turns on stimulatory G protein	Secretory diarrhea with ion loss
Pertussis toxin	*Bordetella pertussis*	Turns off inhibitory G protein	Loss of fluids and electrolytes, lymphocytosis, mucus secretion in respiratory tract
Inhibition of Protein Synthesis			
Diphtheria toxin	*Corynebacterium diphtheriae*	Adenosine diphosphate ribosylates EF-2	Cell death leading to disease symptoms
Exotoxin A	*Pseudomonas aeruginosa*	Adenosine diphosphate ribosylates EF-2	Cell death
Shiga toxin	*Shigella dysenteriae*	Cleaves 28S recombinant RNA	Cell death; watery diarrhea, hemolytic-uremic syndrome
Altered Transmission of Nerve Impulses			
Botulinum toxin	*Clostridium botulinum*	Prevents release of acetylcholine	Flaccid paralysis
Tetanus toxin	*Clostridium tetani*	Prevents release of neurotransmitters from inhibitory neurons	Spastic paralysis

---

BOX 7-4 EXAMPLES OF ENCAPSULATED BACTERIA

Gram-Positive Bacteria
Bacillus anthracis
Bacillus subtilis
Staphylococcus aureus
Streptococcus agalactiae (group B)
Streptococcus pneumoniae
Streptococcus pyogenes (group A)

Gram-Negative Bacteria
Bacteroides fragilis
Campylobacter fetus
Escherichia coli
Haemophilus influenzae
Klebsiella pneumoniae
Neisseria gonorrhoeae
Neisseria meningitidis
Pseudomonas aeruginosa
Salmonella species
Yersinia pestis

Bacteria escape phagocytes by preventing uptake, detoxifying or preventing production of reactive oxygen species, or preventing lysosome function.

4. Reduction of phagocytic cell function
   - Inhibition of phagocytosis by antiphagocytic capsule and certain cell surface proteins (e.g., M protein of *S. pyogenes*)
   - Reduction in phagolysosomal killing of phagocytosed bacteria by capsules, inhibition of phagosome-lysosome fusion (*M. tuberculosis*), and catalase detoxification of peroxide (*S. aureus*)
   - Killing of phagocytic cells by exotoxins (e.g., streptolysins of *S. pyogenes*, lethal toxin of anthrax, and α toxin of *C. perfringens*)

5. Inactivation of antibody
   - Immunoglobulin A (IgA)-degrading proteases produced by some bacteria permit them to colonize mucosal surfaces: *N. gonorrhoeae, N. meningitidis, S. pneumoniae,* and *Haemophilus influenzae.*
   - IgG-binding surface proteins (e.g., protein A of *S. aureus*) protect bacterial cells from antibody action.
6. Inhibition of complement action
   - Antigen in LPS of gram-negative bacteria may protect cells from complement-mediated lysis by preventing access to the membrane.
7. Antigenic variation by DNA rearrangement involving homologous recombination
   - *Salmonella* species: two flagellar variants
   - *Borrelia* species: variants of outer membrane protein
   - *N. gonorrhoeae:* variants of pilus protein

> Bacteria escape antibody control by changing their antigens, by inactivating the antibody, or by hiding within cells.

IV. Antibacterial Immunopathogenesis
- Host immune responses cause the disease for some bacteria.

A. Inflammation
1. Complement, neutrophils, macrophages, and other responses to bacteria lead to inflammation.
2. Cell-mediated immune responses induced to intracellular infections (*M. tuberculosis*) may lead to granulomas.

B. Bacteria that induce tissue-damaging immune responses
- More common for viruses than for bacteria
1. *Chlamydia* species (lymphogranuloma venereum)
2. *Treponema* species (syphilis)
3. *Borrelia* species (Lyme disease)

C. Cross-reacting antibacterial antibodies
- Rheumatic fever, a sequela to streptococcal infections, is caused by antibodies to M protein that cross-react with and initiate damage to the heart.

D. Deposition of immune complexes
- Poststreptococcal glomerulonephritis results from accumulation of antigen-antibody complexes in the glomeruli of the kidneys.

E. Sepsis
- Bacterial cell wall components activate TLRs and induce systemic release of tumor necrosis factor-α, IL-1, and IL-6, which activate acute phase responses.

F. Superantigens
- Activate T cells to release large amounts of cytokines (cytokine storm) to cause sepsis-like pathogenesis

CHAPTER 8

DIAGNOSIS, THERAPY, AND PREVENTION OF BACTERIAL DISEASES

I. Laboratory Identification of Bacteria

- Most medically important bacteria can be classified as gram-positive or gram-negative and further identified based on their shape and various metabolic properties as summarized in Figure 8-1.

A. Gram staining

1. Protocol
   - Step 1: treat smear with crystal violet primary stain.
   - Step 2: add iodine solution, which precipitates primary stain within the peptidoglycan layer of the cell wall.
   - Step 3: rinse with solvent that dissolves the outer membrane and washes out the crystal violet from the thin peptidoglycan layer of gram-negative bacteria but not from the thick peptidoglycan layer of gram-positive bacteria.
   - Step 4: counterstain with red safranin, which is taken up by gram-negative organisms, allowing them to be visualized.

Purple is positive; red is negative

2. Results
   - Purple (positive reaction): organisms with thick peptidoglycan cell wall
   - Red (negative reaction): organisms with thin peptidoglycan layer and an outer membrane

Gram variability occurs with old culture and β-lactam–treated bacteria.

   - Gram-variable or gram-resistant: modified cell wall old cultures or cells treated with β-lactam antibiotics in which the peptidoglycan is weakened—therefore, poor or no color retention; modified cell wall (Box 8-1)

B. Growth and isolation of bacteria

1. Culture media
   - Most bacteria will grow on blood agar or other nonselective media.
     a. Table 8-1 lists common media used to isolate or identify particular bacteria.
   - Selective medium inhibits growth of some bacteria (e.g., EMB agar inhibits gram-positive bacteria).
   - Differential medium incorporates an identifying test.
     a. MacConkey agar is both selective (inhibits gram-positive bacteria) and differential (tests for lactose use).

MacConkey agar distinguishes normal flora enterobacteria (lactose positive—purple colonies) from Salmonella, Shigella, Pseudomonas and other genera (lactose negative—gray colonies)

   - Special medium incorporates particular metabolites or provides specific culture conditions required by certain bacteria.
2. Colony characteristics (Table 8-2)

C. Biochemical tests

1. Metabolic tests for fermentation of various sugars and production of byproducts (e.g., acid or gases)
   - Lactose fermentation differentiates the more and less pathogenic Enterobacteriaceae.
     a. Lactose fermenting includes more benign *Escherichia coli* and *Klebsiella* species.
     b. Nonlactose fermenting includes more pathogenic *Shigella* and *Salmonella* species.

Neisseria species fermentation: meningitidis has an *m* and a *g* for maltose and glucose. Gonorrhoeae has only a *g* for glucose.

   - Glucose and maltose fermentation differentiate *Neisseria* species.
     a. *Neisseria meningitidis* ferments both maltose and glucose. *Neisseria gonorrhoeae* ferments glucose but not maltose.

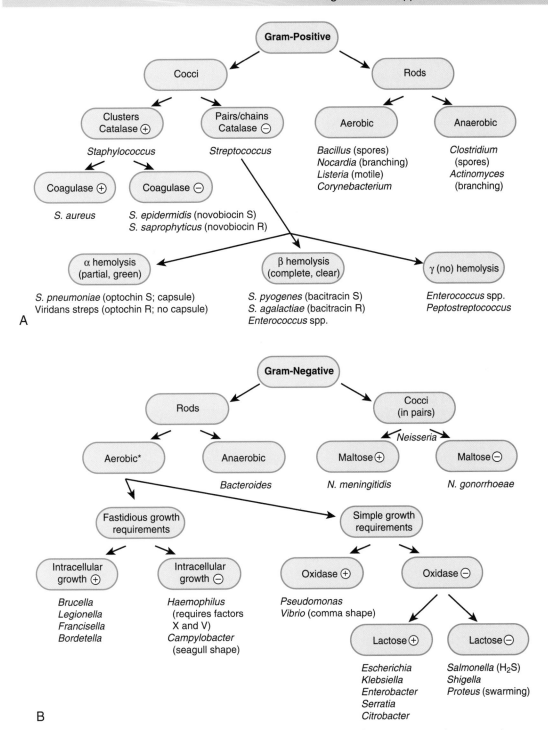

8-1: Laboratory algorithms for identifying medically important gram-positive (**A**) and gram-negative (**B**) bacteria. Catalase, coagulase, and oxidase: +, organism produces the enzyme; −, it does not. Maltose and lactose: +, organism ferments the sugar; −, it does not. S, sensitive to indicated drug; R, resistant to drug. *Facultative aerobic

BOX 8-1	GRAM-RESISTANT ORGANISMS

***Mycobacterium* and *Nocardia*:** waxlike outer layer; visualized with acid-fast stains
***Mycoplasma*:** no cell wall
***Rickettsia, Coxiella, Chlamydia*:** intracellular bacteria
***Treponema*:** thin, spiral organisms visualized by dark-field microscopy and fluorescent antibody staining
***Borrelia*:** thin, spiral organisms that take Giemsa or Wright stain

TABLE 8-1 Media for Isolating or Identifying Selected Bacteria

MEDIUM	BACTERIA	COMMENTS
Selective/Differential Media		
Mannitol salt agar	*Staphylococcus aureus*	High salt inhibits growth of other bacteria
MacConkey agar	Gram-negative enteric rods	Pink/purple colonies (lactose positive): *Escherichia coli*, *Klebsiella* species Colorless colonies (lactose negative): *Salmonella, Shigella, Proteus* species
Eosin methylene blue agar	Gram-negative enteric rods	Red-black colonies: *E. coli* Purple colonies: *Klebsiella* species Colorless colonies: *Salmonella, Shigella* species
Hektoen enteric agar	Gram-negative rods	Yellow-red colonies: *E. coli, Klebsiella* species Green colonies: *Shigella* species Green colonies, black center (H_2S): *Salmonella* species
Special Media		
Chocolate agar	*Neisseria* and *Haemophilus* species	Medium supplies factors V (NAD) and X (hemin)
Löwenstein-Jensen agar	Mycobacteria	Slow growing; colorless or buff-colored colonies: *Mycobacterium tuberculosis, Mycobacterium leprae*
Tellurite agar	*Corynebacterium diphtheriae*	Gray-to-black colonies
Thayer-Martin medium	*Neisseria gonorrhoeae*	Selective chocolate agar medium
Buffered charcoal yeast extract agar	*Legionella* species	

TABLE 8-2 Significant Colony Characteristics

CHARACTERISTIC	BACTERIA IDENTIFIED
Hemolysis in blood agar (diagnostic feature of streptococci)	
Green zone around colony (α hemolysis)	Viridans streptococci (catalase negative; Optochin resistant) *Streptococcus pneumoniae* (catalase negative; Optochin sensitive)
Clear zone around colony (β hemolysis)	*Staphylococcus aureus* (catalase positive; coagulase positive) *Streptococcus pyogenes* (catalase negative; bacitracin sensitive) *Streptococcus agalactiae* (catalase negative; bacitracin resistant)
Swarming	*Proteus mirabilis, Proteus vulgaris*
Pigment Formation*	
Yellow colonies	*S. aureus*
Blue-green colonies	*Pseudomonas aeruginosa*
Red colonies	*Serratia marcescens*

*Only certain species form pigments.

2. Tests for enzymes
- Catalase test: + reaction = bubbles (gas formation)
  a. Distinguishes staphylococci (positive) from streptococci (negative)
- Coagulase test: + reaction = precipitate/gel formation
  a. Distinguishes *Staphylococcus aureus* (positive) from *Staphylococcus epidermidis* (negative)
- Oxidase test: + reaction = blue color
  a. Positive for *Pseudomonas, Neisseria,* and *Vibrio* species (positive reaction)

D. Immunologic tests (see Chapter 3)
1. Detection of surface antigens is useful in identifying some bacteria and distinguishing between strains (serotypes) of a species that have one or more unique antigens.
2. For example, serotypes of *Escherichia coli* possess different O antigens. The O157:H7 serotype are enterohemorrhagic *E. coli* strains.

E. Antibiotic sensitivity assays
1. Serial dilution assay
- Quantitative determination of drug concentration that inhibits growth or kills an organism in culture
  a. Minimal inhibitory concentration (MIC): lowest concentration of a drug that inhibits growth of an organism

b. Minimal bactericidal concentration (MBC): lowest concentration of a drug that kills an organism

2. Kirby-Bauer assay
   - Semiquantitative method used to evaluate sensitivity of an organism to achievable blood levels of an antibiotic
   - Is not useful for infections of central nervous system or bone
   - Diffusion of antibiotic from impregnated disk inhibits growth of susceptible bacteria plated on agar.
   - Diameter of zone of growth inhibition surrounding disk is basis for rating an organism as sensitive, intermediate, or resistant to tested antibiotic.
3. E-test uses a graduated diffusion method to give MIC values for bacteria grown on agar plates.

II. Antimicrobial Drugs
A. Overview
1. Most antimicrobials are inhibitors of essential enzymes or disrupters of membranes (Fig. 8-2; Table 8-3).
2. Antibiotic resistance can arise by several different mechanisms (Box 8-2; see Table 8-3).
   - Antibiotic resistance provides a selective advantage to bacteria.
   - Genes for antibiotic resistance are often on plasmids or transposons and are transmissible.
3. Major antibiotic targets:
   - Peptidoglycan-synthesizing enzymes (cell wall synthesis)
   - Bacterial ribosome (protein synthesis)
   - Bacterial membrane
   - Topoisomerase (nucleic acid synthesis)
   - Enzymes involved in synthesis of folic acid and mycolic acid

B. Inhibitors of peptidoglycan synthesis
- Continued degradation of peptidoglycan in the absence of synthesis prevents growth and eventually leads to cell lysis.
1. Penicillins, cephalosporins, monobactams, and carbapenems inhibit the cross-linking of peptidoglycan chains (Fig. 8-3).
   - These drugs, which only act on growing cells, contain a β-lactam ring essential for their activity.
   - Smaller and more hydrophilic β-lactam drugs can enter gram-negative bacteria through porin channels in the outer membrane, but bulky or hydrophobic drugs are excluded.

Margin notes:

MIC: lowest concentration that inhibits growth. MBC: lowest concentration that kills.

Kirby-Bauer method only for achievable blood levels of antibiotic.

Bactericidal drugs kill bacteria: penicillins, cephalosporins, vancomycin, polymyxins, aminoglycosides, quinolones, and metronidazole.

β-Lactam drugs inhibit cross-linking of peptidoglycan.

Outer membrane is a barrier to large or hydrophobic antimicrobials.

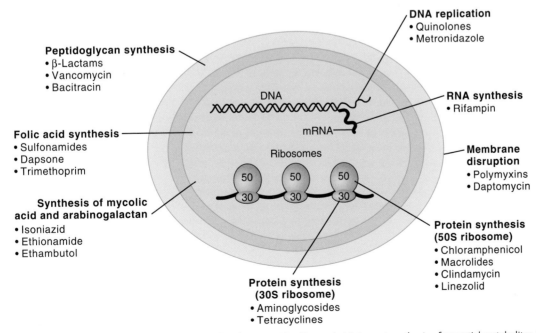

8-2: Primary cellular processes that are targets of antibiotic activity. Drugs that interrupt synthesis of essential metabolites in the cytoplasm are referred to as antimetabolites mRNA, messenger RNA.

TABLE 8-3 **Properties of Common Antibiotics**

DRUG	TARGET PROCESS OR STRUCTURE	RESISTANCE	SPECTRUM*
Inhibitors of Peptidoglycan Synthesis			
β-*Lactams*			
Penicillins	Cross-linking of peptidoglycan	β-Lactamase inactivation of drug	Broad but varies with specific drug
Cephalosporins		Target site mutation	
Carbapenems		↑ Target enzymes	
Monobactams		↓ Permeability [Gm(−)]	
Glycopeptides			
Vancomycin	Elongation and cross-linking of peptidoglycan	Target site mutation ↓ Permeability [Gm(−)] ↑ Number of targets Altered binding site (enterococci)	Gm(+) bacteria (staphylococci) site
Bacitracin	Recycling of bactoprenol	Target site mutation	Gm(+) bacteria
Membrane Disrupters			
Polymyxins	Outer and cytoplasmic membrane	—	Gm(−) bacteria
Daptomycin	Cytoplasmic membrane		*Staphylococcus aureus*
Inhibitors of Protein Synthesis			
Aminoglycosides			
Streptomycin	Assembly of subunits (bind 30S ribosomal subunit); misreading of mRNA	Enzymatic inactivation of drug	Broad but varies with specific drug
Gentamicin		Target site mutation	Gm(−) bacteria
Kanamycin		↓ Drug uptake	
Tetracycline *Doxycycline, etc.*	Chain elongation (binds 30S subunit)	↓ Drug uptake ↑ Drug export	*Chlamydia* and *Rickettsia* species, *Mycobacterium pneumoniae*, *Vibrio cholerae*, and others
Macrolides, etc.[†]			
Erythromycin	Chain elongation (binds 50S subunit)	Target enzyme mutation	*Legionella, Mycoplasma, Chlamydia* species
Azithromycin			
Clarithromycin			
Clindamycin	Chain elongation (binds 50S subunit)	Target site mutation	Anaerobic bacteria Gm(+) bacteria
Chloramphenicol	Chain elongation (binds 50S subunit)	Enzymatic inactivation of drug	—
Linezolid	Blocks formation of initiation complex (binds 50S subunit)	—	Enterococci and other Gm(+) bacteria
Inhibitors of Nucleic Acid Synthesis			
Quinolones	Topoisomerase	Target site mutation ↓ Permeability [Gm(−)]	Gm(+) and Gm(−) bacteria
Rifampin	RNA polymerase	Target enzyme mutation	*Mycobacterium* species; prophylaxis for *Haemophilus influenzae* and *Neisseria meningitides*
Metronidazole	Disrupts DNA	Aerobic bacteria	Anaerobic bacteria; *Clostridium difficile*
Antimetabolites			
Sulfonamides[‡]	Folic acid synthesis	Target site mutation ↓ Need for folic acid	Gm(+) and Gm(−) bacteria
Dapsone Trimethoprim			
Isoniazid	Mycolic acid synthesis	Target enzyme mutation	*Mycobacterium* species
Ethionamide Ethambutol	Arabinogalactan synthesis	Target enzyme mutation	*Mycobacterium*

Gm(−), gram negative; Gm(+), gram positive.
*Only a general guide to spectrum of these drugs.
[†]Refers to ketolides and azalides.
[‡]Sulfonamides are analogs of PABA, a substrate for dihydropteroate synthase. Dapsone also inhibits this enzyme. Trimethoprim inhibits dihydrofolate reductase, another enzyme in the pathway synthesizing folic acid.

BOX 8-2 MECHANISMS OF ANTIBIOTIC RESISTANCE

Some bacteria are naturally resistant to certain drugs, whereas others acquire a mutation in the target gene or acquire plasmid containing genes conferring antibiotic resistance. Resistance mechanisms can be classified into five main types:
- Inactivation of drug by bacterial enzymes (e.g., cleavage of β-lactams and acetylation of aminoglycosides)
- Low permeability to drug (e.g., outer membrane of gram-negative bacteria and alteration in transport protein or porin)
- Alteration in target protein that reduces binding of drug
- Overproduction of target protein or structure
- Metabolic bypass of target pathway

These mechanisms increase the minimal inhibitory concentration of a drug (perhaps to toxic levels) or eliminate its effectiveness entirely.

Penicillins   **Cephalosporins**

8-3: General structures of penicillins and cephalosporins, the most important classes of β-lactam antibiotics. The presence of a hydrophilic R$_1$ group, as in ampicillin, increases activity against gram-negative bacteria. The *arrow* indicates the bond that is broken during hydrolysis by β-lactamase.

- β-Lactamase, an enzyme that cleaves the β-lactam ring, inactivates these drugs.
  a. Many bacteria carry the β-lactamase gene on plasmids, allowing for easy spread of resistance through a bacterial population and even to related strains.
  b. Effectiveness of β-lactamase–susceptible antibiotics is increased by coadministration of penicillin analogs (e.g., sulbactam) that inhibit the β-lactamase.
  2. Vancomycin inhibits elongation of peptidoglycan chains and their cross-linking.
  - "Grabs" onto the D-ala-D-ala of the peptidoglycan precursor
  - Is effective against gram-positive bacteria but too bulky to pass through the outer membrane of gram-negative bacteria
  3. Bacitracin prevents reuse of the bactoprenol carrier that functions in assembly of peptidoglycan from smaller precursors.
  - Stops synthesis of peptidoglycan, teichoic acid, lipopolysaccharide, and capsules, all of which require bactoprenol for their production
  - Is used in most topical antibiotic ointments

C. Peptide antibiotic disrupters of bacterial membranes
  1. Polymyxins and daptomycin have cyclic peptides and a fatty acyl side chain.
  2. Polymyxins (colistin) are especially effective against gram-negative bacteria, disrupting both the outer membrane and the cytoplasmic membrane.
  3. Polymyxins are used in most topical antibiotic ointments.
  4. Daptomycin disrupts membranes of *S. aureus*.

D. Inhibitors of nucleic acid synthesis
  1. Quinolones inhibit bacterial topoisomerase, which is essential for maintaining the proper DNA structure for transcription and replication.
  - Resistance arises from mutation in topoisomerase, preventing binding of drug, or in porin, reducing entry of drug into gram-negative bacteria.
  - Broad-spectrum drugs, especially for gram-negative organisms: ciprofloxacin and norfloxacin
  - Extended-spectrum drugs for gram-positive organisms (pneumococci): moxifloxacin, gemifloxacin
  2. Rifampin inhibits synthesis of messenger RNA (mRNA; transcription) by binding to the bacterial RNA polymerase.
  - Resistance occurs readily because of mutations in RNA polymerase.

β-lactamase gene can be carried on a plasmid to spread resistance. β-lactamase inhibitors can be given with β-lactam antibiotics.

The peptidoglycan cross-linking reaction of methicillin-resistant *S. aureus* is not inhibited by β-lactam antibiotics. Intermediate resistance to β-lactams and vancomycin result from thicker cell walls (more drug targets to act on).

Vancomycin-resistant enterococci do not use D-ala-D-ala in the cross-linking of peptidoglycan and lack the vancomycin-binding target.

E. Inhibitors of protein synthesis

1. Several groups of antibiotics prevent initiation of protein synthesis or peptide bond formation (i.e., chain elongation), or they cause misreading of the mRNA (see Table 8-3).
2. Resistance results from enzymatic inactivation of the antibiotic or its target site, mutation of the target site, or altered transport of the drug.

F. Antimetabolite drugs

Bacteriostatic drugs inhibit bacterial growth: macrolides, clindamycin, chloramphenicol, sulfonamides, and trimethoprim.

- These drugs inhibit cytoplasmic enzymes involved in the biosynthesis of essential bacterial metabolites.
1. Inhibitors of folic acid synthesis
   - Sulfonamides and dapsone inhibit dihydropteroate synthase.
   - Trimethoprim and methotrexate inhibit dihydrofolate reductase.
2. Inhibitors of mycolic acid, an essential component of the mycobacterial cell wall: isoniazid, ethionamide.

III. Antibacterial Vaccines

A. Passive immunization

1. Refers to treatment with antibody usually in the form of gammaglobulin from immune serum
2. Confers immediate, relatively short-term protection
3. Used in treatment of tetanus, botulism, rabies, and diphtheria
4. Used for prevention of hepatitis A and B, varicella, and other virus infections

Passive immunization uses antibody as an antimicrobial.
The mother is the best and most common source of passive immunization.

B. Active immunization

1. Refers to treatment with various types of agents that can induce an immune response (Table 8-4)
2. Confers long-term protection
3. Types of active immunization
   - Killed cells
   - Live, attenuated cells
   - Inactivated toxins (toxoids)
   - Capsular polysaccharides
     a. Conjugation to a carrier protein enhances immune response by promoting T cell involvement.

TABLE 8-4 **Bacterial Vaccines**

BACTERIUM	DISEASE	VACCINE TYPE
Commonly Used Vaccines		
Corynebacterium diphtheriae	Diphtheria	Toxoid (inactivated exotoxin)
Clostridium tetani	Tetanus	Toxoid (inactivated exotoxin)
Bordetella pertussis	Pertussis	Acellular extracts of killed cells
Haemophilus influenzae (type b)	Meningitis, epiglottitis	Capsular polysaccharide plus protein carrier (Hib vaccine)
Streptococcus pneumoniae	Pneumonia, otitis media, sinusitis	Capsular polysaccharide with or without conjugated protein
Limited-Usage Vaccines*		
Neisseria meningitidis (types A and C)	Meningitis	Capsular polysaccharide
Vibrio cholerae	Cholera	Killed cells
Salmonella typhi	Typhoid	Killed cells, polysaccharide
Bacillus anthracis	Anthrax	Killed cells
Yersinia pestis	Plague	Killed cells
Coxiella burnetii	Q fever	Killed cells
Francisella tularensis	Tularemia	Live, attenuated cells
Mycobacterium tuberculosis	Tuberculosis	Live, attenuated BCG cells[†]

*These vaccines are usually administered only to those at high risk for exposure to the indicated organisms.
[†]Bacillus Calmette-Guérin (BCG) is an avirulent strain of *Mycobacterium bovis*. This vaccine is not recommended in the United States.

CHAPTER 9
GRAM-POSITIVE COCCI

I. *Staphylococcus* Species
- Three staphylococcal species commonly cause human disease: *S. aureus* (most virulent), *S. epidermidis*, and *S. saprophyticus*.

A. Shared staphylococcal properties
1. Gram-positive cocci in grape-like clusters
2. Catalase positive; growth in 7.5% salt
3. Ubiquitous distribution; part of normal flora; responsible for many nosocomial infections

B. Coagulase-positive staphylococci *(S. aureus)*
- *S. aureus* is normal flora of skin and the anterior nares.
1. Pathogenesis
   - Table 9-1 summarizes the major contributors to the virulence of *S. aureus*.
2. Diseases caused by *S. aureus* (Box 9-1)
   - Toxin-mediated diseases
     a. Food poisoning, toxic shock syndrome (TSS), scalded skin syndrome
   - Community-acquired methicillin resistant *S. aureus* (CA-MRSA) carries resistance plasmids that also have the Panton valentine leukocidin gene and may be more virulent.
   - Inflammatory diseases mediated by pyogenic and necrotic activities of *S. aureus*
     a. These suppurative (pus-forming) infections range from benign skin lesions (e.g., folliculitis, furuncles, and carbuncles) to life-threatening systemic diseases (osteomyelitis, pneumonia, and endocarditis) and bacteremia.
3. Transmission of *S. aureus*
   - Person-to-person contact and via fomites
   - Endogenous spread via blood or aspiration of nasal secretions
   - Ingestion of preformed enterotoxins in food
     a. *S. aureus* can multiply and make toxin in salted and smoked meats (cold cuts), as well as creamy foods (potato or egg salads), if they are unrefrigerated for extended periods. Reheating does not destroy the heat-stable enterotoxins.
4. Treatment
   - Most staphylococci produce penicillinase (a β-lactamase) and are commonly treated with a penicillinase-resistant β-lactam penicillin derivative, such as nafcillin, oxacillin, or methicillin.
   - MRSA strains (hospital acquired) are treated with vancomycin, linezolid, daptomycin, tigecycline, trimethoprim sulfa, or clindamycin.
   - CA-MRSAs are becoming more common.
     a. Treatment is with trimethoprim-sulfamethoxazole.
   - Methicillin- and vancomycin-resistant *S. aureus* was acquired from an *Enterococcus* plasmid.

C. Coagulase-negative staphylococci (*S. epidermidis* and *S. saprophyticus*)
1. These bacteria are normally benign colonizers of the skin.
2. They are less virulent than *S. aureus*, although their virulence factors are similar (*except* for lack of coagulase).
3. *S. epidermidis* can adhere to artificial heart valves, vascular catheters, shunts, and prosthetic joints, colonizing the implant area and causing tissue destruction mediated by degradative enzymes.
   - Vancomycin is the drug of choice.
4. *S. saprophyticus* is a frequent cause of urinary tract infections (UTIs) in sexually active young women.
   - Treatment: oral cephalosporin or amoxicillin clavulanate

TABLE 9-1 **Major Virulence Factors of** *Staphylococcus Aureus*

FACTOR	BIOLOGIC ACTIONS
Surface Components	
Capsule	**Antiphagocytic**
Protein A	**Inhibits complement fixation, opsonization,** and **ADCC** by binding Fc portion of IgG; very important **virulence factor**
Lipoteichoic and teichoic acids	Promote **adherence** to mucosal surfaces and persistence in tissues by binding to fibronectin
Enzymes	
Catalase	**Reduces phagocytic killing** by converting H_2O_2 to H_2O
Coagulase	Helps **encase infection** by forming fibrin layer around abscess
Degradative enzymes	Promote **tissue destruction** and bacterial spread
Penicillinase (β-lactamase)	Confers **antibiotic resistance** by cleaving β-lactam ring of penicillins
Toxins	
Leukocidins (cytolytic)	Damage and lyse leukocytes limits host response; releases **tissue-damaging substances**
Enterotoxins (A-E)	Act as superantigens; responsible for **gastrointestinal food poisoning**
Exfoliative toxins (A, B)	Cause splitting of cell junctions (desmosomes) in epidermis; responsible for **scalded skin syndrome**
Toxic shock syndrome	Acts as superantigen; promotes massive cytokine release, causes **toxic shock syndrome**

ADCC, antibody-dependent cellular cytotoxicity.

BOX 9-1 *STAPHYLOCOCCUS AUREUS* DISEASES: QUICK CASES

Toxin-Mediated Diseases

Food poisoning due to enterotoxin (A-E): Individual with severe nausea, vomiting, and diarrhea developing 4 hours after eating potato salad and ham sandwiches at a picnic in July. Complete recovery after bed rest for 2 days and drinking plenty of fluids

Scalded skin syndrome due to exfoliative toxin: Young child with blister-like lesions widely disseminated over the body. Large areas of desquamated epithelium but no scarring

Toxic shock syndrome due to TSST-1 (superantigen): Young woman with rapid onset of fever, diarrhea, desquamating rash, multisystem organ involvement, kidney failure, shock with generalized flushing of the skin and mucous membranes. Examination shows a tampon lodged in her vagina.

Toxic shock syndrome due to TSST-1: Child or adolescent develops shock with multiorgan failure and generalized flushing of the skin and mucous membranes within days of sustaining a deep wound.

Suppurative Infections

CA-MRSA: A high school football player with necrotizing fasciitis is treated with clindamycin. Other members of the team also have skin infections (boils and abscesses).

Carbuncle: Diabetic patient whose blood glucose is under poor control with a large swollen area of redness on one leg

Endocarditis: Recent onset of fever, petechial lesions, and detection of a new heart murmur in a patient with an intravascular catheter

Impetigo: Child with honey-colored or clear crusts over ruptured pustules (usually bullous lesions) on the face; intense itching

Osteomyelitis and septic arthritis: Child with fever and localized pain and swelling below the right knee following orthopedic surgery; positive blood culture for *S. aureus*

Pneumonia: Individual suddenly develops fever, difficulty breathing, and empyema (intrapleural abscesses) soon after recovering from influenza.

Wound infection: Elderly man with fever and redness and swelling at the site of recent surgery

---

Trigger words:

S. pyogenes: Bacitracin (A disk-group A) sensitivity, β hemolysis, gram-positive cocci in chains, necrotizing fasciitis, pus, streptolysin O and S

II. *Streptococcus* Species

- Most common streptococcal pathogens in humans are *S. pyogenes*, *S. agalactiae*, viridans group, and *S. pneumoniae*.

A. Shared streptococcal properties

1. Gram-positive spherical or football-shaped cocci in pairs or chains
2. Catalase negative
3. Species-dependent hemolysis in blood agar (Table 9-2)
4. Lancefield classification
   - Groups based on serologic identification of group-specific C-carbohydrates on cell wall

TABLE 9-2 **Streptococcal Hemolysis**

HEMOLYTIC REACTION	ORGANISM	DIFFERENTIATING PROPERTY
α (Incomplete) hemolysis	*S. pneumoniae*	Optochin sensitive
(greenish zone around colony)	Viridans streptococci	Optochin resistant
	Enterococcus (some)	—
β (Complete) hemolysis	*S. pyogenes* (group A)	Bacitracin sensitive
(clear zone around colony)	*S. agalactiae* (group B)	Bacitracin resistant
γ (No) hemolysis	*Enterococcus* (some)	—

B. Group A streptococci (*S. pyogenes*)
  1. Identification
     - β-Hemolytic
     - Sensitive to bacitracin (A disk)
     - Hyaluronic acid–containing capsule
        a. Spreading factor that helps bacteria extend through subcutaneous tissue (cellulitis)
     - Antibodies to streptolysin O appearing 3 or 4 weeks after primary infection
        a. Antistreptolysin O titer is useful in the diagnosis of acute rheumatic fever.
     - Anti-DNase B antibodies
        a. Useful in the diagnosis of acute rheumatic fever, streptococcal skin infections (e.g., scarlet fever), poststreptococcal glomerulonephritis
  2. Pathogenesis
     - Table 9-3 summarizes the major contributors to the virulence of *S. pyogenes* and other group A streptococci.
  3. Group A streptococcal diseases (Box 9-2)
     - Localized suppurative diseases: pharyngitis (strep throat), skin infections, postsurgical cellulitis, puerperal (at childbirth) sepsis
     - Toxin-mediated diseases
        a. Streptococcal TSS, scarlet fever
     - Nonsuppurative autoimmune sequelae
        a. Acute glomerulonephritis, rheumatic fever (Box 9-3)
  4. Transmission of *S. pyogenes*
     - Pharyngitis is spread primarily by respiratory droplets.
        a. Most common in fall and winter
        b. Children 5 to 15 years of age are most susceptible.
     - Skin infections are commonly spread by contact of skin breaks with an infected person, fomite, or insect vector.
     - Other diseases are complications of primary *S. pyogenes* infection.
  5. Treatment
     - *S. pyogenes* is sensitive to penicillin G.

S. pyogenes: causes pharyngitis, scarlet fever, toxic shock, rheumatic fever, acute glomerulonephritis

Group A streptococci must be treated to prevent sequelae.

Sequelae of group A streptococci are rheumatic fever and acute glomerulonephritis.

TABLE 9-3 **Major Virulence Factors of Group A Streptococci**

FACTOR	BIOLOGIC ACTIONS
Surface Components	
Capsule	**Nonimmunogenic** and **antiphagocytic**
M protein	**Inhibits opsonization; immunogenic**
F protein, lipoteichoic acid	Mediate **adherence** to mucoepithelium by binding to fibronectin
Enzymes	
C5a peptidase	**Reduces inflammatory responses** mediated by C5a
DNase	Aids in bacterial spread by reducing viscosity of abscess material
Hyaluronidase	Promotes **tissue destruction** and bacterial spread
Streptokinase	Promotes **bacterial spread** into tissue by breaking down blood clots
Streptolysin O and S	Lyse blood cells and platelets; stimulate **release of lysosomal enzymes**
Toxins	
Pyrogenic/erythrogenic exotoxins	Some act as superantigens
	Other activities

BOX 9-2 GROUP A STREPTOCOCCAL DISEASES: QUICK CASES

Suppurative Infections

Erysipelas: Elderly woman or young child with well-demarcated swollen, erythematous area on face; has fever, headache, and swollen lymph nodes

Impetigo: Child with honey-crusted skin lesions over face or trunk, itching, and possible regional lymphadenopathy. *S. pyogenes* is the second most common cause of impetigo.

Pharyngitis: Child with fever, inflamed throat with possible exudates, general malaise, cervical lymphadenopathy, and no coryza (acute rhinitis); often indistinguishable from viral infection

Pyoderma: Young child (2-5 years) with multiple 1- or 2-mm abscesses over the body, palpable regional lymphadenopathy, and evidence of skin abrasions or insect bites. Most commonly occurs during warm, humid weather and among children in close contact with each other (e.g., in day care centers)

Necrotizing fasciitis: Patient with rapidly expanding area of erythema, bulla formation, and anesthesia around a recent wound on the arm, which leads to tissue destruction; accompanied by fever and other evidence of systemic toxicity (possible shock and multisystem organ failure)

Toxin-Mediated Diseases

Scarlet fever: Child with strawberry tongue and diffuse sandpaper-like erythematous rash over the body within 24 to 48 hours after onset of streptococcal pharyngitis. Rash fades in 5 to 7 days with desquamation.

Streptococcal toxic shock syndrome: Adult man with cellulitis, shock, multisystem organ failure, and generalized skin flushing

Autoimmune Sequelae

Acute glomerulonephritis: Child or teenager with hematuria, red blood cell casts, proteinuria, hypertension, and periorbital edema with history of recently treated skin infection

Rheumatic fever: Child with fever, heart failure, migrating inflamed joints that are not symmetrically involved, and a history of a recent sore throat (see Box 9-3)

BOX 9-3 REVISED JONES CRITERIA FOR DIAGNOSIS OF RHEUMATIC FEVER

Diagnosis requires evidence of preceding group A streptococcal infection (throat culture, positive test for group A antigen, or increased anti–group A antibody titer) plus the presence of two major criteria or one major and two minor clinical or laboratory criteria.

Major Criteria
Carditis
Chorea
Erythema marginatum
Polyarthritis
Subcutaneous nodules

Minor Criteria
Clinical Findings
Fever, arthralgia

Laboratory Findings
↑ Red blood cell sedimentation rate
↑ C-reactive protein
Prolonged P-R interval on electrocardiogram
Increased ASO, DNase B antibodies

Group A streptococci are still sensitive to penicillin.

- Treatment of group A pharyngitis prevents potential sequelae (e.g., rheumatic fever and glomerulonephritis).
- C. **Group B streptococci (*S. agalactiae*)**
  - *S. agalactiae* is a normal inhabitant of the gastrointestinal and lower genital tracts.
  1. Identification
     - β-Hemolytic
     - Resistant to bacitracin
     - Positive CAMP test in which group B hemolysin enhances β hemolysis by *S. aureus*

2. Pathogenesis
  - Antiphagocytic capsule is immunogenic.
  - Anticapsular antibodies are important in host defense.
  - Hemolysins and various degradative enzymes mediate cellular and tissue destruction.
3. Group B streptococcal diseases
  - Early-onset neonatal disease begins within 7 days of birth.
    a. Acquired in utero or at delivery (infection in mother's vagina)
    b. Most common in premature infants
    c. High mortality rate
    d. Symptoms: bacteremia, pneumonia, meningitis
  - Late-onset neonatal disease begins 1 week to 3 months after birth.
    a. Acquired postpartum
    b. Low mortality rate (<20%)
    c. Symptoms: bacteremia, meningitis
  - Postpartum sepsis is usually acquired via wound inflicted during parturition.
    a. Symptoms: endometritis, fever, chills, wound infection, possible UTI
  - Wound infections occur in other adults, especially immunocompromised patients.
4. Treatment
  - Penicillin G alone or in combination with aminoglycosides
  - Passive immunization in serious cases

> Group B streptococci acquired at birth cause bacteremia, pneumonia, and meningitis within first week.

D. **Viridans streptococci (*S. mutans, S. sanguis*)**
  - These constitute a major part of normal flora of the mouth and teeth.
1. Identification
  - α-Hemolytic
  - Resistant to Optochin
  - No Lancefield antigens
2. Viridans streptococcal diseases
  - Streptococcal endocarditis occurs most commonly in patients with damaged heart valves, to which bacteria adhere.
    a. Symptoms include prolonged fever, heart murmur, microembolization (vegetations), immunocomplex disease (e.g., glomerulonephritis, splinter hemorrhages under nails)
    b. Bacteria enter the bloodstream during dental work or after oral trauma, causing transient bacteremia that can initiate disease.
  - Dental caries are caused primarily by *S. mutans*.
    a. Adheres to tooth enamel and erodes teeth by converting sucrose to acetic and lactic acids
3. Treatment of streptococcal endocarditis
  - Penicillin
  - Antibiotic prophylaxis of at-risk individuals (e.g., patient with valvular heart disease who has dental work)

> Viridans streptococci cause dental plaque, caries.
>
> Damaged heart valves are a risk factor for viridans strep endocarditis.

E. ***S. pneumoniae* (pneumococcus)**
  - *S. pneumoniae* is normally present in the throat and nasopharynx.
1. Identification
  - α-Hemolytic
  - Sensitive to Optochin (P disk)
  - No Lancefield antigens
  - Positive quellung reaction (capsular swelling in the presence of specific anticapsular antibody)
2. Pathogenesis
  - Aspiration of nasopharyngeal secretions into lower airways leads to rapid growth of pneumococci in alveolar spaces.
    a. Reduced clearance of airways due to disruption of ciliated epithelium in upper respiratory tract by viral infection or smoking promotes aspiration.
  - Antiphagocytic capsule is required for virulence (See Box 9-4).
  - Pneumolysin (similar to streptolysin O) lyses cells.
  - Pneumococcal immunoglobulin A (IgA) protease cleaves secretory IgA, increasing adherence to mucosal surfaces.
  - Neuraminidase (spreading factor) promotes bacterial spread into tissue.
3. Pneumococcal diseases
  - Typical community-acquired pneumonia
    a. Marked by abrupt onset, high fever (102° to 105°F), rigor, productive cough, and pleuritic chest pain from pleural inflammation from either bronchopneumonia (patchy pneumonia) or lobar pneumonia (involvement of one or more lobes)

> **Trigger words:**
> *S. pneumoniae:* α-hemolytic, capsule, gram-positive diplococci, meningitis, otitis media, P disk (Optochin) sensitive, polysaccharide vaccine, pneumonia
>
> Strep **p**neumo; Optichin sensitive (P-disk; **p**neumoniae) Quellung reaction indicates capsule on *S. pneumoniae.*

S. pneumoniae and *Haemophilus influenzae*: most common bacterial causes of acute otitis media and sinusitis

S. pneumoniae, *H. influenza*, *Neisseria meningitidis*, and *Cryptococcus neoformans* (yeast) have capsules and cause meningitis.

- Bacteremia, found in 25% to 30% of pneumonia patients, may lead to pneumococcal meningitis.
  a. *S. pneumoniae* is the leading cause of bacterial meningitis in people older than 18 years.
- Most common cause of acute otitis media and sinusitis
- Most common cause of sepsis in children with sickle cell disease and dysfunctional spleen
  a. Functioning spleen is required for normal elimination of bloodborne *S. pneumoniae*
- Most common cause of spontaneous peritonitis in children with nephrotic syndrome and ascites
4. Epidemiology of pneumococcal infection
- Transmission of pneumococci occurs via aerosol droplets from infected person followed by aspiration into lower airways. Infection is most common in winter and spring.
- At-risk groups include young children, elderly people, asplenic patients (Box 9-4), and other immunocompromised individuals.
5. Prevention and treatment
- Polysaccharide capsular vaccines (with or without conjugated protein) for at-risk populations and children
- Increasing pneumococcal resistance to penicillin, especially in isolates from children attending day care centers
  a. Macrolides (erythromycin), cephalosporins, and fluoroquinolones are effective alternatives to treatment with penicillin for pneumonia, otitis media, and sinusitis.
- Cefotaxime or ceftriaxone for meningitis

III. *Enterococcus (E. faecalis, E. faecium)*
- These organisms are normal flora of the large bowel and feces. Antibiotic resistance is common among enterococci and contributes to their pathogenicity.

A. **Identification**
1. Gram-positive cocci in twisted chains
2. Catalase negative
3. Bacitracin resistant
4. Variable hemolysis
5. Bile and salt tolerant (growth in media containing 6.5% NaCl)

Enterococci grow in bowel and resistant to bowel conditions: bile and salt.

B. **Enterococcal diseases**
- Risk factors include catheterization and administration of broad-spectrum antibiotics.
1. UTIs, particularly in hospitalized patients
2. Endocarditis (similar to viridans streptococci)
3. Wound infections

C. **Treatment**
1. Ampicillin can be used for sensitive strains
2. Combination of an aminoglycoside and vancomycin for resistant strains.
- Vancomycin-resistant enterococci (VRE) have a substitute for the D-Ala-D-Ala in peptidoglycan that is the target for vancomycin.

Enterococci are inherently resistant to many antibiotics.

Chapter 10
Gram-Positive Toxigenic Rods

I. Bacillus Species
- Bacilli are large, gram-positive, aerobic, spore-forming rods that produce exotoxins.

A. Bacillus anthracis
- *B. anthracis* is nonmotile (unlike other bacilli) and forms Medusa's head colonies on blood agar.

1. Pathogenesis
   - Capsule composed of glutamic acid polymer prevents phagocytosis and antibody plus complement lysis.
   - Anthrax toxin causes localized edema and cell death; highly toxic.
   - Spores are extremely stable and can survive many years in soil, wool, hair, and animal hides.

2. Diseases caused by *B. anthracis*
   - Anthrax is an occupational disease of individuals who handle wools, furs, and hides.
     a. Cutaneous anthrax results from inoculation of spores or bacteria from soil or animal products into a superficial wound or abrasion.
        - Marked by initial itching papule at inoculation site; ulcer with vesicles that can lead to necrosis with massive edema, septicemia, and possible death
        - Most common form of anthrax in humans
     b. Pulmonary anthrax is due to inhalation of spores from contaminated items such as wool, fur, and hides.
        - Virus-like respiratory illness with high mortality rate owing to respiratory failure
     c. Gastrointestinal anthrax results from ingestion of bacteria in contaminated meat.
        - Rare in humans, but seen in developing countries

3. Prevention and treatment
   - Vaccination of animals and proper disposal of infected animals are important in controlling anthrax.
   - Human vaccination is restricted to at-risk individuals (fur and wool handlers, military) and those living where disease is endemic.
   - Prompt therapy is essential to reduce risk for death: amoxicillin if penicillin sensitive, otherwise ciprofloxacin (a fluoroquinolone).

B. Bacillus cereus
- *B. cereus*, a ubiquitous soil organism found in grains, vegetables, and dairy products, is the most common pathogenic bacilli.

1. *B. cereus* food poisoning
   - Emetic form is caused by preformed heat-stable enterotoxin ingested in reheated foods (e.g., rice and beans).
     a. Rapid onset (similar to *S. aureus* food poisoning); nausea, vomiting, and abdominal cramps developing within 1 to 5 hours after eating toxin-containing food
   - Diarrheal form is caused by heat-labile enterotoxin produced by bacteria multiplying in the gastrointestinal (GI) tract following ingestion of contaminated meat, vegetables, or sauces.
     a. Slow onset (similar to *Clostridium perfringens* food poisoning); diarrhea and severe cramps developing 10 to 15 hours after eating bacteria-containing food

Trigger words:
Bacillus anthracis: bioterror; eschar; fur; Medusa's head colonies; sheep, goat, goat hair; spore; toxin; wool-sorters' disease

B. anthracis: only organism with a polypeptide capsule

Anthrax: contact with *B. anthracis* spores or bacteria → painless ulcer; possible progression to septicemia and death. Inhalation of spores → life-threatening pulmonary illness.
Spores of *B. anthracis* are potential biologic warfare agents owing to their stability and ability to cause fatal disease (pulmonary anthrax).

Cutaneous anthrax is an occupational hazard for goat and sheep fur handlers.

Anthrax vaccine is for at-risk individuals.

Trigger words:
B. cereus: heat-labile toxin—diarrhea; heat-stable toxin—vomiting; rice, preformed toxin; 3-hour gastroenteritis

B. cereus: heat-stable toxin → rapid onset of emetic gastroenteritis; heat-labile toxin → slow onset of diarrheal gastroenteritis

2. Prevention and treatment
   - Refrigeration of foods after cooking
     a. Spores survive initial cooking and will germinate into toxin-producing vegetative cells if foods are not refrigerated properly. Later reheating inactivates heat-labile toxin but does not affect vegetative cells or heat-stable toxin.
   - Supportive therapy (e.g., replenish fluids and electrolytes)

C. **Bacillus subtilis and other Bacillus species**
   - These organisms are opportunistic pathogens in immunocompromised patients.

II. **Clostridium Species**
   - Four clostridial species are important human pathogens: *C. botulinum, C. difficile, C. perfringens,* and *C. tetani.*
   - Clostridia are gram-positive, anaerobic (or aerotolerant), spore-forming rods that produce potent exotoxins.

A. **C. perfringens**
   - *C. perfringens* is found worldwide in soil, water, and sewage; normal inhabitant of the GI tract.
   1. Identification
      - Large, boxcar-shaped, aerotolerant, rapidly growing rods
      - Double zone of hemolysis on blood agar
      - Positive Nagler reaction (characteristic diffuse zone around colonies grown on egg yolk agar)
      - Subtypes A to E defined based on production of major toxins
   2. Pathogenesis
      - Type A *C. perfringens* is most virulent in humans.
        a. Alpha toxin (phospholipase C and lecithinase), produced by all types, causes lysis of blood cells and endothelial cells, leading to increased vascular permeability, hemolysis, and tissue destruction.
        b. Hyaluronidase, collagenase, and other degradative enzymes cause tissue destruction.
        c. Heat-labile enterotoxin disrupts ion transport in ileum, leading to watery diarrhea (food poisoning).
        d. Beta and iota toxins have necrotizing activity.
   3. Diseases caused by *C. perfringens* (Box 10-1)
      - Food poisoning (type A)
      - Gas gangrene (myonecrosis)
        a. Diabetic patients and others with poor circulation are at high risk for developing gangrenous infections. Prognosis is poor, with a mortality rate of 40% even with treatment.
      - Necrotizing enterocolitis (type C)
      - Cellulitis and fasciitis
   4. Treatment of gas gangrene
      - Proper wound care and prophylactic antibiotics to prevent infection by *C. perfringens*
      - Rapid, aggressive treatment including surgical débridement, high-dose penicillin plus clindamycin, and, in some cases, amputation

Clostridium versus *Bacillus:* both clostridia and bacilli are gram-positive, spore-forming rods that produce potent exotoxins. Clostridia are anaerobes; bacilli are aerobes.

Trigger words:
C. perfringens: boxcar shaped, diarrhea, double zone of hemolysis, gas gangrene, lecithinase, toxins

C. perfringens destroys tissues with many degradative enzymes, e.g., alpha toxin.

Gangrene is a combination of tissue degradation and gas production in anaerobic tissue.

BOX 10-1 DISEASES CAUSED BY *C. PERFRINGENS*: CLINICAL FEATURES

Clostridial food poisoning: Abdominal cramps and **watery diarrhea,** without fever, nausea, or vomiting. Moderately rapid onset **8** to **24** hours after ingestion of meat contaminated with **enterotoxin**-producing *C. perfringens* **type A.** The disease is **self-limited,** with symptoms usually resolving within 1 day of onset.

Gas gangrene (myonecrosis): Sudden onset of intense pain and swelling in wound area, mild fever, and **rapid heartbeat** developing within 1 week after surgery or trauma to affected area. **Bronze discoloration of skin,** hemorrhagic bullae, tissue necrosis involving muscle, **gas production** from bacterial growth, and **brownish discharge** are evident.

Necrotizing enterocolitis: Abdominal pain, vomiting, and **bloody diarrhea** beginning approximately 1 day after ingestion of contaminated meat. Necrosis of intestinal wall due to **beta toxin** (*C. perfringens* **type C**) may lead to **peritonitis.**

Anaerobic cellulitis and fasciitis: Destruction of skin tissue similar to gas gangrene, but without involvement of muscle, in area of devitalized tissue. Most common in individuals with **poor circulation.**

B. *C. tetani*

- *C. tetani* is present in soil, water, and sewage; part of the normal flora of many animals
1. Identification
   - Small rods with tennis racquet shape due to the presence of terminal spore
   - Strict anaerobe that is very sensitive to oxygen
2. Pathogenesis
   - Tetanospasmin, an A-B type neurotoxin, blocks release of inhibitory neurotransmitters (e.g., γ-aminobutyric acid and glycine), resulting in spastic paralysis due to unregulated excitatory synaptic activity (Fig. 10-1A).
     a. Binding of B subunit to peripheral neurons at the site of infection promotes uptake of A subunit, which then travels to the central nervous system and exerts a blocking effect at inhibitory synapses.
   - Spore formation permits survival in unfavorable conditions.
3. Diseases caused by *C. tetani*
   - Infection is acquired via entry of spores from contaminated materials (e.g., dirty nails and splinters) into a cut or stab wound.
   - Generalized tetanus: onset usually within 1 week of exposure
     a. Spasms of masticatory muscles (trismus, lockjaw), drooling, sweating, irritability, persistent back spasms (opisthotonos), and sardonic grin (risus sardonicus)
     b. High mortality rate in unvaccinated individuals
   - Localized tetanus: later onset and less serious unless progresses to generalized form
     a. Twitching and spasm of muscle groups near site of wound

Trigger words:
C. tetani: A-B toxin, diphtheria, lockjaw, sardonic grin, twitching spasms

Tetanus toxin inhibits release of inhibitory neurotransmitters in the central nervous system → spastic paralysis.

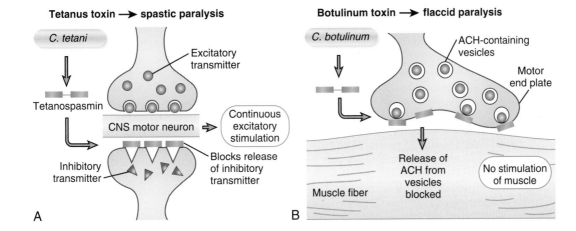

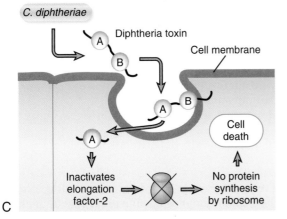

10-1: Action of dimeric A and B exotoxins produced by *Clostridium tetani* (**A**), *Clostridium botulinum* (**B**), and *Clostridium diphtheriae* (**C**). The B subunit binds to the surface of target cells, promoting entry of the A subunit, which inhibits some vital cell functions. *Pseudomonas aeruginosa* toxin works in a similar manner. Tetanus toxin acts at inhibitory synapses in the central nervous system (CNS); botulinum toxin acts on peripheral motor neurons at the junction with muscle cells. ACH, acetylcholine.

4. Prevention and treatment
- Vaccination with tetanus toxoid (formaldehyde-inactivated toxin) administered as part of the DPT or DT vaccine
  a. Booster shots required every 10 years and recommended after probable exposure
- Treatment for unvaccinated individuals
  a. Supportive care (e.g., muscle relaxants, oxygen) to reduce spasms and maintain breathing until circulating toxin is metabolized
  b. Passive immunization with human antitoxin immunoglobulin to neutralize circulating tetanospasmin
  c. Débridement of the primary wound and penicillin therapy to eliminate clostridial cells

C. *C. botulinum*
- Botulinum toxin in patient specimens or food is detected by immunoassay.
1. Pathogenesis
- Botulinum toxin, an A-B type neurotoxin, blocks release of acetylcholine at cholinergic synapses, leading to flaccid paralysis (Fig. 10-1B).
  a. B subunit binds to nerve cells; internalized A subunit exerts neurotoxic effect. Recovery period is prolonged because nerve endings affected by toxin must regenerate.
- Spores are heat resistant, but the toxin and bacteria are not.
2. Diseases caused by *C. botulinum*
- Classic food-borne botulism results from ingestion of preformed toxin, most commonly present in improperly prepared home-canned foods.
  a. Variable onset of symptoms, including weakness and dizziness; blurred vision, fixed and dilated pupils; dry mouth; flaccid paralysis; and death from respiratory paralysis
  b. Spores that survive the canning procedure may germinate and produce toxin in sealed, anaerobic containers.
- Infant botulism is associated with ingestion of honey contaminated with *C. botulinum*, which colonizes the GI tract and produces toxin in vivo.
  a. Most common form of botulism in the United States, primarily affecting infants younger than 1 year of age.
  b. Initial nonspecific symptoms (e.g., failure to thrive and constipation) may progress to flaccid paralysis (floppy baby syndrome) and respiratory arrest (in 1% to 2% of patients).
- Wound botulism results from skin inoculation and local in vivo production of toxin, leading to disease clinically similar to food-borne botulism.
3. Prevention and treatment
- Proper canning techniques and adequate heating of home-canned food, which inactivates any toxin present
- Administration of trivalent antitoxin against the major toxin types (A, B, and E) as early as possible in all forms of botulism
- Emptying of stomach contents, respiratory support, and penicillin (in infant and wound botulism)

D. *C. difficile*
- *C. difficile* is part of normal intestinal flora in some individuals.
- Toxin in stool samples is detected by immunoassay or by its ability to kill cultured cells (cytotoxicity test).
1. Pathogenesis
- Resistance to certain antibiotics may permit overgrowth or acquisition of *C. difficile* in patients receiving these drugs for other infections.
- Enterotoxin (toxin A) promotes fluid secretion and intestinal hemorrhage (similar to cholera toxin).
- Cytotoxin (toxin B) damages mucosal membranes by depolymerizing cellular cytoskeleton.
- Adhesion factor binds to human colon cells.
- Spores are insensitive to oxygen and resistant to many disinfectants, including alcohol-based hand cleaners, making their elimination from hospital environments difficult.
2. Pseudomembranous colitis due to *C. difficile*
- Patients on antibiotic therapy develop profuse, foul-smelling, liquid, sometimes bloody diarrhea. Leukocytes in the stool, fever, and abdominal pain may also be present.

Margin notes (left column):

Tetanus toxoid vaccine is part of DPT
Antitoxin treatment to neutralize tetanospasmin.

Trigger words:
C. botulinum: A-B toxin, botulism, floppy baby, food-borne, honey, spores, strict anaerobe

Botulinum toxin blocks release of acetylcholine at neuromuscular junction → flaccid paralysis.

Floppy baby syndrome results from ingestion of honey containing botulinum spores.

Trigger words:
C. difficile: antibiotic associated, pseudomembranous colitis, spores, toxins A and B

Antibiotic treatment eliminates competing bacterial growth in the gut and allows *C. difficile* to grow.

C. difficile is resistant to alcohol hand cleaners.
C. difficile is a common nosocomial infection, especially for patients taking broad-spectrum antibiotics.

BOX 10-2   RESPIRATORY DIPHTHERIA

Onset of diphtheria is sudden, with a sore throat, low-grade fever, and exudative pharyngitis. The exudate develops into a **thick pseudomembrane** consisting of dead cells, bacteria, and fibrin. This can cover the nasal mucosa, tonsils, uvula, and palate, and it may extend into the respiratory tract. Patients often have a **bull-neck appearance** owing to the pseudomembrane. Serious cases are marked by **obstruction of the airways** and **systemic effects** due to spread of diphtheria **exotoxin** to distant organs.

Immunity to diphtheria can be determined by the **Schick test** for antitoxin-neutralizing antibodies. After intradermal injection of diphtheria toxin, immune individuals develop no skin reaction. Localized edema and necrosis occur in nonimmune individuals, who are susceptible to *C. diphtheriae* infection.

- Disease can be acquired endogenously or exogenously via spores, which are often spread nosocomially on hands of hospital workers or fomites.
- Discontinuation of causative antibiotic therapy is sufficient treatment in mild cases. More serious cases may also require treatment with metronidazole, vancomycin, or even bacitracin.
  a. The presence of antibiotic-resistant spores may lead to relapse.

III. *Corynebacterium diphtheria*
  - *C. diphtheriae* is the only significant human pathogen in the genus *Corynebacterium*.

  A. Identification
  - Small, club-shaped, gram-positive, non–spore-forming rods with metachromatic granules
  - Black colonies on tellurite agar

  B. Pathogenesis
  1. Diphtheria toxin, an A-B type exotoxin, inhibits protein synthesis in mammalian cells, leading to cell death and disease manifestations (Fig. 10-1C).
  2. Lysogenic bacteriophage (β-prophage) carries toxin gene.
     - No phage = no toxin = no disease

  C. Diseases caused by *C. diphtheriae*
  1. Respiratory diphtheria is acquired by inhalation of respiratory droplets from infected individuals, including asymptomatic immunized carriers (Box 10-2).
  2. Cutaneous (wound) diphtheria is acquired by skin contact and entrance of organism via breaks in the skin.
     - Initial papule develops into chronic, nonhealing ulcer; systemic effects, if present, usually are mild.
  3. Systemic toxemia can cause damage to distant organs (e.g., myocarditis, neuropathy, and renal tubular necrosis).

  D. Prevention and treatment
  1. Vaccination with diphtheria toxoid as part of the mixed DPT or DT vaccines
     - Booster is required every 10 years.
  2. Passive immunization with antitoxin early in the course of the disease to neutralize circulating toxin
  3. Penicillin or erythromycin given to patients, carriers, and close contacts to eliminate bacteria

Trigger words:
C. diphtheriae: A-B toxin; DPT vaccine; pseudomembrane.

Diphtheria toxin inhibits protein synthesis by adenosine diphosphate ribosylation of EF-2, which inactivates the elongation factor.

The toxin gene for diphtheria is on a lysogenic bacteriophage.

Diphtheria toxoid vaccine in DPT

CHAPTER 11

ENTEROBACTERIACEAE

I. Defining and Differential Properties of Enteric Bacteria

A. Identification

1. Structure
   - All Enterobacteriaceae are gram-negative rods, which contain lipopolysaccharide (LPS) in their cell envelope.
   - Most have flagella and are motile.
   - *Shigella* species are nonmotile.
   - Some have capsules.
2. Biochemical and growth properties
   - All ferment glucose and are oxidase negative.
   - Lactose-fermenting genera are generally benign
   - Non–lactose-fermenting genera may be more pathogenic.
   - All are facultative anaerobes, permitting survival in the gastrointestinal (GI) tract.
   - Growth on differential media distinguishes Enterobacteriaceae from gram-positive organisms and from each other (Table 11-1).
3. Serologic classification
   - Based on O antigen (polysaccharide portion of LPS), K (capsular) antigen, and H (flagellar) antigen

B. Virulence factors

Endotoxin reactions accompany infections by Enterobacteriaceae, especially bacteremia.

Adhesins on fimbriae prevent bacteria from being washed away and promote urinary tract infections.

1. Endotoxin, a part of the LPS produced by all Enterobacteriaceae, is responsible for many of the systemic manifestations of infection.
2. Exotoxins, produced by some species and strains, cause diarrhea.
3. Adhesins and fimbriae on some species promote adhesion to the colon, bladder, or other tissues.
4. Intracellular growth (*Shigella*, *Salmonella* and *Yersinia* species and enteroinvasive *Escherichia coli*) protects organisms from host defenses.
5. Antibiotic resistance develops rapidly and often is encoded on plasmids, which can be transferred to related bacteria.
6. Capsule on *Klebsiella* and *Salmonella* species is antiphagocytic.
7. The genes for many of the virulence factors are clustered and coordinately controlled within pathogenicity islands.

C. Distribution and infection (Table 11-2)

1. Enterobacteriaceae are found worldwide in soil, water, and vegetation.
2. They are part of the normal intestinal flora of animals and humans.

TABLE 11-1 **Colony Morphology of Important Enterobacteriaceae**

	LACTOSE FERMENTERS		LACTOSE NONFERMENTERS	
MEDIUM	*ESCHERICHIA COLI*	*KLEBSIELLA* SPECIES	*SALMONELLA* SPECIES	*SHIGELLA* SPECIES
MacConkey agar	Purple, pink	Pink	Colorless	Colorless
Eosin–methylene blue agar	Red, black	Purple	Colorless	Colorless
Hektoen enteric agar	Yellow, orange	Yellow-orange	Blue-green with black center (H_2S)	Green, blue-green
Salmonella-shigella agar	Pink	Pink	Colorless with black center (H_2S)	Colorless

TABLE 11-2 **Medically Important Enterobacteriaceae**

ORGANISM	DISEASES
Lactose Positive	
Escherichia coli	Diarrhea, sepsis, urinary tract infection, neonatal meningitis
Klebsiella, Serratia, Citrobacter, Enterobacter species	Opportunistic infections (e.g., pneumonia, sepsis, neonatal meningitis)
Lactose Negative	
Salmonella species	Diarrhea, typhoid fever, bacteremia; localized infections in bone, meninges, liver
Shigella species	Dysentery
Proteus species	Urinary tract infection
Yersinia species	Plague, diarrhea, mesenteric lymphadenitis

3. Human pathogens
   - *Salmonella, Shigella,* and *Yersinia* species are invasive and always associated with disease in humans.
   - Disease is acquired from animal reservoirs or human carriers.
4. Opportunistic organisms
   - *E. coli* and *Klebsiella, Enterobacter,* and *Proteus* species, and other enteric bacteria are generally noninvasive and part of the normal flora in humans.
   - Disease occurs when these organisms are introduced into normally sterile sites.
   - Immunocompromised and debilitated patients are at greatest risk for disease. Some strains have acquired specific virulence factors that increase their pathogenicity.

II. Lactose-Fermenting Enterobacteriaceae
   A. *E. coli*
      1. Pathogenesis
         a. Endotoxin is present in all strains
         b. Noncytotoxic enterotoxins: enterotoxigenic strains (ETEC)
            1) Heat-labile (LT) enterotoxin causes increased cyclic adenosine monophosphate (cAMP) levels, leading to altered electrolyte transport and diarrhea.
               - Mechanism similar to that of cholera toxin.
            2) Heat-stabile (ST) enterotoxin stimulates cyclic guanosine monophosphate (cGMP) production, leading to fluid loss and diarrhea.
         c. Enterohemorrhagic strains (EHEC)
            - Verotoxin is the same as Shiga toxin and cytotoxic to intestinal villi and colon epithelial cells
         d. Enteroinvasive strains (EIEC)
            - Invasion and destruction of colonic epithelial cells
         e. Enteropathogenic strains (EPEC) and enteroaggregative strains (EAEC)
            - Adherence to mucosa of small intestine (plasmid mediated) and disruption of microvilli structure.
         f. Uropathogenic stains (UPEC)
            - *P. fimbriae*–mediated adherence to uroepithelium
      2. Diseases caused by *E. coli*
         - Gastroenteritis
            a. Clinical manifestations are strain specific (Table 11-3).
         - Hemolytic-uremic syndrome
            a. Complication of gastroenteritis caused by EHEC (e.g., strain O157:H7), which occurs primarily in children
            b. Associated with ingestion of contaminated undercooked hamburgers and other beef products
            c. Marked by acute renal failure, thrombocytopenia, and microangiopathic hemolytic anemia
         - UTI
            a. Cystitis and pyelonephritis are common presentations.
         - Neonatal meningitis
            a. Associated with strains that have KI (capsular) antigen
         - Septicemia
            a. Organisms enter from urinary or GI tracts.
            b. *E. coli* is the most common gram-negative agent of septicemia (Box 11-1).

Salmonella, Shigella, and *Yersinia* species, cannot ferment lactose, are not normal flora and always cause disease and must be treated.

Trigger words:
E. coli: diarrhea; EIEC, EHEC, ETEC, EAEC, EPEC; gram-negative rod; lactose positive; neonatal meningitis; O157:H7; oxidase negative; urinary tract infection (UTI)

E. coli: lactose-fermenting, strain-specific virulence factors

E. coli: diarrhea, UTIs, neonatal meningitis, septicemia, hemolytic-uremic syndrome

E. coli (UPEC) is a primary cause of UTIs.

E. coli and group B streptococci are the most common causes of neonatal meningitis.

O157:H7 refers to the O-antigen serotype of the LPS that is on the bacteria that carry the plasmid for the verotoxin Shiga toxin.

TABLE 11-3 **Gastroenteritis Caused by** *Escherichia coli*

E. COLI STRAIN	SITE OF ACTION	CLINICAL FEATURES	PATHOGENESIS
Enterotoxigenic (ETEC)	Small intestine	Watery diarrhea, cramps, nausea, and low-grade fever in **travelers** and **infants**	Enterotoxins promote increased cyclic adenosine monophosphate or cyclic guanosine monophosphate, leading to fluid and electrolyte loss
Enteroaggregative (EAEC)	Small intestine	Persistent **infant diarrhea,** sometimes with gross blood, low-grade fever	Aggregative adherence to mucosa prevents fluid absorption
Enteropathogenic (EPEC)	Small intestine	Copious watery infant diarrhea with fever, nausea, vomiting, and nonbloody, mucus-filled stools	Adherence and destruction of epithelial cells
Enteroinvasive (EIEC)	Large intestine	Fever, cramping, watery diarrhea followed by development of **dysentery** with scant, bloody stools	Invasion and destruction of epithelial cells lining the colon
Enterohemorrhagic (EHEC)	Large intestine	Severe abdominal cramps, initial watery diarrhea followed by grossly **bloody diarrhea,** little or no fever (hemorrhagic colitis); **hemolytic-uremic syndrome** associated with strain **O157:H7**	Cytotoxic verotoxin (Shiga toxin) inhibits protein synthesis

---

BOX 11-1 ENDOTOXIN-MEDIATED TOXICITY WITH SEPTICEMIA

When gram-negative bacteria enter the bloodstream, they release blebs of outer membrane filled with LPS. **Endotoxin,** the lipid A portion of LPS, activates complement and binds to toll-like receptors on macrophages, endothelial cells, and epithelial cells, leading to release of a wide variety of cytokines and other mediators. These mediators and complement components cause the clinical manifestations of **bacterial sepsis,** including the following:

- Fever
- Leukopenia followed by leukocytosis
- Thrombocytopenia
- Disseminated intravascular coagulation
- Decreased peripheral circulation and perfusion to major organs
- Shock
- Death

- Spontaneous peritonitis in adults with cirrhosis and ascites
3. Transmission
   - Endogenous spread of normal flora (e.g., self-inoculation, perforation of bowel)
   - Nosocomial spread from infected individuals
   - Ingestion of contaminated food or water
4. Treatment
   - Antibiotic choice depends on the site of infection and on susceptibility of the organism.

B. *Klebsiella pneumoniae*
   1. Pathogenesis
      - Prominent capsule hinders phagocytosis and is important for virulence.
   2. Diseases
      - Primary lobar pneumonia results from aspiration of organisms into the lungs.
         a. Alcoholic patients and individuals with compromised pulmonary function are at highest risk for developing *Klebsiella* species infection.
         b. Most common pneumonia in nursing homes
      - Bacteremia and UTI also can be caused by *Klebsiella* species.

C. *Enterobacter, Citrobacter,* and *Serratia* species
   1. These species rarely cause primary infection in healthy individuals, but the immunocompromised are at risk for nosocomial infection.
   2. Multiple antibiotic resistance is common, especially in *Enterobacter* species.

III. **Non–Lactose-Fermenting Enterobacteriaceae**
   A. *Salmonella* species
      - *Salmonella* species are carried in the GI tract of many animals but are not part of the normal human flora. Numerous serotypes are recognized based on surface antigens.
      1. Pathogenesis
         - Antiphagocytic capsule

Trigger words:
K. pneumoniae: aspiration, capsule, currant jelly (blood) sputum, pneumonia

K. pneumoniae: lung infection most common in alcoholic patients and those with poor pulmonary function

Trigger words:
Salmonella species: dairy foods, motile, nonbloody diarrhea, nonlactose fermenter, raw eggs and chicken

- Intracellular growth and replication
- Endotoxin and exotoxins (serotypes causing enteritis)
- Animal reservoirs

2. *Salmonella* species diseases
- Enteritis (*Salmonella enteritidis* and other serotypes)
  a. Incubation period is 6 to 48 hours.
  b. Spontaneous resolution usually occurs within 2 to 7 days.
  c. Symptoms include nausea, vomiting, and nonbloody diarrhea.
    - Abdominal pain, low-grade fever, and headache are also common.
  d. Symptomatic treatment, including rehydration, is sufficient.
- Typhoid (enteric) fever *(Salmonella typhi)*
  a. After incubation period of 10 to 14 days, initial symptoms include steadily increasing fever, headache, myalgia, malaise, and anorexia.
  b. Invasion of M cells in Peyer patches results in gastrointestinal symptoms (necrosis, hemorrhage, and perforation of intestinal wall) after the second week of illness.
- Bacteremia releases endotoxin causing fever and other systemic symptoms.
- Localized infections in other sites (e.g., osteomyelitis, meningitis)

3. Transmission
- Fecal-oral route (all serotypes)
- Ingestion of large numbers of organisms in contaminated water and food
  a. Dairy products, raw eggs, and improperly cooked chicken and turkey are common reservoirs of salmonellae except for *S. typhi.*
  b. Reptiles (e.g., pet turtles) are common carriers.
- Asymptomatic carriers *(S. typhi)*
  a. Some individuals who recover from typhoid fever continue to carry *S. typhi* for months (gallbladder is a common reservoir).
  b. Contamination of food or water by salmonellae shed from carriers can spread disease ("typhoid Mary").

B. **Shigella species**
- All four *Shigella* species are pathogenic in humans and cause similar disease manifestations.

1. Pathogenesis
- Invasion of colonic mucosa and replication within mucosal cells
- Shiga toxin *(Shigella dysenteriae)*
  a. A-B type toxin that cleaves 28S recombinant RNA, thereby inhibiting protein synthesis
- Very high infectivity
- No animal reservoirs

2. Shigellosis (bacillary dysentery)
- Initial symptoms include profuse watery diarrhea, abdominal cramps, and fever.
- Tenesmus and the presence of blood, mucus, and polymorphonuclear leukocytes in stool are indicative of invasion of the bowel wall (ulcerative colitis).
- Severity and incidence vary with causative species.
  a. *Shigella sonnei*
    - Relatively mild but most commonly encountered disease
    - Prevalent among children in day care centers and those in long-term care facilities
  b. *Shigella flexneri*
    - Severe disease
    - Mostly in male homosexuals
  c. *S. dysenteriae*
    - Severe disease, but rare except where epidemic

3. Transmission
- Fecal-oral route via hands (most common route)
- Ingestion of food or water contaminated from human source (less common route)

4. Treatment
- Rehydration for diarrhea is often necessary.
- Antimotility agents (e.g., clotrimazole) may prolong disease.

C. **Yersinia pestis**
- *Yersinia pestis* is carried by numerous small animals, including domestic cats, and can be transmitted to humans via flea vectors.

1. Pathogenesis
- Antiphagocytic capsule
- Intracellular growth

Virulence factors of *Salmonella* species include capsule, intracellular growth, endotoxins, and exotoxins.

Salmonella species: recovery from typhoid confers immunity, whereas that from *salmonellal enteritis* does not.

Enteritis: most common form of salmonellosis

Enteritis: excessive fluid and electrolyte loss may be life threatening, especially for infants, elderly people, and immunocompromised patients.

Enteritis: antibiotic therapy prolongs carrier state.

Asymptomatic carriers spread *S. typhi.*

S. typhi invades the gut, establishes bacteremia, and establishes carrier state in gallbladder to release bacteria into stool.

S. typhi only infects humans.

S. typhi is more likely to be isolated from blood than stool during first 2 weeks.

Trigger words:

Shigella species: gram-negative bacillus, lactose negative, no hydrogen sulfide, Shiga toxin, watery, bloody diarrhea

Shigella species: always spreads from human source through food, fingers, feces, flies, or fomites.

Salmonella versus *Shigella* species:

- *Salmonellae:* motile, spread from infection site, can be transmitted from animal reservoirs
- *Shigellae:* nonmotile, do not disseminate widely, have no animal reservoirs
- *Shigellae:* much more virulent (10^1 organisms) than salmonellae (10^5 organisms)

Shigella causes bloody, watery diarrhea owing to invasion of bowel.

Y. pestis is transmitted by flea bite or aerosol.

- Exotoxin
- Ability to disseminate from infection site

2. Diseases caused by *Y. pestis*
- Bubonic plague
  a. Acquired from bite of infected flea
  b. Prairie dogs are reservoir for the pathogen.
  c. Incubation period of 7 days
  d. High fever, painful bubo (inflamed, swollen lymph node) in groin or axilla, conjunctivitis, bacteremia that can lead to death in untreated patients (mortality rate > 75%)
- Pneumonic plague
  a. Acquired by inhalation of infectious droplets from another patient
  b. Incubation period of 2 to 3 days
  c. Fever and malaise, followed 1 day later by respiratory problems that usually lead to death in untreated patients (mortality rate > 90%)
- Bioterror agent

3. Prevention and treatment
- Effective pest control, isolation of infected patients, and vaccination with formalin-killed vaccine (effective against bubonic plague)
- Streptomycin, gentamicin, tetracycline, or chloramphenicol as soon as possible for both forms of plague

D. ***Yersinia enterocolitica***
- *Y. enterocolitica* is carried in livestock, rabbits, and rodents and transmitted to humans in contaminated food, water, or blood products.

1. Enterocolitis (most common disease)
- Bloody diarrhea, fever, and abdominal pain usually last 1 or 2 weeks. Chronic form may last more than 1 year.

2. Mesenteric lymphadenitis
- Enlargement of mesenteric lymph nodes can mimic acute appendicitis (pseudoappendicitis).
- Most common in young children

3. Transfusion-related septicemia
- *Y. enterocolitica* can grow at low temperatures and multiply to toxic levels in refrigerated blood stored for several weeks.

E. ***Proteus mirabilis***
1. Part of normal flora of the human GI tract (unlike other non–lactose-fermenting Enterobacteriaceae)
2. Swarming growth on agar
3. Strong urease activity
4. Common cause of UTIs
- Marked by elevated urine pH due to urease action and often by formation of renal stones (magnesium ammonium phosphate; "staghorn calculus")
- Ammonia smell of urine

Trigger words:

Y. pestis: plague, rodent and animal host, fleas, buboes

Buboes are inflamed swollen lymph nodes.

Plague can be spread by vector or by aerosol.

Trigger words:

P. mirabilis: elevated urine pH, swarmer, urease, UTI

P. mirabilis are motile swarmers.

CHAPTER 12

GRAM-NEGATIVE COCCI AND COCCOBACILLI

I. *Neisseria* Species
- *Neisseria meningitidis* and *Neisseria gonorrhoeae* are strict human pathogens; other *Neisseria* species are commonly present on mucosal surfaces.

A. Shared *Neisseria* properties
1. Structure
   - Gram-negative, nonmotile, coffee bean–shaped diplococci
   - Loosely attached outer membrane that is readily shed, releasing lipooligosaccharide (LOS) into the host
     - a. LOS contains lipid A (endotoxin) and core oligosaccharide found in lipopolysaccharide (LPS), but it lacks strain-specific O antigen found in LPS of most gram-negative bacteria (see Chapter 6, Fig. 6-6).
     - b. LOS is readily shed and induces endotoxemia.
   - Capsule
2. Growth and biochemical characteristics
   - Oxidase positive and catalase positive
   - Sugar fermentation
     - a. *N. meningitidis* uses <u>m</u>altose and glucose.
     - b. *N. gonorrhoeae* uses <u>g</u>lucose only.
   - Intracellular growth
     - a. Both *N. meningitidis* and *N. gonorrhoeae* can grow within cells and survive destruction by phagocytes.
   - In vitro growth on complex chocolate agar in an atmosphere containing additional CO_2

B. *N. meningitidis*
1. Classification
   - Serogroups based on the polysaccharide capsule
     - a. Most common = A, B, C, Y, and W135
   - Serotypes based on the outer membrane protein
   - Immunotypes based on LOS
2. Pathogenesis
   - *N. meningitidis* enters the respiratory tract, invades mucous membranes, and spreads via the bloodstream.
     - a. Present in the posterior nasopharynx
   - Antiphagocytic capsule is important for virulence.
   - Released endotoxin induces fever and increases vascular permeability, potentially leading to shock and petechiae (capillary leakage in skin).
3. Meningococcal diseases
   - Meningococcal infection is most common in children younger than 5 years of age and in those with deficiency of terminal complement components (C5-C9).
   - Meningitis
     - a. *N. meningitidis* most common cause from 1 month to 18 years of age
     - b. Acute onset of fever, headache, and stiff neck
   - Acute meningococcemia
     - a. Septicemia with or without meningitis

N. meningitidis has an *m* and a *g* and ferments maltose and glucose. Gonorrhoeae and glucose only have *g*.

Neisseria are often seen as gram-negative intracellular diploids within phagocytes.

Trigger words:
N. meningitidis: chocolate agar, endotoxin, gram-negative diplococci in cerebrospinal fluid, lipooligosaccharide, meningitis, oxidase positive, petechiae, purpura, septic shock, Thayer-Martin agar, Waterhouse-Friderichsen syndrome

N. meningitidis capsule and endotoxin (LOS) release are virulence factors.

Deficiency in C5-C9 is risk factor for neisserial infections.

b. Characterized by fever, shock, and generalized hemorrhage ranging from petechiae to purpura

c. Can be rapidly fatal (mortality rate of 25% or higher) if not treated promptly

- Waterhouse-Friderichsen syndrome
  a. Complication of meningococcemia
  b. Marked by overwhelming disseminated intravascular coagulation and bilateral hemorrhagic adrenal infarctions with septic shock, acute hypotension, tachycardia, and petechiae
- Chronic meningococcemia
  a. Milder disease characterized by persistent (for weeks) bacteremia
  b. Low-grade fever, arthritis, and petechial skin lesions
- Mild febrile disease with pharyngitis, pneumonia, arthritis, or urethritis

4. Transmission of *N. meningitidis*
   - Person-to-person spread from infected persons
   - Inhalation of aerosol droplets (often from asymptomatic posterior nasopharyngeal carriers)

5. Prevention
   - Breastfeeding infants for the first 6 months of life
   - Active immunization of children older than 2 years of age with a polyvalent conjugate, anticapsular vaccine (not effective against serogroup B)
   - Postexposure prophylaxis with rifampin, quinolones, or sulfonamides (only if the organism is proved susceptible)

6. Treatment
   - Penicillin is the drug of choice.
   - Alternatives include broad-spectrum cephalosporins (ceftriaxone), chloramphenicol, and sulfonamides (if susceptible).
   - Antibiotics must be released from mucosa into secretions to eliminate carrier state.
     a. Gonococci ferment glucose only, are transmitted by sexual contact, and cause infection primarily in sexually active adults.
     b. Meningococci ferment maltose and glucose, are transmitted by aerosols, and cause infection primarily in young children.

C. *N. gonorrhoeae*

1. Thayer-Martin medium (selective chocolate agar)
   - Used for isolating *N. gonorrhoeae* in specimens from nonsterile areas, such as the cervix and urethra
   - Contains vancomycin (kills gram-positive bacteria), colistin (kills gram-negative bacteria except *Neisseria* species), and nystatin (kills fungi)

2. Pathogenesis
   - Pili (fimbriae) and outer membrane protein II (OMPII) promote adherence to and invasion of mucosal cells.
   - IgA protease cleaves secretory IgA, reducing host defense to gonococcal infection.
   - Endotoxin causes fever, vascular permeability, inflammation, and tissue destruction.
   - Antibiotic resistance, especially due to β-lactamase, is common.
   - Antigenic variation of surface proteins permits escape from antibody response.

3. Gonococcal diseases (Box 12-1)
   - Sexually active individuals with multiple partners are at greatest risk for *N. gonorrhoeae* infection, which is spread primarily by sexual contact.
   - Acute gonococcal infection (gonorrhea)

N. meningitidis can cause Waterhouse-Friderichsen syndrome.

Facultative intracellular bacteria: *N. meningitidis*, *N. gonorrhoeae*, *B. pertussis*, and *L. pneumophila*. Resolution of intracellular infections depends on an effective cell-mediated immune response.

Treatment of neisserial meningitis may exacerbate conditions due to release of cell wall activators of toll-like receptors and activation of macrophages.

Trigger words:
N. gonorrhoeae: chocolate agar, gram-negative diplococci, oxidase positive, STD, Thayer-Martin medium, urethritis

N. gonorrhoeae virulence factors include pili, OMPII, immunoglobulin A (IgA) protease, antigenic variation, and endotoxin release.

BOX 12-1 *NEISSERIA* SPECIES INFECTIONS: QUICK CASES

Meningococcal meningitis: Young child with sudden onset of fever, petechiae or purpura (black and blue marks) on the skin, malaise, and stiff neck. The cerebrospinal fluid contains intracellular gram-negative diplococci.

Gonorrhea (local infection): Sexually active man with green-yellow discharge from the urethra has difficulty urinating. Discharge contains gram-negative intracellular diplococci.

Disseminated gonococcal infection: Sexually active woman with painful, inflamed joint and pustules on the right wrist. Aspirate of the knee and pustule contained gram-negative intracellular diplococci.

PID: Sexually active woman who develops fever, abdominal pain, cervical tenderness, and vaginal discharge following unusually severe and prolonged menstrual period. An intrauterine device (IUD) had been inserted into the patient several years ago.

a. Males
- Urethritis with purulent urethral discharge, dysuria (painful urination)

b. Females
- Cervicitis with vaginal discharge, dysuria, abdominal pain, fever

- Pelvic inflammatory disease (PID)
  a. Infection of the uterus, fallopian tubes (salpingitis), and/or ovaries
  b. An ascending infection that may result in infertility and predisposes to ectopic pregnancy
  c. Pus collecting under the right diaphragm causes scar tissue formation between the diaphragm and liver surface causing pain with movement (Fitz-Hughes-Curtis syndrome)

- Neonatal conjunctivitis resulting from infection during delivery by infected mother
  a. Markedly decreased with the use of erythromycin eyedrops administered at birth

- Disseminated diseases
  a. Female dominant disease
  b. Septic arthritis, dermatitis-arthritis syndrome, bacteremia (skin lesions, fever, joint pain), endocarditis
  c. Deficiency of a terminal complement component (C6-C9) predisposes to disseminated disease.

- Anorectal gonorrhea in homosexual men
- Gonococcal pharyngitis

4. Treatment
- Gonococcal urethritis and cervicitis: treatment should be directed against *C. trachomatis* as well as *N. gonorrhoeae* because dual infection is common.
  a. Antigonococcal drugs include cefixime, ceftriaxone, and azithromycin.
  b. Antichlamydial drugs include tetracycline, doxycycline, ofloxacin, and azithromycin.
- Disseminated or bacteremic illness: prolonged therapy with penicillin or ceftriaxone is required.

II. *Bordetella pertussis*

A. Identification
1. Small, gram-negative, oxidase-positive, encapsulated coccobacillus
2. Growth on Bordet-Gengou agar

B. Pathogenesis
1. Filamentous hemagglutinin binds to ciliated epithelial cells, particularly in the nasopharynx and trachea.
2. Survival within phagocytic cells protects *B. pertussis* from circulating antibodies and permits long-term carriage within the lungs.
3. Several exotoxins and endotoxins mediate disease manifestations and increase virulence of *B. pertussis* (Table 12-1).

C. Pertussis (whooping cough)
1. Occurs primarily in unvaccinated children and adults with waning immunity
2. Transmitted by inhalation of infectious aerosols
3. Toxin inhibits signal transduction by chemokine receptors, which prevents lymphocytes from entering lymph nodes, leading to profound lymphocytosis.
4. Disease progresses from common cold–like to paroxysmal to convalescent stages (Fig. 12-1).

D. Prevention and treatment
1. Inactivated whole cell vaccine administered as part of the DPT (diphtheria-pertussis-tetanus) vaccine or multivalent acellular vaccine (DTaP) (at 2, 4, 6, and 16 months and at 5, 11, 19, and 65 years of age)

N. gonorrhoeae: causes sexually transmitted diseases, PID; conjunctivitis in newborns

Most common causes of PID: *N. gonorrhoeae* (acute, high fever) and *Chlamydia trachomatis* (subacute, often undiagnosed)

Neonatal gonococcal and chlamydial conjunctivitis can be prevented by application of erythromycin or silver nitrate to eyes of newborns.

Trigger words:
B. pertussis: Bordet-Gengou agar, DPT vaccine, whooping cough

B. pertussis virulence factors are adherence and toxins.

B. pertussis causes whooping cough.

Immunization is part of DPT, and boosters must be given later in life.

TABLE 12-1 *Bordetella pertussis* Toxins

TOXIN	BIOLOGIC EFFECTS
Pertussis toxin (A-B type exotoxin)	Toxic A subunit enters cell and **ADP-ribosylates inhibitory G protein,** turning it off. The subsequent **increased cAMP level** leads to loss of fluids and electrolytes, lymphocytosis, and massive **mucus secretion** in the respiratory tract.
Adenylate cyclase toxin	Enters host cells and **increases cAMP** production, which blocks immune effector function and prevents clearance of the bacteria
Tracheal cytotoxin	Inhibits and **damages ciliated tracheal cells**
Endotoxin	Causes fever and other **pyrogenic responses**

ADP, adenosine diphosphate; cAMP, cyclic adenosine monophosphate.

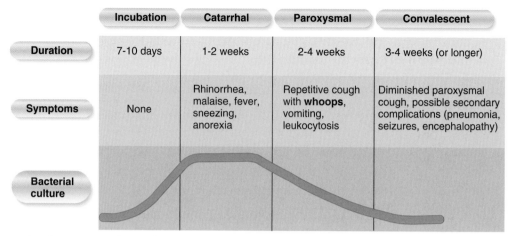

	Incubation	Catarrhal	Paroxysmal	Convalescent
Duration	7-10 days	1-2 weeks	2-4 weeks	3-4 weeks (or longer)
Symptoms	None	Rhinorrhea, malaise, fever, sneezing, anorexia	Repetitive cough with **whoops**, vomiting, leukocytosis	Diminished paroxysmal cough, possible secondary complications (pneumonia, seizures, encephalopathy)
Bacterial culture				

12-1: Clinical presentation of *Bordetella pertussis* disease (whooping cough). Contagion parallels the bacterial culture curve.

2. Macrolide (or similar) antibiotic early in disease and for nonimmune individuals who have been exposed
3. Prophylactic macrolide (or similar) antibiotic for close contacts of patient with symptoms
   - Because peak contagiousness with *B. pertussis* usually occurs before disease is recognized, prophylaxis of contacts helps prevent spread of whooping cough.

III. *Haemophilus* Species

- ***Haemophilus influenzae*** and ***Haemophilus ducreyi*** are the most medically important *Haemophilus* species.

A. **Shared properties of *Haemophilus* species**
1. Small, gram-negative coccobacillus
2. Obligate parasites found on mucous membranes of humans and some animals
3. Factor X (hemin) and/or factor V (NAD) required for growth

B. ***H. influenzae***
1. Pathogenesis
   - Antiphagocytic capsule is critical virulence factor.
     a. *H. influenzae* type b (Hib), the most virulent of the six capsule types, invades the mucosa, enters the blood, and spreads throughout the body, causing systemic diseases.
     b. Nonencapsulated *H. influenzae* is part of the normal flora of the upper respiratory tract and may cause localized opportunistic infections.
   - Endotoxin induces inflammation and contributes to the symptoms.
2. Diseases caused by *H. influenzae*
   - Systemic infection primarily affects unimmunized young children and is spread by respiratory droplets.
   - Meningitis in infants (3 to 18 months of age)
     a. Mild respiratory disease of short duration is followed by bacteremia and then meningitis.
       - Encapsulated strains cause meningitis
     b. Rare due to immunization
   - Epiglottitis in children (2 to 4 years of age)
     a. Cellulitis and swelling of the epiglottis can block breathing.
     b. Inspiratory stridor
     c. Lateral radiograph shows swelling of the epiglottis ("thumbprint" sign).
     d. Rare, due to immunization
   - Cellulitis in the cheek of very young children
     a. Infection begins in buccal mucosa and spreads to the face and neck, causing swelling, blue-red patches on skin, and fever.
   - Arthritis affecting single large joints in children younger than 2 years of age
   - Otitis, sinusitis, and bronchitis are caused by encapsulated and nonencapsulated strains of *H. influenzae* in adults as well as children.
     a. Pulmonary disease is most common in elderly people, individuals with a complement deficiency, and asplenic patients.
3. Prevention and treatment
   - Hib vaccine, consisting of type b capsular carbohydrate conjugated to diphtheria toxoid protein, as part of childhood immunization schedule

Trigger words:
H. influenzae: capsule, epiglottitis, Hib, meningitis, otitis, X and V factors

Virulence factors of *H. influenzae* are endotoxin release and capsule.

H. influenzae and *Streptococcus pneumoniae:* two most common causes of otitis media and sinusitis. Both can also cause meningitis in infants (primarily *H. influenzae*) or adults (primarily *S. pneumoniae*).

a. The Hib vaccine is so successful that it has practically eliminated *H. influenza* B from pediatrics.
- Prompt treatment with a broad-spectrum β-lactamase–resistant cephalosporin (e.g., ceftriaxone) for serious infections
- Rifampin prophylaxis for close contacts

C. ***H. ducreyi***
1. Causes chancroid, a sexually transmitted disease (STD) that is symptomatic in males but usually asymptomatic in females
2. Characterized by a painful ulcer that develops on the genitalia or the perianal region 5 to 7 days after exposure; usually accompanied by inguinal lymphadenopathy

IV. ***Legionella pneumophila***
A. **Identification**
1. Slender, gram-negative, facultatively intracellular, pleomorphic coccobacillus
2. Poorly staining with Gram stain
- Best seen with Dieterle silver stain or fluorescent stain
3. Cysteine and iron salts required for growth
4. Usually cultured on supplemented BCYE agar (buffered charcoal yeast extract agar)
5. Urine antigen test excellent screen

B. **Pathogenesis**
1. Intracellular infection is established in alveolar macrophages and monocytes following inhalation of legionellae.
- Coating of bacteria with C3b promotes their phagocytosis by macrophages.
- Inhibition of phagolysosome fusion by legionellae protects them against intracellular killing in macrophages.
2. Degradative enzymes produced by bacteria eventually kill infected cells.

C. **Diseases caused by L. pneumophila (Table 12-2)**
1. Legionnaires disease
- Atypical pneumonia (unlike pneumococcal pneumonia) marked by fever, chills, headache, and dry, nonproductive cough; possible multiorgan involvement; potentially fatal
2. Pontiac fever
- Self-limited febrile illness without pneumonia

D. **Transmission**
1. Water sources (e.g., air-conditioning cooling towers, mist, condensers, and water systems; and lakes and streams) are natural reservoirs of legionellae.
2. Inhalation of aerosols causes human infection.
- Showers, mist in grocery produce area; rainforest exhibitions; outdoor restaurants on hot days
3. There is no person-to-person spread.

E. **Prevention and treatment**
1. Hyperchlorination of water supplies and heating of water reduce *L. pneumophila* populations.
2. Macrolides (erythromycin, azithromycin), or fluoroquinolones, are antibiotics of choice for treating legionnaires disease.
- Fluoroquinolones, rifampin, and doxycycline are also effective.
- Most strains are resistant to β-lactam antibiotics.

The Hib vaccine consists of capsular carbohydrate conjugated to protein.

Haemophilus ducreyi: chancroid, STD. Must exclude other diseases marked by genital ulcers, such as primary syphilis and herpes simplex disease.

Chancroid (H. ducreyi) is painful, but chancre (syphilis) is not.

Trigger words:
L. pneumophila: air-conditioning, atypical pneumonia, charcoal yeast agar (BCYE agar), warm mist, shower and other lukewarm water sources

L. pneumophila grow intracellularly in phagocytes and even ameba.

L. pneumophila: atypical pneumonia, particularly in individuals older than 55 years, smokers, and patients with chronic obstructive pulmonary disease

Legionella is spread by aerosols from water sources, such as showers and air-conditioning cooling towers.

Common source (e.g., air conditioner), not person-to-person spread, for legionella.

TABLE 12-2 **Comparison of Diseases Caused by *Legionella pneumophila***

CHARACTERISTIC EPIDEMIOLOGY	LEGIONNAIRES DISEASE	PONTIAC FEVER
Presentation	Epidemic, sporadic	Epidemic
Infection rate	<5%	>90%
Person-to-person spread	No	No
Time of onset	Epidemic disease in late summer and fall; endemic disease throughout the year	Throughout the year
Clinical Manifestations		
Incubation period	2-10 days	1-2 days
Pneumonia	Yes	No
Resolution	Requires antibiotic therapy	Self-limited
Mortality rate	15%-20% (untreated); higher with late diagnosis	<1%

I. *Pseudomonas aeruginosa*

- *P. aeruginosa* is the most common clinically significant pseudomonad.

A. Identification
1. Gram-negative, oxidase-positive, aerobic rods with one to three flagella
2. Nonfermenting
3. Positive nitrate reduction test
4. Simple growth requirements
5. Characteristic fruity odor
6. Blue-green pigment (pyocyanin) or other diffusible pigments produced by many strains

B. Pathogenesis
1. Pili promote adherence to respiratory epithelium.
2. Capsule is antiphagocytic and promotes adherence to tracheal epithelium.
3. Exotoxin A inhibits protein synthesis by adenosine diphosphate (ADP)-ribosylation of elongation factor-2 (EF-2), similar to diphtheria toxin (see Chapter 10, Fig. 10-1C).
4. Biofilm production occurs when sufficient bacteria trigger quorum sensing.
5. Other virulence factors include the endotoxin exoenzyme S, which prevents phagocytic killing; degradative enzymes that damage host tissues; and antibiotic resistance.

C. Diseases caused by *P. aeruginosa*
- *P. aeruginosa* causes a wide variety of opportunistic infections, most commonly in hospitalized, immunocompromised, and debilitated individuals.
1. Urinary tract infection (UTI)
   - *P. aeruginosa* is a common cause of UTI, especially in patients with indwelling catheters who are on antimicrobial therapy, which selects for drug-resistant strains.
2. Burn wound infection
   - Colonization of burn wounds followed by vascular damage, tissue necrosis, and bacteremia
3. Ear infections
   - Otitis externa (swimmer's ear)
     a. Usually benign but extremely painful
   - Malignant external otitis
     a. Serious disease marked by pain, swelling, and purulent discharge from the external auditory canal
     b. Invasion of underlying tissue can lead to cranial nerve damage, bacteremia, and sepsis.
     c. Elderly and diabetic patients are most susceptible.
4. Skin infections
   - Vesicular and pustular lesions; cellulitis, abscesses, and subcutaneous infections
     a. Ecthyma gangrenosum
        - Focal skin lesions that are characterized by vascular invasion by the bacteria, resulting in hemorrhage and necrosis (central dark area of lesions)
        - Usually seen in patients with neutropenia
     b. Folliculitis
        - Infection of areas with a high concentration of apocrine sweat glands (external ear, areola, nipple)
        - Acquired by immersion in contaminated hot tubs, whirlpool baths, or swimming pools

5. Pulmonary infections
   - In cystic fibrosis patients, *P. aeruginosa* and *Staphylococcus aureus* are the most common causes of chronic pulmonary infection, which exacerbates the underlying disease and is difficult to eradicate.
   - In neutropenic and other immunocompromised individuals, *P. aeruginosa* acquired from contaminated respiratory therapy equipment can cause diffuse, bilateral bronchopneumonia.
6. Keratitis (fulminating ulceration of the cornea)
   - Initial trauma to the eye followed by exposure to *P. aeruginosa* can lead to eye-threatening panophthalmitis without prompt treatment.
7. Disseminated infections of the immunocompromised host (e.g., transplant patient).
   - Hard to treat septicemia and tissue infections.
8. *P. aeruginosa* osteomyelitis
   - Most often due to puncture of foot through athletic shoes

D. Transmission
   - *P. aeruginosa* is ubiquitous in the environment and in moist reservoirs (e.g., respiratory and dialysis equipment, cut flowers, sinks, and bars of soap) throughout hospitals and other institutions.
   1. *P. aeruginosa* is resistant to soap, many disinfectants, and many antibiotics but sensitive to drying.
   2. Infection usually begins at sites where moisture accumulates.

E. Treatment
   - Aminoglycoside (or fluoroquinolone) + antipseudomonal β-lactam antibiotic, depending on the susceptibility of the isolate

II. *Burkholderia* Species
A. *Burkholderia cepacia* complex
   1. Lung infections in cystic fibrosis or CGD patients
   2. Opportunistic urinary tract infections and catheter associated
   3. Susceptible to trimethoprim sulfamethoxazole

III. *Vibrio* Species and Related Bacteria
   - *Vibrio*, *Aeromonas*, and *Plesiomonas* species are all gram-negative, oxidase-positive motile rods that are salt tolerant or salt requiring.

A. *V. cholerae*
   1. Identification
      - Comma-shaped rods grow in freshwater ponds and brackish water (e.g., where rivers empty into ocean).
      - They can be cultured on most media used for stool culture (e.g., blood agar and MacConkey agar).
   2. Pathogenesis
      - Pili and other adhesins permit *V. cholerae* to adhere tightly to the mucosal epithelium.
      - A-B type exotoxin ADP-ribosylates stimulatory G protein, leading to increased cyclic adenosine monophosphate (cAMP) level within mucosal cells and secretion of ions and fluid (Fig. 13-1).
   3. Cholera
      - Rapid onset occurs 2 or 3 days after inoculation.
      - Initial clinical manifestations are vomiting and severe watery diarrhea with mucous flecks (rice-water stools), leading to dehydration (volume depletion) and electrolyte imbalance.
      - Complications in untreated patients include shock, acidosis, cardiac arrhythmia, and renal failure; there is a high mortality rate.
   4. Transmission
      - Fecal-oral route spreads *V. cholerae* via water, fish, and shellfish.
        a. Large inocula are required to establish infection; thus, direct person-to-person spread is unlikely.
      - Carriers who have recovered from cholera may shed organisms and are an important reservoir of *V. cholerae* in endemic regions.
   5. Prevention and treatment
      - Good public sanitation measures are important in reducing contamination of water sources with cholera-containing feces.
      - Vaccination is largely ineffective, providing only short-term protection against the least serious strain of *V. cholerae*.
      - Supportive care with fluid and electrolyte replacement is required.
        a. Tetracycline, ciprofloxacin, or erythromycin reduce the duration of symptoms.

Pseudomonas and *Burkholderia* (related to *Pseudomonas*) species with *S. aureus* establish chronic infection of lungs of cystic fibrosis patients.

P. aeruginosa osteomyelitis: puncture of foot through athletic shoes

P. aeruginosa is ubiquitous and may be spread in contaminated soap.

Trigger words: *Burkholderia* species: chronic granulomatous disease (CGD), cystic fibrosis, *Pseudomonas*-like

Trigger words: *Vibrio cholerae*: A-B toxin, comma (S) shaped, rice-water diarrhea, shellfish

Virulence factors of *V. cholera* are pili and A-B toxin.

Cholera toxin "turns on" G_s (on) protein in intestinal epithelium; pertussis toxin "turns off" G_i (off) protein in respiratory epithelium. Both result in increased adenylate cyclase activity and rising intracellular cAMP level.

V. cholerae: causes severe diarrhea (by secretory mechanism) with rice-water stools, high mortality rate

V. cholerae is concentrated by filter-feeding shellfish and then ingested. Contaminated water is usually the source of a cholera outbreak.

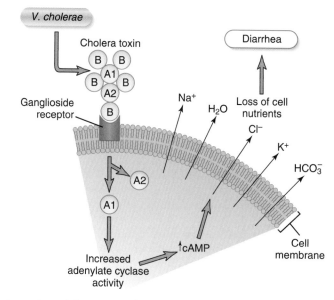

13-1: Mechanism of cholera toxin, an A-B type toxin. The B subunit, comprising five identical peptides, binds to the GM1 ganglioside receptor on the membrane of intestinal cells. The A subunit consists of two peptides: A1, with toxin activity, and A2, which is a linking molecule to the B subunit. After the A subunit enters the cell, the A1 peptide is activated and adenosine diphosphate (ADP)-ribosylates stimulatory G protein, leading to increased adenylate cyclase activity. The resulting increase in intracellular cyclic adenosine monophosphate (cAMP) mediates the active secretion of electrolytes and water into the lumen of the intestine.

B. Other *Vibrio* species, *Aeromonas* species, and *Plesiomonas* species (Table 13-1)
- *Vibrio vulnificus* commonly enters through cuts, causing wound infection that may develop into serious septicemia, especially in immunocompromised patients with preexisting disease.

IV. *Campylobacter* and *Helicobacter* Species

A. Identification
- Organisms in these genera are gram-negative, oxidase-positive motile rods that are microaerophilic and have complex growth requirements.

B. *Campylobacter jejuni*
1. Identification
   - Seagull-shaped rod with a single flagellum
   - Selective medium (Campy plate) used for isolation from stool specimens
2. Pathogenesis
   - *C. jejuni* invades and destroys mucosal surfaces of the jejunum, ileum, and colon.
   - Endotoxin, enterotoxins, and cytotoxins are produced, but their role in pathogenesis is ill defined.
   - Organisms are inactivated by gastric juices and sensitive to complement- and antibody-mediated killing.
   - High infectivity
3. Acute enteritis caused by *C. jejuni*
   - Profuse watery or bloody diarrhea, malaise, fever, abdominal pain, and cramps are common symptoms.
   - Disease is usually self-limited, but symptoms usually last for at least 1 week.

Trigger words:
C. jejuni: bloody diarrhea; thin, curved gram negative; undercooked poultry

Virulence factors of *C. jejuni* are endotoxins, cytotoxins, and invasion.

Bacteria causing bloody diarrhea: *C. jejuni*, *Shigella* species, *Yersinia enterocolitica*, and *Escherichia coli* (enterohemorrhagic and enteroinvasive strains). Except in young children, *C. jejuni* is the primary cause of bloody diarrhea in the United States.

TABLE 13-1 *Vibrio cholerae* and Related Organisms

ORGANISM	SOURCE OF INFECTION	DISEASE MANIFESTATIONS
V. cholerae	Ingestion of contaminated water, raw fish, or shellfish	Severe, watery diarrhea with rice-water stools
V. parahaemolyticus	Ingestion of contaminated shellfish	Explosive, watery diarrhea, cramps, nausea; self-limited
V. vulnificus	Exposure to contaminated seawater or raw oysters	Wound infection with swelling, erythema, pain; eventual tissue necrosis and septicemia
Aeromonas hydrophila and *Plesiomonas* species	Ingestion of or exposure to contaminated water or food	Watery or bloody diarrhea, cramps, vomiting; wound infection; systemic disease in immunocompromised patients

4. Association with Guillain-Barré syndrome
5. Transmission and incidence
   - Infection is commonly acquired by ingestion of contaminated food (especially poultry), milk, or water.
   - Asymptomatic human carriers and animal reservoirs (puppies) promote the spread of *C. jejuni.*
   - The incidence of *C. jejuni* enteritis peaks in young adults.
   - Lack of gastric acids and hypogammaglobulinemia increase risk for *C. jejuni* infection and severity of disease.
6. Treatment
   - Macrolides or quinolones and rehydration as needed

C. **Helicobacter pylori**
   - Curved rod with multiple flagella
   1. Pathogenesis
      - Neutralization of local stomach acid by urease-produced ammonia (NH_3) promotes initial colonization.
      - Rapid penetration of gastric mucus in mucus barrier is facilitated by multiple flagella.
      - Localized tissue damage by mucinase and cytotoxin stimulates infiltration of inflammatory cells.
        a. Increases the risk for developing a low-grade gastric malignant lymphoma
      - Increased secretion of gastrin and gastric acid stimulated by infection promotes gastric metaplasia, which increases the risk for developing gastric cancer.
   2. Diseases caused by *H. pylori*
      - Most common cause of stomach and duodenal ulcers
      - Chronic atrophic gastritis of pylorus and antrum with possible progression to gastric adenocarcinoma
      - Low-grade gastric malignant lymphoma
   3. Tests to identify *H. pylori*
      - *Campylobacter*-like organism (CLO) test
        a. Detects urease in a gastric biopsy
        b. 95% sensitivity and specificity
      - Serologic tests
        a. Remains positive over time
        b. Limits usefulness for detection of recurrences
        c. Limits usefulness for success of treatment
      - Radiolabeled urea breath test
        a. Excellent sensitivity and specificity
      - Stool antigen test
        a. Cheapest test
        b. Excellent sensitivity and specificity
        c. Excellent to detect active disease
        d. Excellent to detect success of treatment
   4. Transmission
      - *H. pylori* is ubiquitous and acquired by ingestion, poor sanitation, and person to person.
      - The prevalence of infection is relatively low during childhood but rises to 40% to 50% in older adults.
   5. Treatment
      - Triple-drug therapy continued for 2 weeks is commonly used.
        a. Bismuth salt + metronidazole + amoxicillin (or tetracycline)
        b. Bismuth salt + ranitidine + clarithromycin
        c. Proton pump inhibitor (e.g., omeprazole) + amoxicillin + clarithromycin

Trigger words:
H. pylori: gastric or duodenal ulcer, urease, urease breath test

Virulence factors of *H. pylori:* urease production of ammonia neutralizes stomach acid, flagella, mucinase, cytotoxin.

Stool antigen detection and urea breath test to detect the presence of *H. pylori* in the stomach; enzyme-linked immunosorbent assay to determine seropositivity.

CHAPTER 14

MYCOPLASMAS, FILAMENTOUS BACTERIA, AND *BACTEROIDES*

I. *Mycoplasma* and *Ureaplasma* Species
   A. **Shared features**
      1. The smallest free-living bacteria capable of passing through a 0.45-μm filter, which retains most other bacteria
      2. Lack peptidoglycan-containing cell wall and thus are very pleomorphic and not visualized with Gram stain
      3. Require sterols for growth
   B. *Mycoplasma pneumoniae*
      1. Identification
         • Slow-growing, obligate aerobe forming granular colonies on Eaton agar
         • Serologic tests for antigen-specific immunoglobulin M (IgM) antibodies
      2. Pathogenesis
         • P1 adhesin protein mediates adherence to respiratory epithelium.
         • Damage to ciliated epithelium by lytic enzymes and hydrogen peroxide (H_2O_2) leads to decreased clearance of upper airways, facilitating the spread of bacteria to the lungs.
         • Superantigen activity is related to systemic symptoms of *M. pneumoniae* infection.
         • Only infects humans
      3. Diseases caused by *M. pneumonia*
         • Transmission
            a. Spread via aerosols from infected persons and asymptomatic carriers
         • Primary atypical ("walking") pneumonia
            a. Interstitial (no alveolar exudate) pneumonia that differs clinically from typical community acquired pneumonia caused by pneumococcus (Table 14-1)
            b. Initial malaise, low-grade fever, and headache followed after 2 to 4 days by nonproductive cough, rales, rhonchi, and myalgia, and, rarely, an IgM-mediated hemolytic anemia
         • Tracheobronchitis

TABLE 14-1 **Mycoplasmal Versus Pneumococcal Pneumonia**

CHARACTERISTIC	MYCOPLASMAL PNEUMONIA	PNEUMOCOCCAL PNEUMONIA
Type of pneumonia	Atypical (interstitial)	Typical (alveolar)
Preceding pharyngitis	Common	Never
Onset	Gradual	Rapid with chills
Fever	Low grade	High
Cough	Nonproductive, paroxysmal	Productive
Sputum	Usually clear	Purulent
Pleuritic chest pain	Absent	Present
Leukocytosis	Absent	Present
Age of highest incidence	Young adults	Older adults
Complications	Otitis media, erythema multiforme, hemolytic anemia, myocarditis, pericarditis, bullous otitis media	Bacteremia, meningitis, otitis media

a. Inflammation of the bronchi marked by nonproductive cough, fever, headache, sore throat, pharyngeal exudates, and cervical lymphadenopathy
- Pharyngitis
   a. May precede pneumonia or constitute milder presentation of *M. pneumoniae* infection
   b. Resembles nonexudative group A streptococcal or viral pharyngitis
- Association with Guillain-Barré syndrome
4. Treatment
- Macrolides, tetracycline, or fluoroquinolones (e.g., levofloxacin)
- No target for β-lactam antibiotics

C. *Mycoplasma hominis* and *Ureaplasma urealyticum*
1. Facultatively anaerobic organisms that form colonies with a fried-egg appearance
2. Cause sexually transmitted genitourinary diseases (nongonococcal urethritis) (Box 14-1)

II. Filamentous Bacteria
- Organisms in the genera *Nocardia* and *Actinomyces* species form long branching filaments looking like fungi (Table 14-2).

A. *Nocardia* species
- Nocardiae are ubiquitous soil organisms that cause exogenous infections primarily in immunocompromised individuals.
1. Identification
- Very slow growing, aerobic, and weakly gram positive
- Partially acid fast owing to the presence of mycolic acids in the cell wall (similar to *Mycobacterium* species)
   a. Sputum, infected tissue, and abscess material show delicate filaments by the acid-fast stain.
2. Nocardioses
- Bronchopulmonary disease
   a. Inhaled organisms (primarily *Nocardia asteroides*) colonize the oropharynx and then are aspirated into the lower airways.
   b. Cough, dyspnea, and fever are usually present and pneumonia with cavitation may develop.
   c. May disseminate to the central nervous system, forming brain abscesses, or to skin.

Mycoplasmas are naturally resistant to β-lactam antibiotics due to lack of cell wall.

M. hominis and *U. urealyticum* are sexually transmitted diseases (STDs).

Trigger words:
Nocardia species: abscess, acid fast, aerobe, filamentous, slow growing, acid fast

Nocardia and *Mycobacterium* species are acid-fast staining bacteria.

Nocardia species: consider nocardiosis in the differential diagnosis of immunocompromised individuals with cavitary pulmonary disease.

BOX 14-1 DISEASES CAUSED BY *MYCOPLASMA* AND *UREAPLASMA*

Mycoplasma pneumoniae
Atypical pneumonia
Tracheobronchitis
Pharyngitis

Mycoplasma hominis
Pyelonephritis
Pelvic inflammatory disease
Postabortal fever
Postpartum fever

Ureaplasma urealyticum
Nongonococcal urethritis

TABLE 14-2 *Nocardia* Versus *Actinomyces*

CHARACTERISTIC	NOCARDIA	ACTINOMYCES
Morphology	Filamentous rods	Filamentous rods
Gram staining	Positive (weak)	Positive
Acid fast	Yes (weak)	No
Growth	Aerobic, slow growing	Anaerobic, slow growing
Part of normal human flora	No	Yes
Common disease manifestations	Lung disease, brain abscess, mycetoma and other skin infections; mostly in **immunocompromised patients**	Abscesses with draining sinus tracts usually **after surgery or trauma;** mycetoma

- Patients with pulmonary nocardia should be screened for central nervous system nocardial infection.
    - Cutaneous infections
        a. Primary infections, acquired through skin wounds, can take various forms.
        b. Mycetoma, often caused by *Nocardia brasiliensis*
            - Painless chronic infection marked by localized subcutaneous swelling, pus formation, and draining sinus tracts
        c. Lymphocutaneous infections
            - Resemble cutaneous infections caused by mycobacteria and the fungus *Sporothrix schenckii*
    3. Treatment
        - Long-term administration of sulfonamides plus surgical intervention
        - Alternative drugs: minocycline, amikacin, or third-generation cephalosporin

Trigger words:
Actinomyces species: anaerobe, draining sinus tracts, filamentous, mycetoma, sulfur granules

B. ***Actinomyces* species**
- They cause endogenous infections when a mucosal barrier is compromised.
    1. Identification
        - *Actinomyces* species are normal colonizers of the upper respiratory tract or the gastrointestinal tract.
        - Slow growing, anaerobic, gram positive, and not acid fast
        - "Sulfur" granules (1- to 5-mm yellow-orange masses of organisms resembling grains of sand) visible in clinical specimens
    2. Actinomycoses
        - *Actinomyces israelii*, which colonizes the oropharynx, is the most common cause of actinomycosis in humans.
        - Cervicofacial disease is marked by tissue swelling, fibrosis, and scarring along draining sinus tracts at the angle of the jaw and neck.
            a. Poor oral hygiene, dental surgery, and oral trauma are risk factors.
        - Abdominal and pelvic infections usually occur following surgery or trauma.
        - Thoracic infection is associated with history of aspiration.
        - Central nervous system infection (abscess and meningitis) usually results from spread from other foci.
        - Mycetoma may represent an exogenous infection caused by soil-borne actinomycetes that enter wounds.

Actinomyces infection of the fallopian tube (salpingitis): risk factor is the use of an intrauterine device.

    3. Treatment
        - Surgical débridement and long-term treatment with penicillin

Trigger words:
Bacteroides fragilis: abscess, foul-smelling, mixed infection

III. ***Bacteroides* Species**
- *B. fragilis* is the most clinically significant of the numerous gram-negative, nonsporulating, anaerobic colonizers of the respiratory, gastrointestinal, and genitourinary tracts (Box 14-2).
    A. **Identification**
        1. Gram-negative, encapsulated, pleomorphic organisms that produce foul-smelling short-chain fatty acids
        2. Broad antibiotic resistance
        3. Weak endotoxin activity

BOX 14-2 NONSPORULATING ANAEROBES

Various nonsporulating anaerobic bacteria are part of the **normal flora** of the human body wherever the oxygen level is low enough for them to multiply. Some of these bacteria can cause endogenous infections when they enter a normally sterile site. Such infections are often **mixed,** involving both **anaerobes** and **facultative gram-negative rods.** Abscess formation at the initial compromised site may be followed by dissemination to other sites. In addition to *Bacteroides* and *Actinomyces,* two other genera of nonsporulating anaerobes associated with human disease are *Propionibacterium* and *Peptostreptococcus.*

Propionibacterium: small **gram-positive rods** that inhabit the skin surface, conjunctiva, external ear, oropharynx, and female genital tract. *Propionibacterium acne* causes **acne,** an infection of sebaceous glands that stimulates an inflammatory response. Treatment includes topical application of **benzoyl peroxide** and antibiotic therapy (**erythromycin** and **clindamycin**). This organism can also cause **opportunistic infections** in those with **prosthetic devices** or **intravascular lines.**

Peptostreptococcus: **gram-positive cocci** that colonize the skin, oral cavity, and gastrointestinal tract. These bacteria can cause a **wide variety of infections,** including aspiration pneumonia, sinusitis, brain abscesses, intra-abdominal sepsis, pelvic infections, and soft tissue infections. Treatment is with **penicillin** or other β-lactam antibiotic.

B. Pathogenesis
1. Antiphagocytic capsule promotes adherence to peritoneal surfaces and abscess formation.
2. Organisms colonizing the bowel spread endogenously to other body sites via the bloodstream and during surgery.
3. Bacterial enzymes promote tissue destruction.

C. Endogenous infections caused by *B. fragilis*
- Surgery and trauma promote endogenous spread of normal colonic flora to sterile sites, where they cause disease.
1. Intra-abdominal infections with abscess formation
2. Suppurative pelvic infections
3. Bacteremia
4. Pleuropulmonary infections

D. Prevention and treatment
1. Prophylactic antibiotics for planned surgical procedures that disrupt the mucosa
2. Surgical intervention (removal of necrotic material, drainage of abscesses) plus antibiotics for established infection
3. Antibiotics include metronidazole, moxifloxacin, and β-lactams with anaerobe activity.

B. fragilis: disease associated with surgery and trauma affecting colonic mucosa

B. fragilis: primary cause of endogenous intraabdominal and pelvic infections and bacteremia

CHAPTER **15**
SPIROCHETES

I. **Shared Spirochetal Features**
   A. **Genera**
   - *Treponema, Borrelia,* and *Leptospira*
   B. **Morphology**
      1. Thin, spiral-shaped bacteria that are surrounded by a mucoid layer
      2. Axial filaments, structurally similar to bacterial flagella, confer motility on these organisms.
   C. **Clinical**
   - Many spirochetal diseases follow a similar clinical course, commonly lasting from months to years if not treated, and induce tissue-damaging immune responses (Box 15-1).
II. *Treponema* **Species**
   - The pathogenic treponemes (*T. pallidum, T. pertenue,* and *T. carateum*) *cannot* be distinguished morphologically or serologically, but they exhibit distinctive clinical manifestations and epidemiology.
   A. **Shared treponemal properties**
      1. Treponemes are shorter than Borreliae and possess three axial filaments.
      2. Anaerobic (or microaerophilic) organisms that cannot be grown in the laboratory
      3. Visualization
      - Because they are so thin, treponemes cannot be seen by light microscopy of Giemsa-stained specimens.
      - Organisms can be visualized by dark-field microscopy or by fluorescence microscopy of specimens stained with fluorescent-labeled antitreponemal antibody.
      4. Serologic tests (Box 15-2)
      - Nontreponemal tests (nonspecific for tissue damage)
         a. VDRL test (Venereal Disease Research Laboratories test)
         b. RPR test (rapid plasma reagin test)
         c. Both decrease in titer after treatment
      - Treponemal tests (specific for antibody to *Treponema* antigens)
         a. FTA-ABS test (fluorescent treponemal antibody absorption test)
         b. MHA-TP (microhemagglutination test for *T. pallidum*)
         c. Confirmatory tests that do not decrease in titer after treatment

Treponemal tests (FTA-ABS) measure antigen; nontreponemal tests (VDRL, RPR) measure released lipid and yield false-positive results.

BOX 15-1 SPIROCHETAL DISEASES

The diseases caused by various spirochetes exhibit a similar clinical course. The **first stage** commonly entails the development of a **characteristic primary lesion** at the site of exposure. The organisms then **disseminate via the blood,** often causing **flu-like manifestations.** The disease then remits for a brief period before **second-stage** signs and symptoms appear. Some diseases exhibit a **third stage,** which may commence after a prolonged latency period. In most spirochetal diseases, the spirochetes persist in patients for long periods. Common spirochetal diseases and their causative agents include the following:

Syphilis: *Treponema pallidum*
Yaws: *Treponema pallidum pertenue*
Pinta: *Treponema carateum*
Lyme disease: *Borrelia burgdorferi*
Louse-borne relapsing fever: *Borrelia recurrentis*
Tick-borne relapsing fever: *Borrelia* species
Leptospirosis: *Leptospira interrogans*

BOX 15-2 SEROLOGIC TESTS FOR *TREPONEMA PALLIDUM* AND OTHER TREPONEMES

VDRL and **RPR** (**nontreponemal tests**) measure antibody that reacts with beef cardiolipin. This **nonspecific anticardiolipin antibody** is induced in response to tissue damage resulting from treponemal infection. These rapid, relatively inexpensive tests are useful **screens** for syphilis and for **monitoring** the effectiveness of **therapy.**

FTA-ABS and MHA-TP (treponemal tests) are specific for antitreponemal antibody but are more expensive than nontreponemal tests and are commonly used to confirm infection. These tests give positive results sooner after infection and remain positive longer (generally for the remaining life of the individual) than nontreponemal tests.

Both types of tests give false-positive reactions in patients with various conditions, including the following:

Nontreponemal tests: acute or chronic illness, collagen-vascular disease, heroin addiction, leprosy, malaria, pregnancy, recent immunization, and viral infection

Treponemal tests: acne vulgaris, crural ulceration, drug addiction, herpes genitalis, mycoses, pregnancy, psoriasis, pyoderma, rheumatoid arthritis, skin neoplasm, and systemic lupus erythematosus

5. Pathogenesis
   - After adherence to skin or mucosal membranes, treponemes produce hyaluronidase, which promotes tissue invasion.
   - Organisms become coated with host fibronectin, which protects them against phagocytosis and immune recognition.
   - Soon after infection, treponemes spread to other skin sites and to other organs via the bloodstream.
   - Host immune response is largely responsible for disease manifestations.

B. Syphilis
   - *T. pallidum* causes syphilis, the most common treponemal disease.
   1. Clinical course of syphilis
      - Primary syphilis
         a. **Chancre,** a painless ulcerated skin lesion, develops at the site of inoculation (usually external genitals, mouth, or anus).
         b. Painless swollen lymph glands (**buboes**) develop 1 to 2 weeks after the appearance of the chancre.
         c. **Spontaneous healing** of the chancre occurs within 3 to 6 weeks but does *not* indicate a cure.
      - Secondary syphilis (bacteremic stage)
         a. Highly contagious, disseminated maculopapular rash develops over the entire body surface.
         b. Flu-like syndrome, with sore throat, headache, fever, myalgia, anorexia, and generalized lymphadenopathy, accompanies the rash.
         c. Treponemes become dormant in liver and spleen.
         d. Condyloma latum
            - Flat lesions in the anogenital area often confused with condyloma acuminata (venereal warts) caused by human papillomavirus 6, 11
         e. Symptoms usually resolve within 6 to 8 months of infection.
      - Tertiary syphilis
         a. Activation of dormant treponemes and their multiplication 3 to 30 years later occur in a small number of untreated cases.
         b. Gummas (destructive granulomatous lesions) form in bone, skin, and other tissues.
         c. Neurosyphilis (tabes dorsalis) and cardiovascular syphilis (aortitis) are life-threatening conditions that may develop.
   2. Transmission of *T. pallidum*
      - Sexual contact during primary stage or skin contact with disseminated rash during secondary stage
      - In utero from infected mother to fetus (congenital syphilis)
      - Transfusion of contaminated blood
   3. Prevention and treatment
      - Use of safe sexual practices can help protect against syphilis.
      - Penicillin is the drug of choice.

C. Yaws
   1. Subspecies *T. pallidum pertenue* causes yaws, which is found in regions of South America, central Africa, and Southeast Asia.

Virulence properties: adherence, hyaluronidase tissue degradation, antiphagocytic coat

The host immune response causes disease.

Trigger words:
T. pallidum: FTA-ABS, gumma, painless ulcer (chancre), palm and sole rash, RPR and VDRL tests, spirochete, STD, strict anaerobe, syphilis, unculturable

T. pallidum: only sexually transmitted treponemal disease
Syphilis is the third most common sexually transmitted disease (STD) in the United States.

Chancre is painless and syphilis; chancroid is painful and *Haemophilus ducreyi.*

Congenital syphilis, acquired from a syphilitic mother during pregnancy, causes severe morbidity and mortality in infants.

- *T. pertenue* causes yaws, and *T. carateum* causes pinta; tropical treponemal diseases; initial skin lesions, spread by nonsexual contact
2. This granulomatous disease is marked early by elevated papilloma-like skin lesions and later by destructive lesions of the skin, lymph nodes, and bones.
3. Transmission is by direct contact with lesions.
4. Treatment is with penicillin.

D. **Pinta**
1. *T. carateum* causes pinta, a skin disease found in Central and South America.
2. Small pruritic papules develop initially and then enlarge into recurrent lesions that cause scarring and depigmentation.
3. Transmission is by direct contact with lesions.
4. Treatment is with penicillin.

III. *Borrelia* **Species**

A. **Characteristics**
1. Bacteria in this genus are larger than treponemes and possess numerous axial filaments.
2. Like treponemes, borreliae are microaerophilic organisms that are difficult to culture.

B. **Lyme disease**
- *B. burgdorferi*, the cause of Lyme disease, is spread by tick vectors.
1. Diagnosis
   - Too few borreliae are present in clinical specimens to visualize the organisms by light microscopy.
   - Enzyme-linked immunosorbent assay or other serologic tests to detect *B. burgdorferi* antibodies become positive 2 to 4 weeks after onset of the initial rash.
   - Because false-positive serologic tests are common, a second test (e.g., Western blot) is needed to confirm *B. burgdorferi* infection.
2. Pathogenesis
   - A tick (bite) deposits borreliae in the skin and blood, and the organisms spread to multiple organs.
   - Host immune response primarily causes disease manifestations.
   - Weak endotoxin-like activity may contribute to disease.
3. Clinical course of Lyme disease (Table 15-1)
   - Like syphilis, Lyme disease follows a three-stage course, although overall its duration in untreated patients is shorter than that of syphilis.
4. Transmission and incidence
   - Natural reservoirs for the ticks that spread Lyme disease are the white-footed mouse and deer.
     a. These ticks also infest pets.
   - In the United States, Lyme disease occurs primarily in the Northeast, upper midwest, and Pacific Northwest.
5. Treatment
   - Doxycycline and amoxicillin are generally effective in treating early-stage Lyme disease.
     a. Early therapy tends to reduce the likelihood and severity of later manifestations.
   - Ceftriaxone is also used to treat later manifestations.

TABLE 15-1 Clinical Course of Lyme Disease in Untreated Patients

STAGE	MAJOR MANIFESTATIONS	PATIENTS AFFECTED	ONSET/DURATION
1	**Erythema chronicum migrans** (≥5 cm) at site of tick bite	Nearly all	Begins 3-30 days after tick bite with appearance of rash; other symptoms may follow. Resolves after 3-4 weeks.
	Systemic symptoms: headache, low-grade fever, chills, myalgia, regional lymphadenopathy	Some	
2	**Severe fatigue** and malaise; **migratory pain** in muscles, joints, and bones; mild hepatitis	50%	Usually begins within 1-4 months after stage 1. Fatigue, malaise, and muscle pain can be prolonged. Cardiac problems last up to 6 weeks; neurologic problems last as long as 9 months.
	Neurologic disorders (meningitis, encephalitis, peripheral neuropathy)	15%	
	Cardiac dysfunction (atrioventricular block with palpitations, myopericarditis, congestive heart failure)	8%	
3	**Migratory polyarthritis** of large joints, arthralgias	60%	Begins 5-24 months after stage 1 and can persist for months to several years.

C. Relapsing fever
1. Etiologic agents
   - Louse-borne (epidemic) relapsing fever is caused by *B. recurrentis*.
     a. This disease typically exhibits a single relapse and is uncommon in the United States.
   - Tick-borne (endemic) relapsing fever is caused by several other *Borrelia* species.
     a. Multiple relapses are common, but the symptoms are less severe than in the epidemic form.
2. Clinical manifestations
   - Febrile (bacteremic) phase is marked by abrupt onset of high fever, shaking chills, headache, and muscle aches and lasts 3 to 7 days.
   - Afebrile phase lasts about 1 week, and then bacteremic symptoms return.
   - Alternating febrile and afebrile phases that characterize relapsing fever result from antigenic variation that occurs during the course of infection.
3. Diagnosis
   - *Borrelia* species that cause relapsing fever can be visualized in blood stained with aniline dyes (Giemsa or Wright stain) soon after infection.
   - Because these organisms undergo extensive antigenic variation within an infected individual, serologic tests are useless in diagnosing relapsing fever.

IV. *Leptospira* Species
A. Characteristics
1. Leptospires, the smallest of the spirochetes, are aerobic organisms with hooked ends that can be visualized by dark-field microscopy.
2. *L. interrogans* is the only species pathogenic in humans.
3. Rats and other rodents and domestic animals (household pets) carry *L. interrogans* and shed organisms in the urine.

B. Leptospirosis
1. Usually a mild flu-like infection, is acquired by contact with contaminated water or the urine or tissues of infected animals
2. Weil syndrome, a severe form of leptospirosis, develops in about 10% of infected patients.
   - Manifestations include headache, rash, jaundice, azotemia, hemorrhages, and vascular collapse.
   - Urine is an excellent body fluid to identify the organisms
3. Treatment is with penicillin or erythromycin.
   - Doxycycline is effective in preventing the disease in individuals exposed to infected animals or water contaminated with urine.

B. recurrentis: spread to humans by ticks carried by white-footed mice and deer

Leptospira interrogans: small spirochete with curled end; only aerobic spirochete that infects humans; no insect vector; mild flu-like disease without jaundice

MYCOBACTERIA

I. Shared Mycobacterial Properties

Mycobacteria are acid-fast bacilli.

Mycobacterial cell wall contains unusual lipids that protect the bacteria from being killed after phagocytosis.

Mycobacteria are slow growing and cultured on Lowenstein-Jensen medium.

Trigger words:

M. tuberculosis: acid fast, caseation, Ghon complexes, granuloma, isoniazid, Löwenstein-Jensen medium, Mantoux reaction, opportunistic disease, PPD

M. tuberculosis is slow growing and uses Löwenstein-Jensen medium.

Infection identified by DTH response to PPD or interferon-γ production in blood test

- Mycobacteria are slow-growing, aerobic, facultative intracellular rods with a lipid-rich cell wall that makes them acid fast.
  ### A. Cell wall components
  - The unusual composition of the mycobacterial cell wall is depicted in Figure 16-1.
  ### B. Mycobacterial diseases (Table 16-1)
  - Most mycobacteria cause chronic diseases that often exhibit a prolonged latent period as well as periods of remission alternating with active disease manifestations.

II. *Mycobacterium tuberculosis*

  ### A. Identification (Box 16-1)
  1. Microscopic detection of acid-fast rods in sputum or biopsy specimen
  2. Isolation by culturing on egg-based Löwenstein-Jensen medium or on special broth media
     - Slow growth of *M. tuberculosis* requires 3 to 6 weeks of incubation.
  3. Serologic tests and DNA probes
  4. Tuberculin skin test
     - Intradermal injection of purified protein derivative (PPD) from cell wall induces a delayed-type hypersensitivity (DTH) response in those who have been previously exposed to *M. tuberculosis* or vaccinated.
     - Positive reaction is indicated by an area of induration (>15 mm for healthy adults) 48 to 72 hours after PPD injection.
       a. Tuberculin skin test is a classic example of a type IV hypersensitivity reaction (DTH).
       b. Skin test reactivity usually develops 3 to 4 weeks after infection.
       c. False-negative results may occur in those with very recent infection, anergic individuals (especially human immunodeficiency virus [HIV]-infected patients), and older people in whom the DTH response has waned.
       d. False-positive results occur in individuals vaccinated with bacille Calmette-Guérin (BCG), the antituberculosis vaccine used in Europe and other countries.

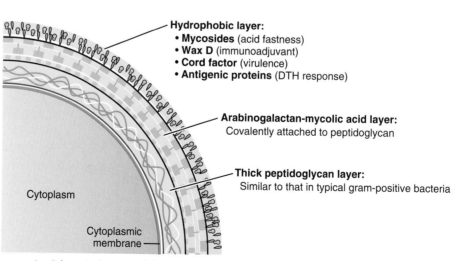

Hydrophobic layer:
- **Mycosides** (acid fastness)
- **Wax D** (immunoadjuvant)
- **Cord factor** (virulence)
- **Antigenic proteins** (DTH response)

Arabinogalactan-mycolic acid layer:
Covalently attached to peptidoglycan

Thick peptidoglycan layer:
Similar to that in typical gram-positive bacteria

Cytoplasm

Cytoplasmic membrane

16-1: Schematic depiction of the mycobacterial cell wall, which consists of three major layers.

TABLE 16-1 **Mycobacterial Diseases**

SPECIES	DISEASE	DISTRIBUTION
Mycobacterium tuberculosis	Classic tuberculosis (TB): pulmonary and extrapulmonary	Highest incidence among young children, elderly people, chronically ill patients, patients in institutions, AIDS patients, and other immunocompromised individuals
Mycobacterium bovis	TB in cattle and humans	Individuals who ingest contaminated milk; rare in the United States (attenuated strain used in BCG vaccine). Intestinal TB in the United States is due to swallowing M. tuberculosis bacilli from a primary site in the lungs; organisms invade Peyer patches in the small intestine.
Mycobacterium leprae	Leprosy (Hansen disease)	Primarily in Asia and Africa
Atypical Mycobacteria		
Mycobacterium avium-intracellulare	Disseminated disease, pulmonary TB, subacute lymphadenitis	Disseminated disease primarily among AIDS patients; others uncommon
Mycobacterium kansasii	TB-like pulmonary disease, osteomyelitis, lymphadenopathy	Individuals with preexisting lung disease or who are immunocompromised
Mycobacterium scrofulaceum	Cervical lymphadenitis (scrofula)	Young children
Mycobacterium marinum	"Fish-tank" granuloma	Pet fish handlers, marine biologists

BOX 16-1 LABORATORY DIAGNOSIS OF MYCOBACTERIAL DISEASE

- Detection
- Skin test (PPD)
- Blood T-cell interferon-γ response to antigen
- Microscopy (acid-fast stain [Ziehl-Neelsen, Kinyoun methods])
- Direct nucleic acid probes
- Culture on Löwenstein-Jensen (egg-based) medium or broth-based media
- Identification
- Morphologic properties
- Biochemical reactions
- Analysis of cell wall lipids
- Nucleic acid probes
- Polymerase chain reaction
- Nucleic acid sequencing

B. Transmission and incidence
1. Humans are the only natural reservoir of *M. tuberculosis*
2. Spread of tubercle bacilli through respiratory droplets is promoted by crowded conditions and coughing.
3. Young children, elderly people, and immunocompromised individuals have the highest risk for developing active tuberculosis (TB).

C. Pathogenesis
- Infection with *M. tuberculosis* may involve any organ, but the lungs are the initial and most common sites affected.
1. Inhaled mycobacteria are engulfed by alveolar macrophages and replicate freely in these cells.
   - Cell wall components prevent bacterial destruction in macrophage lysosomes.
   - Intracellular growth protects mycobacteria from antibody-mediated elimination.
   - Other macrophages are attracted to the site and destroy the infected cells, releasing mycobacteria that can spread through the bloodstream.
2. Sequence of formation of a tuberculous granuloma (type IV hypersensitivity reaction)
   - Tubercle bacilli are phagocytosed by alveolar macrophages.
   - Unactivated macrophages cannot kill mycobacteria.
   - Other macrophages process and present antigen to CD4 T cells in association with class II antigen sites.
   - Macrophages release interleukin-12 (IL-12), which stimulates naïve helper T cells to produce T_H1 class memory cells, and IL-1, which causes fever and activates T_H1 cells.
   - T_H1 cells release IL-2 (stimulates lymphocyte proliferation), interferon-γ (activates macrophages to kill tubercle bacillus, called *epithelioid cells*), and migration inhibitory factor (causes macrophages to accumulate).

Virulence factors: intracellular growth, dormant presence in macrophages, lipid-containing cell wall

- Lipids from killed tubercle bacillus lead to caseous necrosis.
- Activated macrophages fuse, become multinucleated giant cells, and wall off infection.

3. Lack of a host response (e.g., lack of CD4 T cells in acquired immunodeficiency syndrome [AIDS]) leads to dissemination of disease without the formation of granulomas.

D. Clinical course of TB (Fig. 16-2)

1. Primary pulmonary TB
   - Overview
     a. Active disease occurs within 2 years of infection in 5% to 10% of cases (primary) and recurs later in life in a small number of these cases (secondary).
     b. The remainder of infected individuals never develops active TB.
   - Localized infection foci form within lung after inhalation of *M. tuberculosis*.
     a. CD4 T_H1 cell–macrophage response restricts intracellular proliferation of mycobacteria to the mid to lower lung region and encloses them within tubercles.
     b. Subpleural lesion of caseous necrosis is called a *Ghon focus*.
     c. Lymphatic spread to the hilar lymph nodes is called a *Ghon complex*.
   - Clinical manifestations of active TB (Box 16-2)
     a. Nonspecific symptoms include malaise, weight loss, cough, night sweats, and hemoptysis.
     b. Active disease is marked by pneumonitis and hilar lymphadenopathy.
       - Miliary spread may occur.
     c. Calcification of healed primary lesions leaves scars that appear as spots on the lung in radiographs.
     d. Individuals with latent tuberculosis, infection without active disease, are *not* infectious but can develop active TB later in life.

Granulomas: composed of activated macrophages (epithelioid cells), multinucleated giant cells, and CD4 helper T cells

Tuberculosis and AIDS: low CD4 T cell counts typical of HIV-infected patients increase the risk for primary and reactivation tuberculosis and for disseminated infection with rapid progression to death.

Healed primary TB lesions leave scars called Ghon complexes.

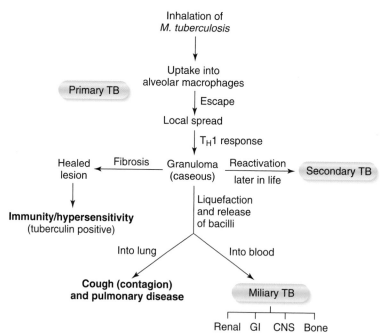

16-2: Pathogenesis and clinical course of tuberculosis (TB) caused by *Mycobacterium tuberculosis*. Secondary tuberculosis can result from reactivation of dormant bacilli within granulomas or from reinfection of hypersensitized host. Primary disease usually occurs in children, and secondary disease usually occurs in adults (especially those who are immunocompromised).

BOX 16-2 TUBERCULOSIS: QUICK CASE

A 17-year-old girl has recent weight loss, night sweats, fever, and cough. PPD test shows redness and swelling and an 18-mm lesion at the site of injection. Radiograph of the chest shows bilateral upper lobe involvement and mediastinal and hilar lymphadenopathy. Sputum contains acid-fast bacilli.

2. Secondary pulmonary tuberculosis
   - Recurrence of clinical manifestations, due to reactivation of dormant tubercle bacilli or reinfection, is most likely in immunocompromised patients.
   - Formation of fibrocaseous cavitary lesions occurs in the apex of the upper lobes.
     a. Danger of hemoptysis
   - Miliary spread in the lungs may occur.
3. Extrapulmonary (miliary) TB
   - Tissue destruction at other sites (e.g., lymph nodes, pleura, genitourinary tract, and the central nervous system) results from hematogenous spread of tubercle bacilli.
   - The kidney is the most common extrapulmonary site.

E. **Prevention**
1. United States
   - Surveillance programs using the PPD skin test (Mantoux test) identify previously infected individuals, followed by chest radiograph of individuals with positive response.
   - Prophylactic isoniazid may be given to those at high risk for developing active disease (e.g., latent TB).
2. Europe and other countries
   - Live, attenuated BCG vaccine is somewhat effective.
   - BCG-immunized individuals test weakly positive in PPD screening programs.
3. Prophylaxis after exposure to drug-resistant TB includes pyrazinamide plus either ethambutol or levofloxacin.

F. **Treatment of active TB**

> Tuberculosis therapy requires long-term combined drug therapy: RESPIre = rifampin, ethambutol, streptomycin, pyrazinamide, isoniazid.

1. Multidrug therapy with isoniazid, rifampin, ethambutol, and pyrazinamide is required to successfully eliminate *M. tuberculosis* in most patients.
   - The duration of treatment and drug combinations depend on the specific case.
2. Multidrug-resistant strains are becoming more common in the United States, especially among immunocompromised patients (e.g., AIDS patients).
   - These patients are treated with some combination of isoniazid, rifampin, pyrazinamide, ethambutol, and streptomycin.

III. **"Atypical" Mycobacteria: Nontuberculosis Mycobacteria (NTB)**
   - Numerous *Mycobacterium* species causing TB-like diseases are classified based on their rate of growth and pigment production.

A. *Mycobacterium avium-intracellulare complex* (MAC)

> MAC is a common opportunistic disease of AIDS patients in terminal stages (CD4 T cells < 50/mL)

1. Major mycobacterial pathogen in AIDS patients, causing disseminated TB-like disease
2. Usually produces asymptomatic infection in healthy adults but may cause pulmonary disease
3. Acquired by ingestion of contaminated food or water or by inhalation
4. MAC are resistant to anti-TB drugs and are treated with clarithromycin or azithromycin plus ethambutol and rifampin.

> MAC are resistant to anti-TB drugs.

B. *Mycobacterium kansasii* and *Mycobacterium scrofulaceum* (see Table 16-1)

IV. *Mycobacterium leprae*
   - *M. leprae* causes leprosy (Hansen disease), which is characterized by skin lesions, nerve damage, and extensive tissue destruction in some cases.

> **Trigger words:**
> *M. leprae:* anesthetic skin lesion, lepromatous leprosy—T_H2, nerve damage; tuberculoid leprosy—T_H1
>
> *M. leprae:* T_H1 response (strong) → tuberculoid, self-limited disease; T_H2 response (weak) → lepromatous, more severe form

A. **Pathogenesis**
   - The type of immune response initiated by a patient determines the outcome of *M. leprae* infection.
1. T_H1 response (DTH, interferon-γ, macrophage activation) → milder tuberculoid leprosy
2. T_H2 response (humoral antibody) → more severe lepromatous leprosy

B. **Clinical presentations** (Table 16-2)
1. Lepromatous leprosy
   - Many skin lesions with large numbers of *M. leprae* at the site of the lesion
   - Nodular lesions on the face ("leonine" facies)
   - Negative lepromin skin test (shows lack of cellular immunity)
2. Tuberculoid leprosy
   - New skin lesions with small numbers of *M. leprae* at the site of the lesion
   - Hypopigmented skin lesions with lack of sensation
   - Autoamputation of digits
   - Positive lepromin skin test (shows intact cellular immunity)
3. Dimorphic leprosy: lesions ranging between the tuberculoid and lepromatous forms

TABLE 16-2 **Clinical and Immunologic Manifestations of Leprosy**

PROPERTY	TUBERCULOID	LEPROMATOUS
Appearance of skin lesions	**Few** erythematous or hypopigmented and atrophic plaques with flat centers and raised demarcated borders	**Many** erythematous macules, papules, or nodules accompanied by extensive tissue damage to nose cartilage, bone, testicles
Histopathology of skin lesions	Granulomatous with **Langerhans cells** and **epithelioid cells** surrounded by lymphocytes	Predominantly **"foamy" macrophages** with few lymphocytes and no Langerhans cells
Nerve involvement	**Early** peripheral nerve damage with complete sensory loss; visible nerve enlargement (ulnar nerve, greater auricular nerve); autoamputation of the digits	**Late** diffuse nerve damage with patchy sensory loss; no nerve enlargement
Acid-fast bacilli	**Few or none present** in skin lesions or nerves	**Abundant** in skin lesions, nerves, and internal organs
Infectivity	**Low**	**High**
IMMUNE RESPONSES		
DTH reaction to lepromin	Yes	No
Immunoglobulin levels	Normal	Hypergammaglobulinemia
Lepromin skin test	Positive (intact cellular immunity)	Negative (absent cellular immunity)

C. Transmission
1. Direct skin contact with lesions on infected people and inhalation of infectious droplets spread *M. leprae* organisms.
2. Asymptomatic carriers and contaminated soil are possible sources of infection.
3. Armadillos are a natural reservoir of *M. leprae* in the United States.

D. Treatment
1. Long-term combination therapy is required to treat leprosy.
2. For tuberculoid form: dapsone + rifampin for 6 months
3. For lepromatous form: dapsone + rifampin + clofazimine for 2 years

CHAPTER 17
CHLAMYDIAE AND ZOONOTIC INTRACELLULAR BACTERIA

I. *Chlamydia* species
- Three chlamydial species are pathogenic for humans: *C. trachomatis*, *C. psittaci*, and *C. pneumoniae* (Table 17-1).

A. Shared chlamydial properties
1. Chlamydiae are very small, obligate intracellular bacteria.
2. They possess a cytoplasmic membrane and outer membrane but lack peptidoglycan layer (unlike gram-negative bacteria) and thus are insensitive to β-lactam antibiotics.
   - Chlamydiae are energy parasites.
3. Morphologic forms
   - Elementary body (EB)
     a. Smaller, extracellular infectious form that is metabolically inert and resistant to harsh conditions
   - Reticulate body (RB)
     a. Larger intracellular form that is metabolically active and replicates within target cells
     b. RBs cannot produce ATP and thus depend on target cells for energy production.
4. Growth cycle (Fig. 17-1)
   - Ingested EB is converted to RB within a cytoplasmic phagosome.
   - RB replication by binary fission produces a large inclusion body containing numerous RBs, most of which are reorganized into EBs.
   - Extrusion of the inclusion body releases infectious EBs into extracellular environment and ruptures the cell.

> Chlamydia cannot make adenosine triphosphate (ATP) and lack peptidoglycan.

> *Chlamydia* species: small, obligate intracellular bacteria existing in two forms: Elementary body Enters cells; Reticulate body Replicates within cells.

TABLE 17-1 **Comparison of *Chlamydia* Species**

PROPERTY	CHLAMYDIA TRACHOMATIS	CHLAMYDOPHILA PSITTACI	CHLAMYDOPHILA PNEUMONIAE
Host range	Humans primarily	Animals primarily; humans occasionally	Humans only
Iodine staining of inclusion bodies	Yes	No	No
Sulfonamide susceptibility	Sensitive	Resistant	Resistant
Diseases	Types A to C: trachoma Types L1 to L3: lymphogranuloma venereum Types D to K: sexually transmitted diseases, infantile pneumonia, conjunctivitis	Psittacosis (parrot fever)	Pharyngitis Bronchitis Pneumonia Sinusitis
Transmission	Sexual contact, in birth canal, contact with body fluids	Inhalation of dried bird feces	Inhalation of aerosols from infected persons

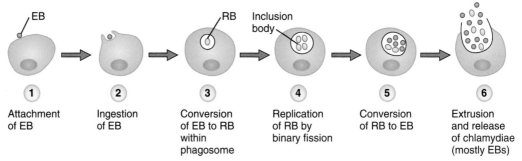

17-1: Growth cycle of *Chlamydia trachomatis*. For each elementary body (EB) that enters a susceptible cell, replication and reorganization yield an inclusion body containing 100 to 500 EBs, which are released from the cell. RB, replication body.

Trigger words:
C. trachomatis: elementary bodies, iodine stain, intracellular inclusion bodies, LGV, PID, reticulate bodies, STD, trachoma, UTI

Virulence factors: adhesion, intracellular growth

Inflammatory reactions are major cause of chlamydial pathogenesis.

C. trachomatis: types D through K = most common cause of sexually transmitted diseases (STDs) in the United States.

Reiter syndrome triad: arthritis, urethritis, uveitis-conjunctivitis

C. trachomatis: most common cause of neonatal blindness worldwide

Lymphogranuloma venereum initially causes small painless lesion at infection site with possible fever, headache, and myalgia but can progress to swollen draining lymph nodes.

B. *C. trachomatis*
- Three major groups of serotypes are associated with different diseases.
  1. Identification
     - Cytologic examination for iodine-staining inclusion bodies
     - Growth and isolation in cell culture
     - Polymerase chain reaction (PCR)
     - Detection of chlamydial antigens or nucleic acid sequences in clinical specimens
     - Serologic tests for antichlamydial antibodies
  2. Pathogenesis
     - Types A through K infect nonciliated epithelial cells of mucous membranes, which have EB-binding receptors on their surface.
       a. These target cells are found in the urethra, vagina, fallopian tubes, anorectal tract, respiratory tract, and conjunctiva.
     - Types L1, L2, and L3 infect macrophages.
     - Destruction of target cells due to bacterial replication and severe host inflammatory reactions cause disease manifestations.
  3. Chlamydial infections caused by types D through K (Box 17-1)
     - Transmitted by sexual contact or during passage through infected birth canal
     - Urogenital infections
       a. Asymptomatic infections are more common in women than in men.
       b. Symptomatic infections produce mucopurulent discharge, with dysuria or pyuria.
     - Systemic infections
     - Ocular and neonatal infections
  4. Lymphogranuloma venereum
     - Caused by types L1 through L3 and transmitted by sexual contact
     - Initial stage
       a. A small, painless lesion appears at the site of infection 4 to 6 weeks after exposure.
       b. Possible accompanying fever, headache, and myalgia

BOX 17-1 INFECTIONS CAUSED BY *CHLAMYDIA TRACHOMATIS*, TYPES D THROUGH K

Urogenital Infections
In women: cervicitis, urethritis, salpingitis, pelvic inflammatory disease
In men: urethritis, epididymitis, proctitis

Systemic Infections
In women: arthritis, dermatitis
In men: Reiter syndrome (nongonococcal urethritis; triad of arthritis, urethritis, uveitis-conjunctivitis)

Ocular and Neonatal Infections
Adult inclusion conjunctivitis: mucopurulent discharge, keratitis, inflammation, potential scarring; spread by autoinoculation or ocular-genital contact
Neonatal conjunctivitis: swelling of eyelids, hyperemia, and **purulent discharge** beginning 2 to 30 days after birth to infected mother. Conjunctival scarring and corneal vascularization develop in untreated infections. **Topical erythromycin,** which is administered routinely to neonates, prevents eye infection.
Infant pneumonia: rhinitis beginning 2 to 3 weeks after birth followed by distinctive **staccato cough;** no fever. Without treatment, infection may develop into diffuse interstitial pneumonia.

- Late stage (untreated)
  a. Painful inflammation and swelling of draining lymph nodes (usually inguinal nodes)
  b. Enlarged nodes may rupture, forming draining fistulas and local ulcers (rectal strictures), especially in women and homosexual men.
5. Trachoma (chronic keratoconjunctivitis)
  - Caused by types A through C and spread by tears, contaminated clothing, and hands (not sexually transmitted)
  - Leading cause of preventable blindness worldwide
    a. Especially prevalent in Africa
  - Early stage
    a. Initial follicular conjunctivitis with diffuse inflammation of the conjunctiva marked by pain, photophobia, and lacrimation
  - Late stage (untreated)
    a. Formation of hard, red papillae and in-turning of eyelids leading to corneal abrasion, ulceration, scarring, and eventually blindness
6. Prevention and treatment
  - Prophylactic topical erythromycin can prevent neonatal conjunctivitis.
  - Safe sex practices and improved personal hygiene can reduce the rate of infection.
  - Tetracycline, erythromycin, or fluoroquinolones are used to treat chlamydial infection.

C. ***Chlamydophila psittaci***
1. *C. psittaci* causes psittacosis (parrot fever).
2. Parrot fever may be asymptomatic or manifest mild flu-like symptoms.
  - May progress to serious interstitial pneumonitis with cyanosis, jaundice, and central nervous system involvement (headache, convulsions, coma)
3. Transmission occurs via inhalation of contaminated dried bird feces.

D. ***Chlamydophila pneumonia***
  - *C. pneumonia*, *Legionella pneumophila*, and *Mycoplasma pneumoniae* can cause atypical pneumonia
1. *C. pneumoniae* causes respiratory tract infections.
2. Clinical manifestations include pharyngitis, sinusitis, bronchitis, or pneumonia, with a persistent cough and malaise.
3. Transmission occurs from person to person through aerosols.
4. Strong association with coronary artery disease

II. **Zoonotic Intracellular Bacteria (Box 17-2)**
A. ***Rickettsia* and Related Species**
1. Rickettsiae are small, gram-negative, nonmotile pleomorphic bacteria that are obligate intracellular parasites.
2. They cause zoonotic diseases and typically are transmitted by insect vectors from various animal reservoirs.
3. Pathogenesis
  - Rickettsiae enter and replicate slowly within host cells, especially endothelial cells.
  - Organisms are continuously shed from infected cells and are also released by cell lysis.
  - Disease manifestations result from destruction of host cells and from systemic responses to cell damage.
4. Rickettsial and related diseases (Table 17-2)
  - The incubation period is 7 to 20 days except for chronic Q fever, which has a prolonged incubation period (months to years).
  - Abrupt onset marks these diseases, except for endemic (murine) typhus and chronic Q fever.
  - Fever, chills, headache, and myalgia are usual initial symptoms; characteristic rash develops in most rickettsial diseases.
5. Geographic distribution in the United States

Topical erythromycin on eyelids of newborn prevents C. trachomatis and Neisseria gonorrhoeae

Trigger words:
C. psittaci: birds, parrots
C. psittaci: only chlamydial species that causes zoonotic disease

Trigger words:
Rickettsia: Obligate intracellular growth, Southeastern Atlantic and south central states, tick, Weil-Felix reaction

Rickettsia, Coxiella, Ehrlichia species: zoonotic disease, insect vectors

Virulence factors: intracellular growth, zoonotic, cytolytic

BOX 17-2 ZOONOTIC INTRACELLULAR BACTERIA

- *Bartonella* species (cat-scratch fever)
- *Brucella* species (undulant fever)
- *Chlamydophila psittaci* (psittacosis-parrot fever)
- *Coxiella burnetii* (Q fever)
- *Francisella tularensis* (tularemia)
- *Listeria monocytogenes* (meningitis, sepsis)
- *Rickettsia* species (Rocky Mountain spotted fever, typhus)

TABLE 17-2 **Common Rickettsial and Related Diseases**

DISEASE	ORGANISM	VECTOR	CLINICAL FEATURES*
Rocky Mountain spotted fever	*Rickettsia rickettsii*	Ticks	Abrupt onset of usual symptoms; **inward-spreading macular rash**
Epidemic typhus	*Rickettsia prowazekii*	Lice	Abrupt onset of usual symptoms plus arthralgia; **outward-spreading macular rash**
Endemic (murine) typhus	*Rickettsia typhi*	Fleas	**Gradual onset** of fever, headache, myalgia, and cough; **maculopapular rash on trunk**
Rickettsialpox	*Rickettsia akari*	Mites	Abrupt onset of usual symptoms; generalized **papulovesicular rash** accompanied by **sloughing**
Q fever (acute)	*Coxiella burnetii*	None	Abrupt onset of usual symptoms; granulomatous hepatitis; **no rash**
Ehrlichiosis	*Ehrlichia* species	Ticks	Abrupt onset of usual symptoms plus anorexia and nausea; possible rash, hepatitis, or other symptoms; inclusion in monocytes
Cat-scratch fever	*Bartonella* species	Cat fleas, lice	Initial papule or pustule at site of cat scratch or bite; then chronic, benign **regional lymphadenopathy with granulomatous abscesses**

*Usual symptoms are fever, chills, headache, and myalgia.

- Rocky Mountain spotted fever, caused by *Rickettsia rickettsii*, usually occurs in the south-eastern Atlantic states and south-central states (not usually in the Rocky Mountains).
- Endemic (murine) typhus, caused by *Rickettsia typhi*, occurs in the southeastern states and near the Gulf of Mexico (especially Texas).
  a. Rats and other rodents are primary reservoirs.
  b. Typhus is spread by the rat and cat flea.

6. Treatment
- Tetracycline or chloramphenicol

B. ***Brucella* species**
1. Four closely related *Brucella* species cause zoonotic disease in humans.
2. Brucella are small, gram-negative, nonencapsulated, facultative intracellular coccobacilli.
3. Pathogenesis
- Phagocytosed brucella are resistant to intracellular killing and survive within neutrophils and macrophages, thereby evading immune control.
- Infected phagocytes carry brucella to the spleen, lymph nodes, bone marrow, and other sites.
- Granulomas form around infection foci as a result of host T_H1 response.
4. Brucellosis (undulant fever)
- Subacute, acute, and chronic forms occur.
- Symptoms include malaise, chills, sweats, fatigue, weight loss, reactive arthritis, and undulating fever pattern.
5. Transmission
- Animal hosts include cattle *(Brucella abortus)*, goats and sheep *(Brucella melitensis)*, and dogs *(Brucella canis)*.
  a. Ingestion of contaminated milk or cheese is a common means of acquiring brucellosis among the general population.
  b. Contact with infected animal hosts and inhalation of airborne brucellae are common transmission routes among farmers, veterinarians, and slaughterhouse workers.
6. Prevention and treatment
- Control of disease in animals and pasteurization of dairy products help prevent human disease.
- Prolonged therapy is required to prevent relapse.
  a. Tetracycline plus streptomycin
  b. Trimethoprim-sulfamethoxazole

C. ***Francisella tularensis***
1. *F. tularensis* is a very small, gram-negative, facultative intracellular coccobacillus that grows slowly on cysteine-containing media.
2. Pathogenesis
- Antiphagocytic capsule present on virulent strains
- Intracellular growth within macrophages
- Very high infectivity (ID_{50} of about 50 organisms)
3. Tularemia

- Incubation period of 3 to 5 days is followed by abrupt onset of fever, chills, malaise, and fatigue.
- Ulceroglandular form: most common presentation in the United States
  a. Skin ulcers at the site of infection
  b. Painful, swollen draining lymph nodes (glandular fever)
- Oculoglandular form: due to direct inoculation of the eye
  a. Painful conjunctivitis that develops into ocular ulcer
  b. Regional lymphadenopathy
- Other: typhoidal (sepsis), pneumonic, gastrointestinal
4. Transmission
- Natural reservoirs for *F. tularensis* include rabbits, many other small wild animals, and ticks.
- Spread to humans occurs by bites from infected ticks, direct contact with infected animals, ingestion of contaminated meat or water, and inhalation of infectious aerosols (e.g., while skinning an infected animal).
5. Prevention and treatment
- Live attenuated vaccine, which reduces severity of disease, for at-risk individuals (hunters, veterinarians)
- Streptomycin for all forms of tularemia

D. *Listeria monocytogenes*
1. *L. monocytogenes*, part of the normal gastrointestinal flora of many animals, is transmitted to humans by ingestion of contaminated food, especially unpasteurized dairy products.
2. Grows in the cold (e.g., ice cream)
3. Identification
- Small, gram-positive, facultative intracellular coccobacillus that does not form spores
- β-Hemolytic, catalase positive, tumbling motility at room temperatures
- Cold enrichment facilitates isolation
4. Pathogenesis
- Intracellular growth in macrophages and epithelial cells protects bacteria from humoral immune response.
- Listeriolysin O (a β-hemolysin similar to streptolysin) lyses phagosome, releasing bacteria into cytoplasm, where they replicate.
- Direct cell-to-cell transfer (actin rockets) permits spread of infection to new cells without exposing bacteria to extracellular antibodies or other bactericidal agents.
5. Listeriosis in adults
- Meningitis and sepsis in immunocompromised individuals
- Mild flu-like illness (fever, chills) with sepsis in pregnant women
6. Neonatal listeriosis
- Granulomatosis infantiseptica: acquired transplacentally in utero
  a. Disseminated abscesses and granulomas in multiple organs
  b. High mortality rate unless promptly treated
- Late-onset disease: acquired at or soon after birth by contact with contaminated body fluids of infected mother
  a. Onset 2 to 3 weeks after birth
  b. Meningitis and sepsis
7. Treatment
- Ampicillin for all listerial infections

Hunters, animal skinners, taxidermists, and rabbit owners are at risk for tularemia.

Trigger words:
L. monocytogenes: baby, cold enrichment, intracellular growth, meningitis, milk products, motility, undercooked meat

Virulence factors: intracellular growth, listeriolysin O, cell-to-cell spread, growth at refrigerator temperatures

Contaminated food is common source of *Listeria* species infection.

Major causes of neonatal meningitis with sepsis: *L. monocytogenes*, *Streptococcus agalactiae* (Group B), and *Escherichia coli*

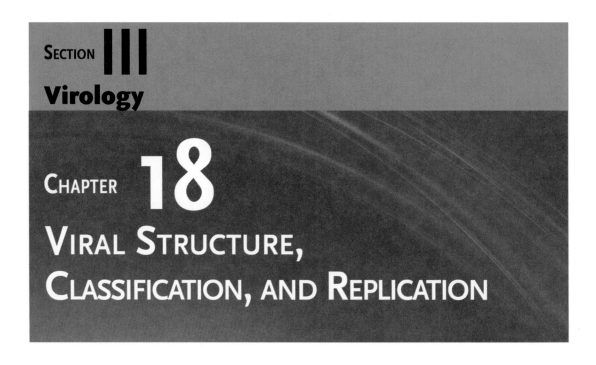

I. Structure and Classification of Viruses

A. Overview

1. A virion, or viral particle, consists of a genome (DNA or RNA) packaged within a protein coat, the capsid, which may or may not be surrounded by a membrane envelope.
2. Essential enzymes or other proteins are carried within some viruses.
3. The major virus families can be classified based on their genome structure, size, and whether they are enveloped or not enveloped.

B. Genome structure

1. DNA genome (Fig. 18-1A)
   - Single-stranded (linear) DNA: parvoviruses
   - Double-stranded DNA
     a. Linear genome: adenoviruses, herpesviruses, and poxviruses
     b. Circular genome: polyomaviruses and hepadnaviruses
2. RNA genome (Fig. 18-1B)
   - Positive-sense (+) RNA
     a. Same sequence as messenger RNA (mRNA)
     b. Directly translated into protein
        - Exception is the retroviruses in which the (+) RNA genome is not translated but is converted into DNA, which then acts as a template for production of mRNA.
   - Negative-sense (–) RNA
     a. Sequence complementary to mRNA
     b. Must be copied into (+) strand to generate mRNAs for protein synthesis
   - Double-stranded (+/–) RNA: copying of (–) strand generates mRNA for protein synthesis
3. Segmented genome
   - Found in the reoviruses, a (+/–) RNA genome, and in three families of (–) RNA viruses (orthomyxoviruses, arenaviruses, and bunyaviruses)
   - Consists of several pieces, or segments, each of which encodes at least one polypeptide
   - May undergo reassortment among genomic segments, yielding new virus strains, particularly in influenza viruses

C. Viral capsid (Fig. 18-3)

- In viruses that lack an outer envelope, the capsid enclosing the genome forms the outer layer of the virion.

1. Shape
   - Icosahedral capsid is found in many simple viruses (e.g., picornaviruses); shape approximates a sphere with 12 vertices.
   - Icosadeltahedral capsid is found in larger viruses (e.g., herpesviruses); shape is similar to a soccer ball.
   - Helical capsid is found inside most viruses with (–) RNA genomes (e.g., paramyxoviruses).

The following characteristics: genome type, enveloped or naked capsid, and relative size (large, medium, or small) allow you to predict many of the properties of the virus.

Parvoviruses: only DNA viruses with single-stranded genome

All (–) RNA viruses are enveloped and must carry their RNA-dependent RNA polymerase as part of the nucleocapsid.

DNA (except pox) and (+) RNA (not retro) do not need to carry a polymerase into the target cell, and their genomes are sufficient to infect a cell.

Reoviruses: double-double: double-capsid/double-stranded, segmented genome

Be able to recognize viruses with characteristic shapes (Fig. 18-2).

An icosahedron or icosadeltahedron is the basic capsid shape and looks like a soccer ball.

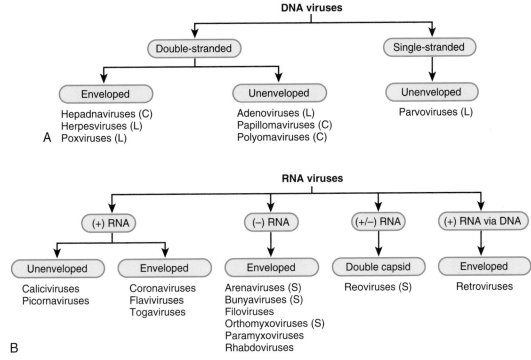

DNA viruses

Double-stranded

Enveloped

Hepadnaviruses (C)
Herpesviruses (L)
A Poxviruses (L)

Unenveloped

Adenoviruses (L)
Papillomaviruses (C)
Polyomaviruses (C)

Single-stranded

Unenveloped

Parvoviruses (L)

RNA viruses

(+) RNA

Unenveloped

Caliciviruses
Picornaviruses

Enveloped

Coronaviruses
Flaviviruses
Togaviruses

(−) RNA

Enveloped

Arenaviruses (S)
Bunyaviruses (S)
Filoviruses
Orthomyxoviruses (S)
Paramyxoviruses
Rhabdoviruses

(+/−) RNA

Double capsid

Reoviruses (S)

(+) RNA via DNA

Enveloped

Retroviruses

B

18-1: Classification of major viral families based on genome structure and virion morphology. **A,** DNA viruses. L, linear genome; C, circular genome. **B,** RNA viruses. S, segmented genome.

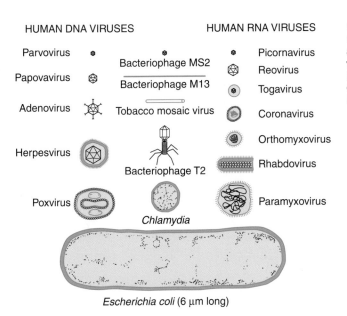

HUMAN DNA VIRUSES

Parvovirus

Papovavirus

Adenovirus

Herpesvirus

Poxvirus

Bacteriophage MS2

Bacteriophage M13

Tobacco mosaic virus

Bacteriophage T2

Chlamydia

Escherichia coli (6 μm long)

HUMAN RNA VIRUSES

Picornavirus

Reovirus

Togavirus

Coronavirus

Orthomyxovirus

Rhabdovirus

Paramyxovirus

18-2: Morphology and relative size of viruses. Herpesvirus, adenovirus, poxvirus, retroviruses, and rhabdoviruses have characteristic shapes, whereas other viruses are distinguished by size, presence of an envelope, or an icosa(delta)hedral capsid. *(Courtesy the Upjohn Company, Kalamazoo, Michigan.)*

   2. Formation
     • Capsids are assembled sequentially from smaller proteins (Fig. 18-4).
   3. Capsid components recognize and bind to cell surface receptors on host cells.
     • Canyon-like clefts within capsid structure (picornaviruses)
     • Fibers that extend from capsid (adenoviruses and reoviruses)
     • Neutralizing antibody is directed against capsid proteins that interact with cell surface receptors.
  D. Viral envelope
     • Important differences between nonenveloped and enveloped viruses are summarized in Table 18-1.

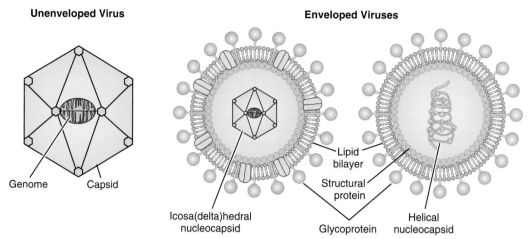

Unenveloped Virus

Genome   Capsid

Enveloped Viruses

Lipid bilayer

Structural protein

Icosa(delta)hedral nucleocapsid

Glycoprotein

Helical nucleocapsid

18-3: Virion structures. Nonenveloped (naked) viruses consist of a genome surrounded by a protein shell, or capsid. Shown here is an icosahedral capsid, the most common type in nonenveloped viruses. Enveloped viruses have a membrane that surrounds the nucleocapsid, which can have an icosahedral, icosadeltahedral, or helical shape. The helical nucleocapsid, found only in most enveloped (−) RNA viruses, is formed by association of viral proteins, including RNA polymerase, with the genome.

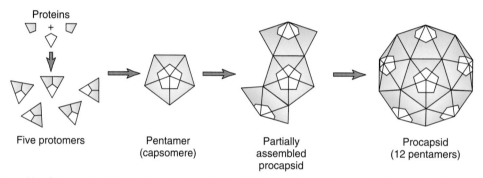

Proteins

Five protomers

Pentamer (capsomere)

Partially assembled procapsid

Procapsid (12 pentamers)

18-4: Assembly of the icosahedral capsid of a picornavirus. Individual proteins associate into subunits, which associate into protomers, capsomeres, and an empty procapsid. Insertion of the (+) RNA genome triggers conversion of procapsid to the final capsid (not shown).

TABLE 18-1   **Nonenveloped (Naked) Versus Enveloped Viruses**

PROPERTY	NONENVELOPED VIRUSES	ENVELOPED VIRUSES
Components	Proteins	Phospholipids, proteins, glycoproteins
Sensitivity to heat, acid, detergent, drying	Resistant (stable)	Sensitive (labile)
Release from host cell	By cell lysis (host cell killed)	By budding (host cell survives) and cell lysis
Transmission or mode of spread	Fomites, dust, fecal-oral	Large droplets, secretions, and organ or blood transplants
Effect of drying	Retain infectivity	Lose infectivity
Survival within gastrointestinal tract	Yes	No (except corona-and hepadna-viruses)
Host immune response (minimal protection)	Antibody response	Antibody and cell-mediated responses (the latter often contribute to pathogenesis)

1. Shape
   • Most enveloped viruses do not have a defined shape. Exceptions are the brick-shaped poxviruses and bullet-shaped rhabdoviruses.
2. Formation
   • Viral envelopes are derived from host cell membranes into which viral structural proteins and glycoproteins are inserted (see Fig. 18-3).
   • Source of envelope:
      a. Intracellular membranes → bunyaviruses, coronaviruses, flaviviruses, herpesviruses, and poxviruses
      b. Plasma membrane → all other enveloped viruses

BOX 18-1   PRINCIPLES OF VIRAL REPLICATION

- Viruses must replicate to survive.
- Viruses require appropriate host cells in which to replicate.
- Replication of all viruses proceeds through the same basic steps, but mechanisms vary depending on the genome structure and whether a virion has an envelope or is nonenveloped.
- Host cell biochemical machinery is appropriated by viruses for their replication.
- Any protein necessary for viral activity that is not produced by host cell must be encoded by viral genome. Examples include **polymerase enzymes** that catalyze synthesis of RNA from an RNA template and **reverse transcriptase** of retroviruses, which synthesizes double-stranded DNA from single-stranded RNA.
- Larger viruses encode nonessential proteins that facilitate replication (e.g., the deoxyribonucleotide-scavenging enzymes of the herpesviruses).

---

3. Viral envelope glycoproteins that promote entry into target cells.
   - Viral attachment proteins (VAPs) (e.g., human immunodeficiency virus [HIV] gp120, influenza HA)
     a. Neutralizing antibody is directed at VAPs
   - Fusion proteins
   - Enzymes (e.g., neuraminidase)

II. **Basic Steps in Viral Replication (Box 18-1; Fig. 18-5)**
   A. **Recognition of target cell**
      - Recognition step determines which cells will be infected (tropism or specificity of a virus) and is a major determinant of disease manifestations resulting from infection.
      1. VAPs or other structures on the virion surface recognize tissue-specific receptors on target cells.
      2. Cell surface virus receptors may be proteins, glycoproteins, or glycolipids. Examples of such receptors and the viruses that bind to them include the following:
         - CD4 molecules on T cells and macrophages: HIV and human T lymphotropic virus
         - CR2 receptor for C3b complement component on B cells and epithelial cells: Epstein-Barr virus
         - Sialic acid side chains on membrane proteins or lipids: influenza viruses; paramyxoviruses (e.g., mumps, measles viruses)
         - ICAM-1 on B lymphocytes, epithelial cells, and fibroblasts: rhinoviruses (common cold viruses)
   B. **Attachment to host cell**
      - Tight association results from multiple interactions between virus and cell surface receptors.
   C. **Entry (penetration) of virion into target cell**
      1. Receptor-mediated endocytosis: most nonenveloped and some enveloped viruses
         - Endocytosed virions generally are released into cytoplasm as a result of decreased pH in endosomal vesicle or lysis of vesicle by virus.
      2. Fusion of viral envelope with cell membrane
         - Some enveloped viruses, including paramyxoviruses, herpesviruses, and retroviruses (e.g., HIV)
      3. Viropexis (direct penetration of cell membrane by virions): reoviruses, picornaviruses
   D. **Uncoating of nucleocapsid to release viral genome and enzymes**
   E. **Synthesis of viral mRNAs (Fig. 18-6)**
      1. Early mRNAs encode enzymes and control proteins required in small amounts (e.g., DNA-binding proteins).
      2. Late mRNAs encode structural proteins required in large amounts (e.g., capsid proteins and glycoproteins).
      3. DNA viruses depend on host cell machinery in the nucleus to make mRNAs from viral genomes.
         - Exception is poxvirus, which uses RNA polymerase carried in virion to make mRNAs from viral genome in the cytoplasm.
      4. RNA viruses use several mechanisms for generating mRNA depending on the structure of the genome, as depicted in Figure 18-6.
         - The RNA-dependent RNA polymerase is carried into the cell as part of the helical nucleocapsid by (–) RNA viruses and makes mRNA in the cytoplasm.
         - The RNA-dependent RNA polymerase of (+) RNA viruses is made after infection of the cell and make a (–) RNA template and then copies new mRNA and new genomes from it.

Viral attachment and recognition: major determinants of host range, tropism, and tissue specificity of a virus.

Neutralizing antibodies are directed at VAPs.

Paramyxoviruses, herpesviruses, and retroviruses enter by fusion at plasma membrane and can also cause syncytia.

Early proteins are enzymes and control proteins. Most late proteins are structural proteins.

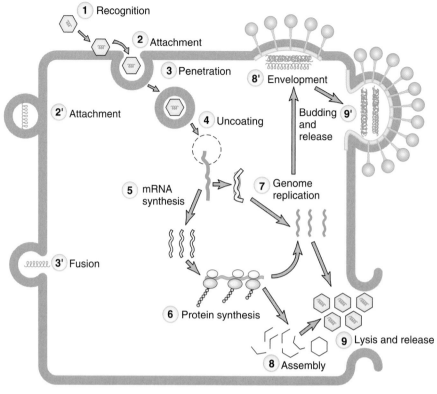

18-5: General scheme of virus replication. Enveloped viruses have alternative means of entry (steps 2' and 3'), assembly (step 8'), and exit from the cell (step 9'). Antiviral drugs inhibit various steps, as indicated at the bottom. Antiviral drugs are described in Chapter 20 and for the relevant virus. mRNA, messenger RNA.

Viruses use cell's ribosomes, posttranslational modification enzymes, adenosine triphosphate (ATP), and metabolites.

DNA viruses replicate in nucleus; RNA viruses replicate in cytoplasm, with exceptions.

F. Synthesis of viral proteins

1. Translation of mRNA into protein uses host cell ribosomes and other synthetic machinery.
2. Posttranslational modifications (e.g., glycosylation, phosphorylation, and proteolytic cleavage) are carried out by host enzymes and occasionally by viral enzymes.

G. Replication of viral genome

1. DNA viruses replicate their genomes in the nucleus using host or virus-encoded DNA polymerases.
   - Exceptions are poxvirus and hepadnavirus (hepatitis B virus), which replicate their genomes in the cytoplasm using viral enzymes.
2. RNA viruses (except retroviruses) use viral RNA-dependent RNA polymerase (replicase) to synthesize complementary (antisense) RNA, which acts as a template for synthesis of new genomes in the cytoplasm.
   - Exception is orthomyxovirus (influenza virus), which is replicated in the nucleus but by viral enzymes.

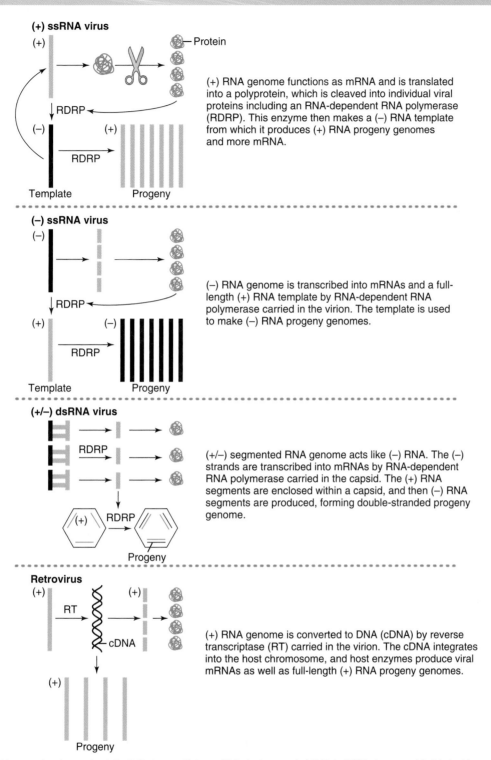

18-6: Macromolecular synthesis in RNA viruses. Virions of (–) single-stranded RNA (ssRNA) viruses and (+/–) double-stranded RNA (dsRNA) viruses carry RNA-dependent RNA polymerase (RDRP), and retroviral virions carry reverse transcriptase (RT). The genome of (+) RNA viruses (except retroviruses) can function directly as messenger RNA (mRNA) and these viruses encode RDRP, but the virions do not carry the enzyme. cDNA, complementary DNA.

3. Retroviruses carry reverse transcriptase, a viral enzyme that converts (+) single-stranded RNA genome into double-stranded DNA, which is integrated into host chromosomal DNA.
   • Transcription of integrated viral DNA (provirus) by host cell enzymes yields new retroviral genomes as well as mRNAs.
4. Hepadnaviruses use the cell's DNA-dependent RNA polymerase to make an overlapping (+) RNA copy of the genome that is encapsidated with a reverse transcriptase that converts it into DNA.

H. Assembly of virions
1. Nonenveloped viruses
   - Procapsid (empty shell) may assemble first and then be filled with the genome.
   - Capsid proteins may assemble around the genome, forming the nucleocapsid.
2. Enveloped viruses
   - Viral glycoproteins are inserted into host plasma membrane or membranes of the rough endoplasmic reticulum, Golgi complex, or nucleus.
   - Nucleocapsid associates with glycoprotein-modified membrane.
     - a. Viral protein (e.g., matrix protein) may line glycoprotein-modified membrane (RNA viruses).
   - Membrane envelopes nucleocapsid (budding out) to form a virion.

I. Release of virions
1. Cell lysis is most efficient but kills the cell.
   - Most naked capsid viruses (but not hepatitis A) and poxviruses
2. Budding from cell surface is next most efficient and does *not* kill the cell, allowing continued virus production.
   - Enveloped viruses that assemble at plasma membrane
3. Exocytosis is least efficient but does not kill the cell.
   - Enveloped viruses that assemble at intracellular membranes, such as flavivirus, arenavirus, hepadnaviruses, and herpesvirus

III. Viral Genetic Mechanisms (Fig. 18-7)
A. Rapid mutation rate
   - Viral polymerases make many mistakes, especially for RNA viruses.

Drug and antibody-resistant strains of HIV result from selection of mutants generated by the error-prone HIV polymerase.

B. Virus selection
   - Antibody and antiviral drugs can select for resistant viruses that can be generated during infection of an individual.

C. Recombination
   - Hybrid viral genomes may result during coinfection of a cell with two strains or types of DNA viruses or HIV.

D. Reassortant
   - Hybrid viruses with new mixtures of gene segments can arise during coinfection of a cell with two strains of influenza or rotavirus.

Pandemic influenza A strains (like A/ Mexico/2009(H1N1) result from a shift in antigen after reassortment of gene segments from multiple strains.

IV. Summary
   - Tables 18-2 and 18-3 summarize the structural properties of viral families and list important human pathogens in each.

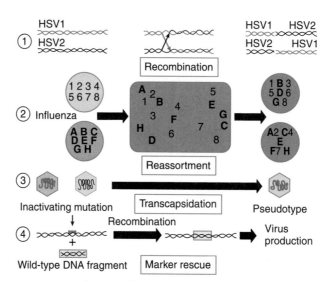

18-7: Gene exchange for viruses. 1. Recombination of two closely related strains or types of viruses (e.g., herpes simplex virus [HSV] or human immunodeficiency virus [HIV]). 2. Reassortment of segmented genomes (e.g., influenza or rotavirus). 3. Transcapsidation/pseudotype (e.g., encapsidation or envelopment of a viral genome in a different virus capsid or envelope). 4. Marker rescue of a inactivating or conditional mutation. *(From Murray PR, Rosenthal KS, Pfaller MA: Medical Microbiology, 6th ed. Philadelphia, Mosby, 2009, Fig. 4-15.)*

TABLE 18-2 **DNA Virus Families**

FAMILY	DNA GENOME	OTHER PROPERTIES	CLINICALLY IMPORTANT MEMBERS
Adenoviridae	DS, linear	Nonenveloped; midsize Icosadeltahedral capsid Encodes DNA polymerase	Adenovirus Possible vector for gene therapy
Hepadnaviridae	DS, partially circular	Enveloped; small Replicates genome via RNA intermediate using viral reverse transcriptase	Hepatitis B virus
Herpesviridae	DS, linear	Enveloped; large Icosadeltahedral capsid Encodes DNA polymerase that replicates genome in nucleus	Epstein-Barr virus Herpes simplex virus 1 Herpes simplex virus 2 Human herpesvirus 6,7 Human herpesvirus 8 Varicella-zoster virus
Papillomaviridae	DS	Nonenveloped; small, icosahedral capsid	Human papillomavirus
Polyomaviridae	DS, circular	Nonenveloped, small Icosahedral capsid	JC, BK virus
Parvoviridae	SS, linear	Nonenveloped; small Icosahedral capsid	B19 parvovirus
Poxviridae	DS, linear	Enveloped; largest virus (brick shaped) Produces mRNA and replicates genome in cytoplasm using viral enzymes	Molluscum contagiosum virus Vaccinia virus (used in vaccines) Variola (smallpox) virus (now eradicated)

DS, double-stranded; mRNA, messenger RNA; SS, single-stranded.

TABLE 18-3 **RNA Virus Families**

FAMILY	RNA GENOME	OTHER PROPERTIES	CLINICALLY IMPORTANT MEMBERS
Arenaviridae	(−) SS, circular, segmented	Enveloped; midsize Helical capsid Carries RDRP in virion	Lymphocytic choriomeningitis virus Lassa fever virus
Bunyaviridae	(−) SS, linear, segmented	Enveloped; midsize Helical capsid Carries RDRP in virion	California encephalitis virus Hanta virus
Caliciviridae	(+) SS, linear	Nonenveloped; small Icosahedral capsid Genome functions as mRNA	Norwalk virus
Coronaviridae	(+) SS, linear	Enveloped; large Helical capsid Genome functions as mRNA	Coronaviruses and severe acute respiratory syndrome virus
Filoviridae	(−) SS, linear	Enveloped; midsize Helical capsid Carries RDRP in virion	Ebola and Marburg viruses
Flaviviridae	(+) SS, linear	Enveloped; small Icosahedral capsid Genome functions as mRNA	Dengue virus Hepatitis C virus St. Louis encephalitis virus Yellow fever virus
Orthomyxoviridae	(−) SS, linear, segmented	Enveloped; large Helical capsid Carries RDRP in virion	Influenza viruses (types A-C)
Paramyxoviridae	(−) SS, linear	Enveloped; large Helical capsid Carries RDRP in virion	Measles virus Mumps virus Parainfluenza virus Respiratory syncytial virus Metapneumovirus
Picornaviridae	(+) SS, linear	Nonenveloped; small Icosahedral capsid Genome functions as mRNA	Coxsackieviruses Echovirus Hepatitis A Poliovirus Rhinoviruses

TABLE 18-3 **RNA Virus Families—Cont'd**

FAMILY	RNA GENOME	OTHER PROPERTIES	CLINICALLY IMPORTANT MEMBERS
Reoviridae	(+/−) DS, linear, segmented	Nonenveloped; midsize Double capsid Carries RDRP in virion	Rotavirus
Retroviridae	(+) SS, linear (two copies)	Enveloped; midsize Helical capsid Reverse transcriptase in virion converts genome to cDNA; host enzymes form viral mRNAs and progeny genomes	Human immunodeficiency virus Human T lymphotropic virus
Rhabdoviridae	(−) SS, linear	Enveloped; midsize, bullet shaped Helical capsid Carries RDRP in virion	Rabies virus
Togaviridae	(+) SS, linear	Enveloped; small Icosahedral capsid Genome functions as mRNA	Rubella virus Eastern, Western, and Venezuelan equine encephalitis viruses

+, Identical to mRNA sequence; −, complementary to mRNA sequence; cDNA, complementary DNA; DS, double stranded; RDRP, RNA-dependent RNA polymerase; SS, single stranded.

CHAPTER 19
VIRAL PATHOGENESIS

I. Factors Affecting Viral Virulence

A. Host range
1. Species that can be infected by a virus
2. Cells must express surface molecules recognized by a viral attachment protein or other structure.
3. Cells must provide compatible biochemical machinery to replicate virus.

B. Routes of viral entry into host cells
- Initial viral replication generally occurs at the site of entry, but some viruses spread to target tissues where major pathologic effects occur.
1. Oral or respiratory routes
   - Most common means of viral entry
   - Many infections remain localized in the respiratory tract.
2. Through breaks in the skin
   - Herpes simplex virus (HSV), human papillomavirus (HPV)
3. Through conjunctiva: adenovirus
4. Through genital tract
   - Hepatitis B virus, HPV, human immunodeficiency virus (HIV), HSV
5. Direct injection
   - Needle/direct transfusion of blood (hepatitis B, C, and D viruses; HIV) or insect bite (arbovirus)

C. Tissue specificity (tropism)
- Consequences of viral infection depend on target organs involved and extent of the damage to these tissues.
1. Local infection without spread (e.g., rhinovirus, other common cold viruses)
   - Viruses that manifest symptoms at the initial site of entry cause diseases with short incubation periods and early prodromes.
2. Viremic spread from viral point of entry (e.g., measles, mumps, and chickenpox viruses) results in diseases with longer incubation periods.
   - Example: varicella-zoster virus (VZV) is acquired by respiratory route and initiates infection in the lungs. Infection spreads through blood to liver and other organs, initiates a secondary viremia, and then reach the skin to cause classic symptoms of chickenpox. Incubation period is 10 to 30 days.
   - Attenuated virus strain that cannot reach or infect its disease-related target organ may lose its virulence (e.g., attenuated live polio vaccine, cannot infect the brain to cause major disease).
   - Virus-specific antibodies can block viremic spread to target tissue.
3. Neuronal spread (e.g., rabies virus, HSV)

D. Support of viral replication by host cells
- To spread and cause disease, a virus must replicate in host cells.
1. Permissive cells possess all the biochemical machinery needed by a virus to enter the cell and replicate, yielding a productive infection.
2. Nonpermissive cells do not support replication, but they may be transformed by DNA tumor viruses (e.g., Epstein-Barr virus and HPV).
3. Semipermissive cells allow some viral functions to occur or support low levels of replication.

Viral disease = viral pathology + immunopathology

Organs damaged by a particular viral infection determine its disease symptoms. Infections involving the central nervous system, lungs, liver, and heart produce the most serious manifestations.

Antibody blocks viremic spread to target tissue.

II. Viral Cytopathogenesis

A. Pathogenic mechanisms

1. Major viral mechanisms for disrupting the structure and functioning of infected cells are summarized in Table 19-1.
2. Appearance of characteristic inclusion bodies in infected cells facilitates laboratory diagnosis of infection by some viruses (e.g., rabies, HSV, and cytomegalovirus).

B. Types of infections

- Classification of viral infections based on the fate of virus-infected cells is shown in Table 19-2.

1. Cytolytic infection
   - Viral replication leads to death of target cell
   - Relatively rapid antibody-mediated immune resolution is common.
2. Chronic infection
   - Continual production of virions or viral components occurs without cell lysis or immune resolution.
3. Latent infection
   - Virus remains dormant within certain cells until reactivated by stress or immunosuppression to become cytolytic or chronic.
4. Immortalizing infection
   - Persistent infection by tumor viruses promotes uncontrolled cell growth, contributing to transformation of infected cells into cancer cells (Fig. 19-1).
   - DNA tumor viruses do not replicate in infected cells (production of virions leading to cell lysis would preclude transformation).
     a. Prevent activity of normal growth-suppressor proteins such as p53 or RB proteins (human papillomavirus, adenovirus)
     b. Act as mitogens to stimulate proliferation (Epstein-Barr virus)
     c. Inhibit apoptosis, or programmed cell death (Epstein-Barr virus)

> DNA tumor viruses (e.g., papillomaviruses, EBV and hepatitis B virus) transform nonpermissive cells (no virions produced), whereas RNA tumor viruses (e.g., human T lymphotropic virus [HTLV]) transform permissive cells (virions produced).

TABLE 19-1 Viral Cytopathogenesis

MECHANISM	REPRESENTATIVE VIRUSES
Inhibition of cellular protein synthesis	Polioviruses, HSV, togaviruses
Inhibition of cellular DNA synthesis; degradation of DNA	Herpesviruses
Alteration of cell membranes	
Glycoprotein insertion	All enveloped viruses
Syncytia (giant cell) formation	HSV, varicella-zoster virus, paramyxoviruses, HIV
Permeability changes	Togaviruses, herpesviruses
Disruption of cytoskeleton	Naked capsid viruses, HSV
Formation of inclusion bodies	
Negri bodies (cytoplasmic)	Rabies
Basophilic (owl's eye) nuclear bodies	Cytomegalovirus
Cowdry type A nuclear bodies	HSV
Nuclear basophilic bodies	Adenoviruses
Acidophilic perinuclear bodies	Reoviruses
Toxicity of virion components	Adenovirus fibers
Immunosuppression	HIV, cytomegalovirus, measles virus, influenza virus

HIV, human immunodeficiency virus; HSV, herpes simplex virus.

TABLE 19-2 Effect of Viral Infection on Target Cells

INFECTION TYPE	VIRAL REPLICATION	CELL FATE	REPRESENTATIVE VIRUSES
Cytolytic	Yes	Death	Polioviruses, togaviruses, herpesviruses, poxviruses
Chronic	Yes	Senescence or immune elimination	Hepatitis B and C viruses, HIV, HTLV
Latent	No	No effect until virus is activated	Herpesviruses, retroviruses
Immortalizing DNA tumor viruses	No	Growth and transformation	HPV, EBV, HHV-8, hepatitis B virus
RNA tumor viruses	Yes	Growth and transformation	Certain retroviruses (HTLV)

EBV, Epstein-Barr virus; HHV-8, human herpesvirus-8; HIV, human immunodeficiency virus; HPV, human papillomavirus; HTLV, human T lymphotropic virus.

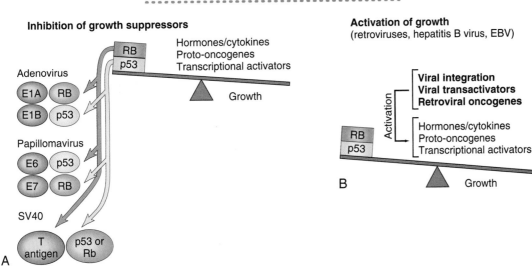

19-1: Mechanisms of viral transformation (immortalization). Cell growth is controlled by the balance of extracellular and intracellular growth activators and growth suppressors such as p53 and RB proteins (*top*). **A,** Some oncogenic viruses tip the balance toward growth by encoding proteins (e.g., E1A, E6, and T antigen) that bind to suppressors, inhibiting their function. **B,** Other oncogenic viruses tip the balance toward growth by various activating mechanisms. EBV, Epstein-Barr virus.

- RNA tumor viruses (retroviruses) replicate in infected cells without killing cells.
  a. Fast-transforming viruses encode proteins (e.g., hormone receptors, protein kinases, and transcription activators) that function in cellular growth-promoting pathways (no human viruses).
  b. Slow-transforming viruses encode proteins that activate expression of host growth-promoting genes (HTLV).

III. Antiviral Host Response and Immunopathogenesis
- Resolution of viral infections requires elimination of extracellular virions and destruction of virus-infected cells.

A. Key components of antiviral response (see Chapter 4, Fig. 4-6)
1. Interferons (IFN-α and IFN-β) secreted by infected cells induce an antiviral state in neighboring noninfected cells, thus limiting spread of infection within host tissues.
   - These cytokines also initiate immune responses (see Chapter 4, Box 4-5).
2. Natural killer cells activated by IFN kill infected cells.
3. Antibodies have a major role in resolution of lytic infections.
   - Antibody can inactivate (neutralize) or help eliminate (opsonize) free virions.
   - Antibody is essential for controlling viruses that are spread by viremia.
4. T_H1 inflammatory and cell-mediated cytolytic responses are essential for resolution of nonlytic and enveloped virus infections because virus may not kill the infected cells.

B. Pathologic effects of antiviral response
- The immune response to viral infections is responsible for many of the clinical manifestations of these infections, especially those that are nonlytic (Table 19-3).

C. Viral escape from immune responses
- Viruses employ various mechanisms to evade or reduce host antiviral responses, thereby increasing their spread and persistence in the host.
1. Formation of syncytia, which permit direct cell-to-cell spread of virions, protecting them from antibody
   - HSV, VZV, paramyxoviruses, retroviruses
2. Initiation of latency in certain cells
   - HSV, VZV, retroviruses
3. Antigenic shift in viral proteins that induce immune response
   - Influenza A virus, HIV

IFN-α and IFN-β mediate flu-like symptoms associated with many viral infections.

Antibody to the viral attachment protein (neutralizing) is protective. T cells recognize peptides from any viral protein if presented by major histocompatibility complex.
Antibody controls viremia and lytic viruses; cell-mediated immunity is necessary for enveloped and nonlytic viruses.

TABLE 19-3 **Antiviral Immunopathogenesis**

PATHOLOGIC EFFECT	IMMUNE MEDIATORS	REPRESENTATIVE VIRUSES
Flu-like symptoms	Interferons, other cytokines	Respiratory viruses, viremia-inducing viruses
Delayed-type hypersensitivity and inflammation	T cells, macrophages, cytokines	Enveloped viruses
Immune complex deposition	Antibody, complement, macrophages	Hepatitis B virus
Hemorrhage	T cells, antibody, complement	Dengue virus
Postinfection cytolysis	T cells	Enveloped viruses

TABLE 19-4 **Incubation Periods of Common Viral Infections**

INCUBATION PERIOD	DISEASE (VIRUS)
Very short (<1 wk)	Acute respiratory disease (adenoviruses), common cold (rhinoviruses), croup and bronchiolitis (parainfluenza virus), influenza
Short (1-3 wk)	Chickenpox, measles, mumps, rubella
Long (4-21 wk)	Hepatitis B, mononucleosis (Epstein-Barr virus), rabies, warts (papillomaviruses)
Very long (1-10 yr)	Acquired immunodeficiency syndrome (human immunodeficiency virus)

4. Lymphocyte destruction or injury
- HIV killing of CD4⁺ T cells

5. Inhibition of IFN antiviral activity
- Adenovirus, hepatitis B virus

6. Inactivation of complement (e.g., HSV)

7. Release from infected cells of viral antigen that can block antibody neutralization of virions
- Hepatitis B surface antigen (HBsAg) of hepatitis B virus

IV. Clinical Course of Viral Diseases

A. Incubation period

> If disease occurs at the same site as infection, there is a short incubation period.
> If virus must travel to cause disease *or* if disease is due to immunopathogenesis, there is a long incubation period.

- Viral infections may be asymptomatic or symptomatic. Site of disease manifestation and time needed for damage to occur determine the incubation period (Table 19-4).
  1. Diseases that manifest at the site of entry generally have incubation periods of less than 1 week.
     - Exception is warts (papillomaviruses), with incubation periods of 7 to 21 weeks.
  2. Diseases that manifest in tissues distant from the site of entry have incubation periods ranging from about 1 week to several months (rabies).
  3. Diseases that result from immunopathogenesis or slow accumulation of tissue damage (e.g., neuronal) may have incubation periods ranging from several weeks (HBV and Epstein-Barr virus) to years (acquired immunodeficiency syndrome [AIDS]).

B. Acute versus persistent infections (Fig. 19-2)

  1. Acute infections
     - Host immune response leads to complete resolution (i.e., elimination of virus).
  2. Persistent (recurrent) infections
     - Only incomplete immune resolution occurs.
     - Latent infections may be preceded by acute disease, often in a different tissue.
     - Chronic infections may exhibit early or late disease manifestations.

C. Conventional slow infections

> Prions: cause progressive neurodegenerative diseases: Creutzfeldt-Jakob disease; Gerstmann-Sträussler-Scheinker syndrome; kuru in humans; and mad cow disease, which may be associated with Creutzfeldt-Jakob disease.

- These infections, which all involve neuronal tissue, are characterized by a very slow increase in viral load over a long period of time and gradual progression once symptoms appear.
  1. Progressive multifocal leukoencephalopathy caused by JC virus usually occurs in immunocompromised individuals.
  2. Subacute sclerosing panencephalitis is a rare late complication due to defective measles virus in the brain.
  3. HTLV-1 initial infection is asymptomatic or causes mononucleosis-like disease, and then 25 to 30 years later, it causes adult acute T cell lymphocytic leukemia (ATLL).

D. Prion-related diseases (Box 19-1)

- These unconventional slow infections include a group of **spongiform encephalopathies** that exhibit rapid progression to death once symptoms appear.

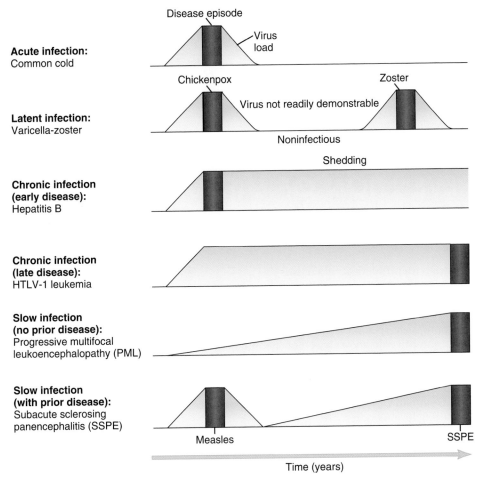

19-2: Diagram depicting acute viral infection and various types of persistent infections. *Dark shaded vertical boxes* indicate periods of symptom manifestations; *light shading* indicates virus load. PML is caused by JC papovavirus. SSPE, a late complication of measles, is due to infection of the brain by defective measles virus.

BOX 19-1 PRIONS

Prions are **filterable infectious agents** consisting of **aggregates of glycoproteins** that may be acquired or inherited. These pathogens (sometimes mistakenly called "slow viruses") lack nucleic acids; are **resistant to inactivation** by disinfectants, proteases, heat, or radiation; and **elicit no host immune response.** Prion protein occurs in a normal form **(PrPc)** and an abnormal form **(PrPSc),** which forms aggregates and causes disease. PrPSc can bind to PrPc on cell surfaces and convert the normal form to the abnormal form.

Diagnosis of prion infection is made on the basis of clinical symptoms and confirmed by histopathology of the brain, including **vacuolation of neurons, amyloid-like plaques,** and **gliosis** with **no inflammation.** Prions cause progressive degenerative neurologic diseases **(spongiform encephalopathies)** that have a **long incubation period** (1 to 30 years) but **progress rapidly** to death after onset. Symptoms include loss of muscle control, shivering, tremors, and dementia.

Human prion diseases include **Creutzfeldt-Jakob disease** and **Gerstmann-Sträussler-Scheinker syndrome,** which may be transmitted by injection, transplantation of infected tissue, or contact with contaminated medical devices. These diseases may also be inherited (the prion gene is on human chromosome 20). **Kuru,** a prion disease that occurs only among certain tribes in New Guinea, is acquired by consumption of or contact with infected tissue during ritual cannibalism. No treatment is available for any prion disease.

I. Laboratory Identification of Viruses

A. Overview

1. Bacterial or fungal etiology for an infection should be excluded before undertaking laboratory analysis for viral infection.
2. Appropriate specimens for analysis are determined by the site of infection and presumptive diagnosis based on symptoms.

B. Microscopic examination of clinical specimens

1. Light microscopy can detect virus-induced histologic changes, called viral cytopathic effects (CPEs), in cells and tissues.
   - Common CPEs include vacuolization, necrosis, syncytia formation, and various types of inclusion bodies.
2. Electron microscopy can visualize virions directly in cells or stool specimens.
   - Direct visualization is most useful for detecting viruses that are produced in abundance and have a characteristic morphology (e.g., rotaviruses).

C. Viral isolation and growth

1. Unlike bacteria or fungi, viruses replicate only within cells and must be isolated and grown in cells that support their replication.
2. Some viruses cannot be grown in the laboratory because no suitable culture system has been developed.

D. Laboratory assays for detecting viral proteins

1. Hemagglutination: viral hemagglutinin (HA) protruding from the surface of some enveloped viruses binds to erythrocytes of specific species, causing them to clump.
   - HA is encoded by influenza, parainfluenza, and mumps viruses and by togaviruses.
   - Hemagglutination inhibition (HAI): specific antibody blocking of hemagglutination can identify the virus strain causing HA. Patient serum that can block HA of a specific strain of virus indicates prior infection with that strain of virus (e.g., influenza A H1N1)
   - Hemadsorption is the binding of certain erythrocytes to viral HA expressed in the membrane of infected cells.
2. Immunologic assays
   - Virus-specific antibody is used to detect free virions and free or cell-associated viral proteins.
     a. Antibody-antigen binding is detected by a probe such as a fluorescent marker, radiolabel, or enzyme (e.g., horseradish peroxidase, alkaline phosphatase, and β-galactosidase) that produces a colored product on addition of substrate.
   - Immunofluorescence (IF) and enzyme immunoassay (EIA) detect viral proteins expressed on the surface of infected cells (see Fig. 5-3).
   - Enzyme-linked immunosorbent assay (ELISA) and radioimmunoassay (RIA) detect and quantitate free virions or viral proteins in a sample.
   - Direct versus indirect assays
     a. For direct assays, antiviral antibody is covalently linked to the probe.
     b. For indirect assays, the probe is linked to a secondary antibody that binds to the primary antiviral antibody after it interacts with viral antigen.

Inclusion bodies useful in viral detection: Negri bodies = rabies virus; owl's-eye nuclear bodies = cytomegalovirus; Cowdry type A nuclear bodies = herpes simplex virus

Hemagglutination detects virus, hemagglutination inhibition (HAI) assay antibody but can also be used to identify a virus strain.

E. **Laboratory assays for detecting viral nucleic acids**
  - Assays for viral nucleic acids are particularly useful in identifying slowly replicating viruses or those that do not have obvious cytopathic effects.
  1. Polymerase chain reaction (PCR) (DNA), reverse transcriptase PCR (RT-PCR) (RNA), and related technologies, which permit amplification of specific nucleic acid sequences, are especially helpful in rapid detection of viruses
      a. RT-PCR converts viral RNA genomes into DNA and then amplifies the sequence.
      b. Quantitative (real-time) PCR determines the number of DNA copies. RNA genomes are converted to DNA with reverse transcriptase and then quantitated.
  2. Southern blotting for DNA and Northern blotting for RNA detect electrophoretically separated genome sequences.
  3. In situ hybridization detects viral DNA or RNA within infected cells.

F. **Serology (history of the infection)**
  1. Serologic testing can determine the type and titer of antiviral antibodies in serum and the identity of viral antigens.
  2. Titers of antibody to key viral antigens indicate the stage of infection with Epstein-Barr virus and hepatitis B virus.
  3. Tests for specific antibody
      - Complement fixation, latex agglutination, ELISA, RIA
  4. Tests for defining serotype of a virus
      - Hemagglutination inhibition, viral neutralization

II. **Antiviral Drugs**
  A. **Overview**
  1. Because viruses use much of the host cell biochemical machinery, they offer fewer targets than bacteria for drugs that are effective antiviral agents but nontoxic to host cells.
  2. The primary potential targets of antiviral drugs are illustrated in Chapter 18, Fig. 18-5.

  B. **Common viruses treatable with antiviral drugs**
  1. The mechanism of action and approved uses of the major types of antiviral drugs are summarized in Table 20-1.
  2. The largest number of approved drugs are nucleoside analogues that disrupt replication of the viral genome in herpesviruses or HIV.

  C. **Mechanisms of viral resistance to drugs**
  1. Mutation in target protein (e.g., polymerase) or activating enzyme (e.g., thymidine kinase of herpes simplex virus) of antiviral drug.
  2. Rapid mutation rate of viruses can facilitate generation of resistance
  3. Resistance is rare when multiple drugs with different mechanisms are used for HIV (highly active antiretroviral therapy [HAART]).

III. **Antiviral Vaccines**
  A. **Passive immunization by administration of immunoglobulin (Table 20-2)**
      - Provides rapid, short-term protection
  1. Rabies gammaglobulin immediately after infection to block progression of the virus
  2. Varicella-zoster gammaglobulin for immunocompromised children (e.g., those with leukemia), postexposure for pregnant women up to 20 weeks, and newborns of mothers with active varicella-zoster virus infection
  3. Hepatitis A virus and hepatitis B virus gammaglobulin to block infection of liver after exposure
  4. Antibodies to respiratory syncytial virus protect early-term babies against life-threatening pneumonia

  B. **Active immunization (Table 20-3)**
  1. Live vaccines
      - Attenuated strains of virus, which will not cause serious disease in immunocompetent individuals
      a. Common vaccines include measles, mumps, rubella, influenza, and varicella-zoster, all of which are recommended for routine administration to young children.
      b. Live vaccines have a small probability of causing disease in immunocompromised individuals.
      c. The live oral polio vaccine (Sabin) is not recommended because of potential for reversion to virulence and production of disease.

PCR is a rapid, specific means to detect and identify DNA viruses.

RT-PCR is a rapid, specific means to detect and identify RNA viruses. Quantitative PCR is used to determine virus load for human immunodeficiency virus (HIV).

A fourfold increase in antibody titer between acute and chronic sera is necessary for a positive test.

Immunoglobulin M (IgM) indicates first time and early in the infection.

Acyclovir and related drugs must be phosphorylated by viral thymidine kinase to act; they are effective only against cells infected with herpesviruses that encode thymidine kinase.

Major viruses treatable with antiviral drugs: herpesviruses (herpes simplex virus, varicella-zoster virus, cytomegalovirus), influenza virus, HIV, respiratory syncytial virus

Live vaccines elicit a better memory response than killed vaccines; they provide longer-lasting immunity.

TABLE 20-1 **Antiviral Drugs***

DRUG	MECHANISM OF ACTION	APPROVED USES
Nucleoside Analogues		
Acyclovir Penciclovir Valacyclovir	Inhibit viral DNA polymerase by causing premature chain termination; activated by viral thymidine kinase	HSV VZV
Famciclovir		
Ganciclovir	Activated by viral kinase and inhibits viral DNA polymerase	
Valganciclovir		CMV
Iododeoxyuridine	Incorporated into viral genome, leading to trifluorothymidine errors in replication and transcription	HSV
Adefovir		HBV
Cidofovir		CMV
Azidothymidine Dideoxycytidine Dideoxyinosine Stavudine	Inhibit viral reverse transcriptase by causing premature chain termination; activated by host cell enzymes	HIV
Lamivudine	HIV, HBV	
Ribavirin	Inhibits GTP-requiring enzymes and induces hypermutation of viral genome	RSV Hepatitis C virus
Non-nucleoside Polymerase Inhibitors		
Phosphonoformate binds to pyrophosphate pocket in polymerase	Herpesviruses	
Nevirapine	Binds outside of active site of polymerase	HIV
Protease Inhibitors		
Saquinavir Ritonavir Indinavir	Bind to and inhibit viral protease, whose activity is needed for assembly of infectious virions	HIV
Other		
Amantadine Rimantadine	Inhibits uncoating of nucleocapsid by blocking H+ channel formed by M2 protein and reducing fusion of viral envelope with endosome membrane	Influenza A virus
Oseltamivir (Tamiflu)	Inhibits neuraminidase and viral release	Influenza A and B viruses
Zanamivir (Relenza)	Inhibits neuraminidase and viral release	Influenza A and B viruses
Phosphonoformate	Binds to viral DNA polymerase and inhibits its activity; requires no activation	CMV
Interferon-α	Induces antiviral state in noninfected cells that interferes with synthesis of viral mRNAs and proteins, thereby limiting spread of infection;	Hepatitis B and C viruses, HPV, also stimulates host immune response

*Viruses against the indicated drugs have been approved for use. A more complete list of anti-HIV drugs is provided in Chapter 26.
CMV, cytomegalovirus; GTP, guanosine triphosphate; HBV, hepatitis B virus; HIV, human immunodeficiency virus; HPV, human papillomavirus; HSV, herpes simplex virus; RSV, respiratory syncytial virus; VZV, varicella-zoster virus.

TABLE 20-2 **Passive Immunization Targets**

VIRUS	RECIPIENT
Hepatitis A	Contacts
Hepatitis B	Potentially infected individuals
Measles	Potentially infected individuals
Rabies	Potentially infected individuals
Respiratory syncytial virus	Premature newborns
Varicella-zoster virus	Immunocompromised children
Cytomegalovirus	Transplant recipients

TABLE 20-3 **Frequently Used Viral Vaccines**

VIRUS	TYPE OF VACCINE	INDICATIONS
Hepatitis A	Inactivated	Travelers
Hepatitis B	Subunit	Newborns, medical personnel, sexually promiscuous individuals, intravenous drug abusers
Human papilloma subunit virus	Young women aged 13-25 years (before sexual activity)	
Influenza	Inactivated	Adults, especially medical personnel and elderly patients
Influenza	Attenuated	Children (>2 yr) and adults (<60 yr)
Measles	Attenuated	Children
Mumps	Attenuated	Children
Polio	Inactivated (Salk vaccine)	Children (recommended)
	Attenuated (Sabin vaccine)	Children
Rotavirus	Attenuated or reassortant	Children
Rubella	Attenuated	Children
Varicella-zoster	Attenuated	Children (stronger form for adults [>60 yrs])

- Virus from another species that elicits a protective response in humans
  - a. Smallpox vaccine is prepared from vaccinia virus. With eradication of this virus, vaccination is no longer necessary.
  - b. Rotavirus vaccines consist of a reassortant (mixture) virus with gene segments from human and animal rotaviruses or an attenuated human rotavirus.
2. Inactivated vaccines
  - Whole viruses that are inactivated by heat or chemicals (e.g., Salk polio vaccine, influenza vaccines)
    - a. Influenza vaccines are prepared from viruses grown in eggs and may cause allergic reactions in some individuals.
  - Viral subunits that form into virus-like particles prepared by genetic engineering (e.g., hepatitis B vaccine, human papillomavirus vaccine).

Inactivated and live influenza vaccines are reformulated every year.

Polio vaccines: Salk = killed (inactivated) vaccine; IPV. Sabin = live (attenuated) vaccine given orally; oral polio virus

CHAPTER 21
NONENVELOPED (NAKED) DNA VIRUSES

Trigger words:
Adenovirus: conjunctivitis,
dense basophilic
intranuclear inclusion
bodies, diarrhea in infant,
hemorrhagic cystitis,
icosadeltahedral capsid
with fibers, infectious
genome, pharyngitis,
poorly chlorinated
swimming pools

Adenoviruses,
papillomaviruses, and
papovaviruses express
early and late proteins.

Adenoviruses,
papillomaviruses, and
papovaviruses inhibit
growth suppressing
p53 and RB proteins to
stimulate cell growth.

Virulence factors
for adenovirus: lytic
replication, persistence in
lymphoid tissue

Rotavirus: primary
cause of gastroenteritis
in infants and young
children; adenovirus:
second most important
cause

I. Adenoviridae
- Midsized viruses with a linear double-stranded DNA genome and naked, icosadeltahedral capsid that has fibers extending from the vertices.

A. Pathogenesis
1. Fibers extending from viral capsid bind to specific receptors on epithelial and other cells.
2. Primary lytic infection with accompanying inflammation occurs in mucous membranes of the respiratory tract, gastrointestinal tract, conjunctiva, and cornea.
3. Persistent, latent infection in lymphoid tissues (e.g., tonsils, adenoids, and Peyer patches) is common.
4. Viremia may occur.

B. Adenoviral illnesses (Table 21-1)
1. Incubation period for acute adenoviral illness is 4 to 9 days, but virions may be released for long periods, even after resolution of symptoms.
2. Acute, self-limited illness is the most common manifestation of adenoviral infection.
3. Infections occur primarily in children, military recruits, and immunocompromised individuals.

C. Laboratory identification
1. Dense, basophilic intranuclear inclusion body within infected cells is diagnostic of adenoviruses.

TABLE 21-1 **Common Illnesses Associated with Adenoviruses**

TYPE OF ILLNESS	CLINICAL FEATURES
Acute febrile pharyngitis	Fever, sore throat, cough, coryza, and other symptoms that may **mimic streptococcal infection** Most common in **young children** (<3 yr)
Acute respiratory disease	Rapid onset of fever, cough, sore throat, rhinorrhea, and cervical adenitis Occurs mostly in **military recruits**
Pharyngoconjunctival fever	Similar to acute pharyngitis but accompanied by **conjunctivitis** ("pink eye") Occurs in **older children,** often in outbreaks associated with use of **poorly chlorinated swimming pools** Preauricular lymphadenopathy important diagnostic finding
Atypical pneumonia	Nonproductive cough with pulmonary infiltrates and effusions Seen in children and adults
Epidemic keratoconjunctivitis	Inflamed pebbled conjunctiva (pink eye) in adults similar to conjunctivitis in children but of longer duration and followed by keratitis Usually associated with irritation to eye by dust or other debris
Gastroenteritis	Diarrhea with possible vomiting primarily in infants and young children due to serotypes 40-42 Other serotypes (e.g., 25-28) cause diarrhea in hospitalized patients.
Acute appendicitis	Lymphoid hyperplasia in appendix compromises blood supply leading to acute inflammation.

2. Adenovirus serotypes can be distinguished by immunoassay, DNA probe, or polymerase chain reaction (PCR) analysis of cultured specimens.
   - Common viruses have the lower serotype numbers; more than 47 serotypes are recognized.

  D. Transmission
1. As naked capsid viruses, adenoviruses are resistant to drying and detergents and are very contagious.
2. Virions are spread via aerosols, fecal-oral route, fomites, and close contact and in inadequately chlorinated swimming pools.

  E. Prevention and treatment
1. Live oral vaccine has been developed for military recruits against adenovirus types 4 and 7.
2. Supportive care is used to treat adenoviral infections.
   - No drug therapy is available.

  F. Adenovirus is used for gene replacement therapy and as a hybrid vaccine.

II. Papilloma and Polyomaviridae (Papova)

  A. Overview
1. The papillomaviruses and polyomaviruses are small, naked, icosahedral capsid viruses with double-stranded DNA genomes. They used to be grouped together as the Papovaviridae.
2. Lytic, chronic, latent, or transforming infections may be established depending on the host cell.

  B. Human papillomaviruses (HPVs)
1. Pathogenesis
   - HPVs infect and replicate in cutaneous and mucosal epithelial tissue.
   - Early viral proteins E6 and E7, which inactivate cellular tumor suppressor proteins (RB and p53 [TP53]), promote hyperplasia of host cells in the basal layer of infected epithelium.
2. Diseases associated with HPVs (Table 21-2)
   - More than 40 HPV serotypes are associated with epithelial lesions in different sites.
   - Clinical features, histology of lesions, and PCR are the usual basis for diagnosis of HPV infection because viruses cannot be isolated in tissue culture.
3. Association with cervical carcinoma: HPV 16, 18, 31, 33
4. Transmission
   - HPV is spread by direct contact with skin warts, through sexual contact with anogenital lesions, and from infected mother to infant during birth.
   - Asymptomatic shedding promotes spread via fomites.
5. Treatment and prevention
   - Warts
     a. Nonsurgical removal and injection with interferon-α
     b. Recurrences are common.
   - Laryngeal papillomas
     a. Surgical removal

Nonenveloped DNA viruses, including adenovirus, are resistant to detergent, acid, and the gut environment.

Adenovirus can be transmitted by aerosols, fecal-oral route, fomites, or close contact.

Adenoviruses (especially serotypes 4 and 7) are used in gene therapy.

Trigger words: Papillomavirus: cervical cancer, CIN, koilocytes, STD, warts

Virulence factors for HPV: immortalizing infection by certain strains, persistence, hidden from immune response

HPVs: benign skin and anogenital warts, cervical intraepithelial neoplasia, and cervical cancer (high-risk types: 16, 18, 31, 33) Sexually transmitted HPV diseases: condyloma acuminata (anogenital warts), HPV-induced cervical dysplasia, HPV-associated cervical cancer

TABLE 21-2 Diseases Caused by Human Papillomaviruses

CONDITION	SEROTYPES*	CLINICAL AND HISTOLOGIC FEATURES
Skin warts	1-4	Benign lesions on **keratinized surfaces** usually of hands and feet (not mucous membranes) Most common in **children** and **young adults** **Hyperplasia of prickle cells** and **hyperkeratosis** seen microscopically
Anogenital wart (condyloma acuminata)	6, 11	Benign growths on **squamous epithelium** of external genitalia and perianal regions Thickened epithelium with fibrous overgrowths
Laryngeal papillomas	6, 11	Benign tumors, can be life threatening in children owing to **airway obstruction** Most common in **children** and **middle-aged adults**
Cervical intraepithelial neoplasia	16, 18	Progressive changes in **cervical mucosa** leading to **dysplasia** and possible **carcinoma in situ** **Koilocytotic cells** (pyknotic nuclei and cytoplasmic vacuoles) seen on Papanicolaou test

*Most common serotypes associated with particular condition; others may also cause similar manifestations.

- Imiquimod
  a. Stimulator of toll-like receptor and inflammation
- Cidofovir
  a. Nucleotide analogue
- Vaccine containing capsid protein formed into virus like particles for HPV 16, 18, 6, 11 or HPV 16, 18 to block HPV infection and papillomas and to prevent cervical carcinoma
  a. Offered before sexual activity to young women aged 11 to 26 years.

C. **Polyomaviruses**
  - BK virus and JC virus, the only human pathogens in this group, are ubiquitous but rarely cause disease in healthy individuals.
  - Polyomavirus genome is circular double-stranded DNA.
  1. Pathogenesis
     - Primary infection of the kidney by BK or JC virus is generally asymptomatic and becomes latent.
     - Reactivation of latent infection may occur in immunocompromised individuals and pregnant women.
  2. Reactivation diseases (in immunocompromised individuals)
     - Progressive multifocal leukoencephalopathy (PML) results from reactivation of JC virus, followed by viremia and spread to the central nervous system.
       a. Patients undergo slow accumulation (*progressive*) of multiple (*multifocal*) neurologic symptoms, including impairment of speech, sight, coordination, and mental abilities leading to paralysis and death.
       b. Brain tissue histology shows abnormal oligodendrocytes near areas of demyelination.
     - Urinary tract infection, which may be severe, and viruria (viral shedding in the urine) result from reactivation of BK virus.
     - BK virus reactivation is prevalent in kidney transplant recipients.

III. **Parvoviridae**
  - This family of very small viruses with a naked, icosahedral capsid and linear single-stranded DNA genome includes only one human pathogen, parvovirus B19.

A. **Pathogenesis**
  1. Initial infection with B19 at the site of entry (usually upper respiratory tract) is followed by viremic spread to rapidly dividing erythroid precursor cells in bone marrow.
  2. Cytolytic replication in erythroid precursor cells and subsequent immune response cause manifestations of B19 infection.

B. **Diseases caused by parvovirus B19**
  1. Erythema infectiosum (fifth disease) is a biphasic disease that occurs mainly in children aged 4 to 15 years.
     - Initial phase, reflecting lytic infection, is marked by nonspecific flu-like symptoms and decreased hemoglobin levels.
     - Immune-mediated phase, beginning 2 to 3 weeks later, is characterized by rash and arthralgia.
       a. Slapped-cheek rash appears first on the face and then spreads to arms and legs.
       b. It lasts 1 to 2 weeks.
  2. Polyarthritis in adults may not be preceded by rash.
     - Predominately affects knees, hands, wrists, and ankles
  3. Aplastic crisis may result from B19 infection in those with sickle cell disease or other chronic hemolytic anemia.
     - Transient reticulocytopenia (7 to 10 days) leads to decreased hemoglobin levels.
     - Symptoms include fever, malaise, itching, chills, possibly arthralgia, maculopapular rash, and joint swelling.
  4. Fetal infection results in stillbirth (hydrops fetalis) but *not* in congenital abnormalities.

HPV vaccine will prevent cervical carcinoma.

Trigger words:
Polyomaviruses: JC virus: opportunistic disease, PML, abnormal oligodendrocytes, demyelination; BK virus: kidney

Virulence factors for polyomaviruses: persistent infection

PML is an opportunistic disease seen in acquired immunodeficiency syndrome (AIDS) patients, transplant recipients, and chronic immunocompromised individuals.

Trigger words:
Parvovirus B19: aplastic anemia, fifth disease, lacy-patterned rash, slapped cheeks, sickle crisis

Virulence factors for parvovirus: lytic infection of erythroid precursor cells.

B19 infects and compromises erythroid precursors leading to transient anemia.

B19 is the only human parvoviral pathogen. B19 erythema infectiosum is one of the five classic childhood rashes with measles, chickenpox, roseola, and rubella.

B19 infection of people with anemia may go into aplastic crisis.

CHAPTER 22
ENVELOPED DNA VIRUSES

I. Herpesviridae
- This family comprises large viruses with an enveloped, icosadeltahedral capsid and a linear, double-stranded DNA genome.
- All three subfamilies (alpha, beta, and gamma) contain significant human pathogens, which can establish primary lytic or persistent infection, as well as latent and recurrent infections (Table 22-1).

A. Herpes simplex viruses type 1 (HSV-1) and type 2 (HSV-2)
1. Pathogenesis
   - Initial infection and viral replication occur in mucoepithelial cells.
   - Characteristic HSV lesions associated with lytic infection are due to virus-induced cytopathic effects and inflammatory reactions.
   - Latent infection, causing no detectable damage, is established in sensory ganglia (neurotropic) innervating the site of the initial lesion.
   - Reactivation of latent HSV may be induced by emotional or physical stress, certain foods, or immune suppression.
     a. After reactivation, virus travels to peripheral tissue and replicates, causing **recurrence** of lesions.

Herpesviruses are large, enveloped DNA viruses that establish lytic and latent infections and are controlled by cell-mediated immunity.

The herpesviruses are ubiquitous.

The herpesvirus genome replicates in the nucleus.

Herpesviruses encode DNA-dependent DNA polymerase

Herpesviruses undergo immediate-early, early, and late stages of protein synthesis.

Trigger words:
Herpes simplex virus: Cowdry type A inclusion bodies, syncytia, destruction of temporal lobe, DNA, encephalitis, enveloped, keratoconjunctivitis, multinucleated giant cells, neonatal HSV, neurotropic, stress-induced recurrence, Tzanck smear, vesicular lesion

HSV virulence factors: lytic-latent infection, immune escape, neuronal infection, syncytia, and cell-to-cell transmission

TABLE 22-1 **Herpesviruses**

VIRUS	DISEASES	MAJOR SITE OF LATENCY	COMMON MODE OF TRANSMISSION
Alpha Subfamily			
HSV-1	Oral herpes, encephalitis, keratoconjunctivitis; also HSV-2 diseases	Sensory ganglia	Direct contact with lesions
HSV-2	Genital herpes, neonatal herpes, meningitis; also HSV-1 diseases	Sensory ganglia	Direct contact with lesions
VZV	Chickenpox (primary), shingles (recurrent)	Sensory ganglia	Aerosols
Gamma Subfamily			
EBV	Infectious mononucleosis; hairy oral leukoplakia (in AIDS); Burkitt lymphoma, nasopharyngeal carcinoma	B cells	Saliva (kissing)
HHV-8	Kaposi sarcoma (in AIDS)	?	Saliva
Beta Subfamily			
CMV	Congenital disease; hepatitis, pneumonia, and retinitis in immunocompromised; heterophile-negative mononucleosis	Monocytes, lymphocytes	Body fluids, transplacental, transplants
HHV-6	Roseola (exanthem subitum)	T and B cells	Aerosols

AIDS, acquired immunodeficiency syndrome; CMV, cytomegalovirus; EBV, Epstein-Barr virus; HHV, human herpesvirus; HSV, herpes simplex virus; VZV, varicella-zoster virus.

HSV-1 (generally above the waist) → herpes labialis (fever blisters and cold sores), gingivostomatitis, temporal lobe encephalitis

HSV-2 (generally below the waist) → herpes genitalis, neonatal herpes (disseminated), meningitis

HSV infection can be detected in a Tzanck or Pap smear by presence of syncytia or Cowdry type A nuclear inclusion bodies.

HSV is spread by mixing and matching of mucous membranes ("4 Ms")

HSV thymidine kinase activates nucleotide analogue antiviral drugs that target HSV polymerase.

Valacyclovir is a derivative of acyclovir, and famciclovir is a derivative of penciclovir.

Trigger words:
Varicella-zoster virus: all stages of lesions at once, chickenpox, Cowdry type A nuclear inclusion bodies, crops of vesicular lesions, dermatome distribution of vesicles, latency, multinucleated giant cells (syncytia), neurotropic, shingles, thymidine kinase, vesicles

Unlike HSV, VZV is transmitted by aerosols and contact, is spread by viremia, and recurs and causes lesions along the entire neuronal dermatome (zoster).

Unlike smallpox, all stages of VZV rash are present at the same time.

2. HSV diseases
   - Overview
     a. Clinical manifestations of HSV infection depend on the tissue infected. Recurrent disease is less severe than primary infection and may be asymptomatic.
     b. HSV-1 and HSV-2 cause disease at the site of infection and cause similar disease presentations.
   - Classic HSV lesions are vesicular with an erythematous base.
     a. Appear about 3 days after exposure and can last up to 2 weeks (primary herpes)
   - Oral herpes (herpes labialis and gingivostomatosis) is caused primarily by HSV-1 in children and also by HSV-2 in young adults.
   - Genital herpes is most commonly caused by HSV-2.
   - Encephalitis and keratoconjunctivitis are usually due to HSV-1.
     a. Meningitis is usually due to HSV-2.
   - Disseminated infection and more severe disease occur in individuals with compromised cell-mediated immunity and in neonates.
3. Laboratory identification
   - Characteristic cytopathic effects are observed in vesicle fluid, biopsy samples from affected tissue (Tzanck smear and Papanicolaou smear), or cultured infected cells.
     a. Rounded cells with extensive cell death
     b. Syncytia (multinucleated giant cells)
     c. Cowdry type A acidophilic nuclear inclusion bodies
   - Immunoassays for type-specific viral antigens can detect and distinguish HSV-1 and HSV-2.
   - Polymerase chain reaction detection of HSV nucleic acids in cerebrospinal fluid is used in diagnosis of encephalitis.
4. Transmission and incidence
   - Direct contact with vesicle fluid or virus-containing mucus (e.g., by kissing, sharing utensils, sexual contact, autoinoculation, and passage through birth canal) spreads HSV.
   - HSV-1 is ubiquitous, and more than 90% of the population is infected in childhood.
   - HSV-2 is usually transmitted sexually and acquired later in life by about 30% of the population.
5. Treatment
   - Acyclovir, penciclovir, famciclovir, and valacyclovir are the most common anti-HSV drugs.
     a. Once activated by viral thymidine kinase, these nucleoside analogues inhibit viral DNA polymerase.
     b. Prophylactic treatment is common.
   - Drug-resistant strains have mutation in thymidine kinase or DNA polymerase.

B. **Varicella-zoster virus (VZV)**
   1. Overview
      - Like HSV, VZV causes vesicular lesions and establishes latency in neurons.
      - VZV differs from HSV in its transmission (aerosols), usual site of entry (respiratory tract), and spread within the body (through lymphatics and the bloodstream).
   2. Chickenpox
      - Primary VZV disease (Fig. 22-1)
      - Skin lesions first appear on the trunk, 10 to 14 days after exposure (maximum, 90 days), and then on the peripheral regions of the body, including the scalp.
        a. Lesions progress from initial macule → papule → vesicle → pustule → crusts.
        b. A thin-walled vesicle on a maculopapular base (dewdrop on a rose petal) is the hallmark of chickenpox.
      - Chickenpox is generally benign and self-limited in otherwise healthy children, but it can be life threatening in immunocompromised children.
        a. Disease is more severe in adults, with significant potential for pneumonia to develop.
      - Respiratory spread before the onset of symptoms is the primary mode of transmission of VZV.
      - Risk for developing Reye syndrome if child takes aspirin
   3. Herpes zoster (shingles)
      - Recurrent VZV disease
        a. Results from reactivation of latent VZV in neurons, often years after primary infection

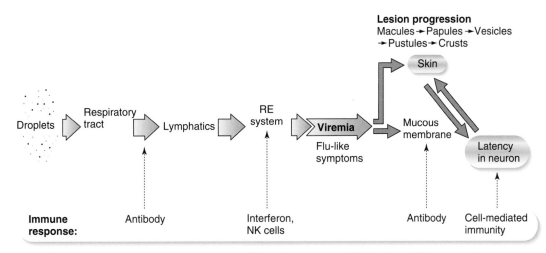

Lesion progression
Macules → Papules → Vesicles
→ Pustules → Crusts

22-1: Pathogenesis and spread of varicella-zoster virus (VZV) within the body. VZV initially establishes lytic infection in mucoepithelial cells of the respiratory tract. Spread of virions by the reticuloendothelial (RE) system and bloodstream to other parts of the body causes flu-like symptoms (fever, malaise, and headache), followed by the appearance of the characteristic skin lesions of chickenpox. Reactivation of latent infection in neurons later in life causes herpes zoster (shingles). The spread of virions can be blocked by various components of the immune response at the indicated stages.

- Shingles usually begins with severe pain along a single dermatome, followed by eruption of a belt of maculopapular lesions on an erythematous base.
- Thoracic and lumbar dermatomes are most commonly involved, but recurrence can occur along the trigeminal nerve or any dermatome.
4. Laboratory identification
- Diagnosis of VZV is generally made on the basis of clinical symptoms.
- Multinucleated giant cells and Cowdry type A nuclear inclusion bodies are present in VZV-infected cells from clinical specimens.
5. Prevention and treatment
- Live attenuated varicella vaccine is recommended for children at 15 months and for nonimmune adults.
- Stronger varicella vaccine is recommended for adults at risk for zoster (>60 years of age)
- Antiviral drugs: acyclovir, famciclovir, or valacyclovir
- Varicella-zoster immunoglobulin is used for immunocompromised children who have been exposed.
C. **Epstein-Barr virus (EBV)**
1. Pathogenesis
- Infects B cells in the oropharynx (e.g., tonsils) after attaching to CD21 (C3d receptor)
a. Initial lytic infection of the B cells leads to shedding of virions into the saliva and surrounding lymphoid tissue.
- Nonproductive infection of B cells induces their proliferation with production of immunoglobulin M (IgM) heterophile antibodies
- Cell-mediated response to EBV-infected B cells is essential for resolving infection and is largely responsible for lymphocytosis and other symptoms associated with acute disease.
- Virus may remain dormant in B cells, causing recurrences
2. Heterophile antibody-positive infectious mononucleosis (Fig. 22-2)
- Disease is milder in children than in adolescents or adults.
a. Symptom triad of lymphadenopathy, splenomegaly, exudative pharyngitis
- Additional findings include extreme fatigue, fever, and headache.
- Serological confirmation (see later)
b. Rash appears if the patient is given ampicillin (*not* an allergic reaction).
c. Saliva containing shed virions is the usual means of spreading EBV, most commonly during kissing or shared drinking glasses, bottles, and so forth.
- Asymptomatic infection or recurrence with virion production in oropharynx is common and promotes transmission.
a. Peak incidence of infectious mononucleosis occurs among adolescents and young adults.
- Much of the population is seropositive by 30 years of age.

VZV: latent infection in neurons; chickenpox (primary) and shingles (recurrent)

Both VZV and HSV produce similar cytopathic effects: multinucleated giant cells (syncytia) and Cowdry type A nuclear inclusion bodies.

Trigger words:
Epstein-Barr virus: ampicillin-induced rash, atypical lymphocytes, B cell, fatigue, heterophile antibody, lymphocytosis, mononucleosis, monospot test, pharyngitis, rash

Virulence factors: lytic, latent, and immortalizing infection of B lymphocytes.

EBV: Infection of B cells causes infectious mononucleosis, immortalizes B cells, and is associated with Burkitt's lymphoma.

EBV laboratory data: atypical lymphocytes, heterophile antibody, hyperplasia, EBV-specific antibodies

EBV is shed into saliva and transmitted by saliva sharing.

EBV symptomatic triad: lymphadenopathy, splenomegaly, exudative pharyngitis

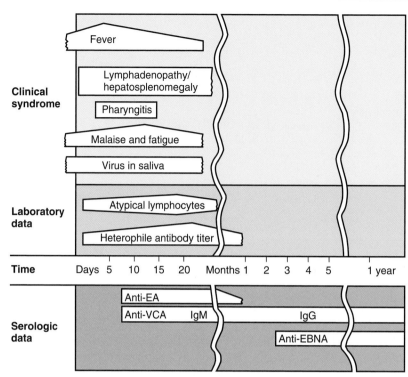

22-2: Clinical course and laboratory findings of primary infection with Epstein-Barr virus (EBV). Infection may be asymptomatic or produce the symptoms of infectious mononucleosis. The incubation period can be as long as 2 months, and resolution takes weeks to months. Early antigen (EA), viral capsid antigen (VCA), and Epstein-Barr nuclear antigen (EBNA) are viral antigens.

3. Laboratory identification
   - Atypical lymphocytes (Downey cells) are antigenically activated T cells on blood smear.
   - Heterophile antibody is detected by heterophile antibody test or enzyme-linked immunosorbent assay.
     a. Heterophile antibody, an early IgM response from EBV-activated B cells, cross-reacts with the Paul-Bunnell antigen on sheep, horse, or bovine (not guinea pig) erythrocytes, causing agglutination.
   - Epstein-Barr nuclear antigen (EBNA) is a late marker of infection present in all infected cells.
   - Antibodies to early antigen (EA) and viral capsid antigen (VCA) are detectable during active infection.
   - Antibodies to EBNA are produced after resolution of infection after release of EBNA due to T cell killing of infected cells.
4. Other diseases caused by EBV
   - Hairy oral leukoplakia
     a. Raised, corrugated white lesions that do not scrape off in mouth, especially on the tongue
     b. Occurs only in immunosuppressed patients, especially patients with acquired immunodeficiency syndrome (AIDS)
   - Neoplasms associated with EBV transforming activity
     a. Burkitt lymphoma (prevalent malarial region of Africa)
        - Infection of B cells by EBV is a contributing factor.
        - Increased mitoses increases risk for a t(8;14) translocation.
     b. Nasopharyngeal carcinoma (prevalent in Asia)
        - Tissue tropism of EBV for oropharynx is a contributing factor.
     c. Primary central nervous system lymphoma in patients with AIDS
   - Mixed-cellularity Hodgkin lymphoma
D. **Cytomegalovirus (CMV)**
   1. Pathogenesis
      - CMV infects most cell types.
      - Initial nonlytic infection primarily of epithelial cells is followed by latent infection of monocytes, macrophages, and lymphocytes.
      - Cytopathic effects detectable in infected cells
        a. Large basophilic (owl's eye) nuclear inclusion body
        b. Hypertrophied (cytomegalic) cells

Monospot test uses horse erythrocytes to detect heterophile antibody associated with infectious mononucleosis.

EBV, human papillomavirus, human T lymphotrophic virus, and hepatitis B virus are associated with human cancers.

Trigger words:
Cytomegalovirus: congenital CMV, intracerebral calcifications, large owl's-eye nuclear inclusion body, mononucleosis-like syndrome, microcephaly, opportunistic disease, swollen *(megalo)* cells

Virulence factors: latent infection of most cells

- Cell-mediated immune response generally controls and resolves infection in immunocompetent individuals.
  a. Immunosuppression allows reactivation of latent infection and subsequent disease manifestations.
2. Diseases due to CMV
  - CMV infection of children and adults is usually asymptomatic.
  - Congenital CMV infection
    a. Virions produced in the mother can cross the placenta and infect the fetus.
    b. Symptoms include rash, periventricular cerebral calcification, hepatosplenomegaly, deafness, microcephaly (small head), and mental retardation.
    c. Most severe manifestations are associated with primary maternal infection during pregnancy.
    d. Less severe manifestations are associated with recurrent infection in a seropositive mother.
  - Opportunistic diseases in immunosuppressed individuals, especially AIDS patients and transplant recipients
    a. Chorioretinitis (blindness), pneumonia, esophagitis, colitis, pancreatitis, hepatitis, or encephalitis may develop.
  - Heterophile antibody-negative mononucleosis syndrome
    a. Mild disease in immunocompetent individuals is usually acquired sexually or from transfused blood.
E. **Other herpesviruses pathogenic in humans**
  1. Human herpesvirus-6
    - Causes roseola (exanthem subitum; sixth disease), a common benign disease of children marked by high fever and later a rash due to an immune response
  2. **Human herpesvirus-8**
    - Associated with Kaposi sarcoma primarily in AIDS patients
F. **Case presentations of common herpes infections (Box 22-1)**

CMV: generally asymptomatic except for congenital disease and in immunosuppressed patients

CMV: most common viral cause of congenital defects: cerebral calcification, deafness, microcephaly, mental retardation

CMV is controlled by an effective cell-mediated immunity but recurs in its absence.

Heterophile-negative mononucleosis is caused by CMV, toxoplasma and occurs during the initial phase of HIV infection.

Roseola is one of the six childhood rashes.

BOX 22-1 HERPESVIRUS INFECTIONS: QUICK CASES

Herpes Simplex Viruses

Primary oral herpes: A 5-year-old boy has an ulcerative rash, with vesicles, around the mouth. Vesicles and ulcers are also present throughout the mouth. Tzanck smear shows multinucleated giant squamous cells and Cowdry type A inclusion bodies.

Primary vaginal herpes: A sexually active woman in her mid-20s has ulcerative lesions on the vagina with pain, itching, dysuria, and systemic symptoms, including fever lasting 10 days. Pap smear shows multinucleated squamous cells and Cowdry type A inclusion bodies.

Encephalitis: A patient has focal neurologic symptoms and seizures. Magnetic resonance imaging shows destruction of the temporal lobe. Erythrocytes are present in the cerebrospinal fluid, and polymerase chain reaction is positive for viral DNA.

Varicella-Zoster Virus

Varicella (chickenpox): A 5-year-old boy develops a fever and maculopapular rash on his abdomen 14 days after a school trip to the local natural history museum. Successive lesions appear for 3 to 5 days, and the rash spreads peripherally.

Zoster (shingles): A 65-year-old woman has a belt of vesicles along the thoracic dermatome and experiences severe pain localized to the region.

Epstein-Barr Virus

Infectious mononucleosis: A 23-year-old college student develops severe malaise, fatigue, fever, swollen glands, and pharyngitis. After treatment with ampicillin, a rash appears. Heterophile antibodies are present, and atypical lymphocytes are noted in the blood smear.

Cytomegalovirus

Congenital cytomegalovirus infection: A neonate exhibits microcephaly, periventricular cerebral calcification, hepatosplenomegaly, and rash. The mother had symptoms similar to mononucleosis during the first trimester of her pregnancy.

Human Herpesvirus-6

Roseola (exanthem subitum): A 4-year-old child experiences a rapid onset of a high fever that lasts for 3 days and then suddenly returns to normal. Two days later, a maculopapular rash appears on the trunk and spreads to other areas of the body.

Smallpox is a large, enveloped, DNA virus with a characteristic boxcar, complex shape.

Poxviruses are an exception; they replicate in the cytoplasm and carry an RNA polymerase.

II. Poxviridae

A. Overview

1. This family consists of large, complex, brick-shaped viruses with a linear, double-stranded DNA genome.
2. Unlike all other DNA viruses, poxviruses replicate in the cytoplasm. Virions carry RNA polymerase for synthesizing messenger RNAs, and virus-encoded DNA polymerase produces progeny genomes.

B. Variola virus

1. Human virus causing smallpox, which is now eradicated
2. Vaccination with vaccinia virus was used in eradication efforts against smallpox.
   - Vaccination of military and health care personnel has been reinitiated because of bioterror threat.
   - Routine vaccination has been discontinued because of risk for serious side effects.
   - Contacts of vaccinated individuals are at risk for disseminated vaccinia.

C. Animal pox viruses (e.g., vaccinia, orf, monkeypox)

   - May cause disease in humans

D. Molluscum contagiosum virus

1. Human virus that causes small raised, umbilicated lesions on the trunk, genitals, and proximal extremities
2. Lesions occur singly or in groups and have a central granular plug containing virions (molluscum bodies)
3. Infection is benign, usually self-limited, and transmitted by close contact or fomites.
4. All populations are susceptible.
5. May be disseminated in human immunodeficiency virus (HIV)

III. Hepadnaviridae

   - The only human pathogen in this family is hepatitis B virus, discussed in Chapter 27.

CHAPTER 23

NONENVELOPED (NAKED) RNA VIRUSES

I. Picornaviridae

- This family of small viruses with a naked, icosahedral capsid and single-stranded (+) RNA genome includes the enteroviruses and rhinoviruses.

A. Enteroviruses: poliovirus, Coxsackie A virus, Coxsackie B virus, echovirus, and hepatitis A virus (see Chapter 27)

- The enteroviruses are acid stable, can survive in the gastrointestinal (GI) tract, and are transmitted primarily by the fecal-oral route.

1. Pathogenesis (Fig. 23-1)

- Initial replication occurs in the mucosa and lymphoid tissues of the pharynx and tonsils and subsequently in the GI tract.
- Viremic spread of virions to target tissues depends on tissue specificity (tropism) of the virus.

   a. Poliovirus binds to receptors on muscle cells and neurons, causing disease in the central nervous system (CNS).

   b. Coxsackie viruses and echoviruses have a broader tissue tropism, causing disease in the CNS, lungs, heart, pancreas, and other tissues.

- Cytolytic replication in target tissues causes direct tissue damage.

Microinjection of picornavirus or calicivirus genome (+RNA) into cells is sufficient for infection.

Picornavirus, calicivirus, and reovirus are resistant to detergent and acid and are transmitted by fecal-oral route.

Virulence of enterovirus lytic infection; certain viruses are neurotropic

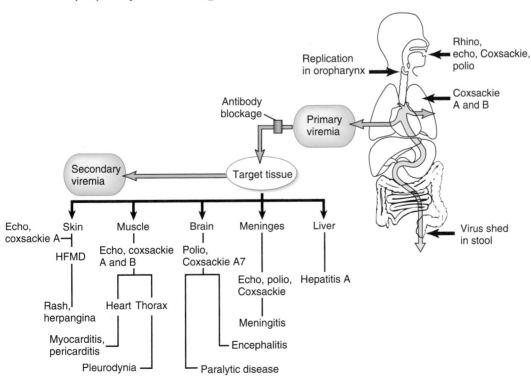

23-1: Pathogenesis of picornaviruses. All of the enteroviruses can be spread by the fecal-oral route but cause different diseases depending on the target tissue that is infected. Some enteroviruses, like the rhinoviruses, can be spread by respiratory means and cause symptoms of the common cold. HFMD, hand-foot-and-mouth disease.

BOX 23-1 ENTEROVIRUS INFECTIONS: QUICK CASES

Poliovirus
Poliomyelitis: A 15-year-old Burmese boy experiences fever, headache, nausea, and a stiff neck for 24 to 36 hours. His condition improves for several days, and the same symptoms return, accompanied by increasing weakness and paralysis of the legs. His medical history indicates that he had *not* been vaccinated against poliovirus.

Coxsackie A Virus
Herpangina: During summer vacation, a 7-year-old child develops a sudden fever accompanied by loss of appetite, sore throat, vomiting, and pain on swallowing. Examination shows discrete vesiculopapular lesions on the tongue and roof of the mouth.
Acute hemorrhagic conjunctivitis: A young girl has swollen eyelids with redness, congestion, and pain in her eyes. Several other children who attend the same nursery school show similar symptoms.

Coxsackie B Virus
Epidemic pleurodynia: A 13-year-old boy suddenly develops a fever and severe paroxysmal chest pain, which lasts for 4 days. He also complains of headache, fatigue, and aching muscles.

Coxsackievirus or Echovirus
Aseptic (viral) meningitis: A 9-month-old girl has a fever and skin rash and is suffering from nausea. She appears listless and has difficulty moving her head from side to side. CSF analysis shows normal glucose, no bacteria, and an increase of proteins and lymphocytes. Within 1 week, the infant is fully recovered.

Trigger words:
Poliovirus: asymmetric flaccid paralysis, fecal-oral, major disease, minor disease, picornavirus

Coxsackie and echoviruses: picornavirus, fecal-oral, Coxsackie B (for Body), myocarditis, pleurodynia; Coxsackie A virus: hand foot and mouth disease, vesicular lesions.

Coxsackie B (B is for body) virus can cause life-threatening pericarditis and myocarditis in infants; it usually causes asymptomatic or mild disease in older children and adults.

2. Diseases due to enteroviruses (Box 23-1)
   - Poliomyelitis
     a. Usually caused by **poliovirus** but also Coxsackie A virus
     b. Abortive poliomyelitis (minor illness)
     c. Nonparalytic poliomyelitis (aseptic meningitis): fever, headache, sore throat, stiff neck, pleocytosis of cerebrospinal fluid (CSF)
     d. Paralytic poliomyelitis (major illness): same symptoms as nonparalytic polio plus flaccid paralysis resulting from destruction of lower motor neurons
        - Paralytic polio is more common when exposure does not occur until late childhood or adulthood.
   - Herpangina and hand-foot-and-mouth disease: Coxsackie A virus
     a. Self-limited diseases of young children marked by vesicular lesions with mild fever
   - Acute hemorrhagic conjunctivitis: Coxsackie A virus
   - Epidemic pleurodynia (Bornholm disease): Coxsackie B virus
     a. Sudden, sharp paroxysmal chest pain with fever, usually seen in adolescents or young adults
   - Aseptic (viral) meningitis with possible rash: Coxsackie viruses, echoviruses
   - Respiratory infection with symptoms of common cold: Coxsackie viruses, echoviruses
   - Fatal neonatal disease: echovirus 11, Coxsackie B virus
3. Laboratory identification
   - Isolation from feces and growth in an appropriate cell culture system (if available)
   - Serologic tests to detect virus-specific immunoglobulin M (IgM) antibody or a fourfold increase in specific IgG antibody
   - Reverse transcriptase–polymerase chain reaction (RT-PCR) to detect virus in CSF, blood, or other clinical samples
4. Transmission
   - All enteroviruses can be spread by the fecal-oral route.
   - Coxsackie viruses and echoviruses are also spread by aerosols.
   - Wild-type polio exists only in Africa and Southeast Asia.
5. Prevention and treatment
   - Polio vaccines are part of the recommended childhood vaccination regimen.
     a. Salk vaccine is formalin-inactivated polio vaccine (IPV).
     b. Sabin vaccine is live oral polio vaccine (OPV).
        - OPV is a mixture of the three poliovirus types.
        - Live vaccine poses a risk for reversion to virulence and a risk in immunocompromised individuals.
     c. Killed (IPV) vaccine is currently recommended where natural polio has been eradicated.
   - Pleconaril, a drug with antienteroviral activity, is available but not yet in common use.

OPV is a live attenuated vaccine that is not recommended for use in the Western Hemisphere.

IPV is recommended.

B. Rhinoviruses
1. Overview
   - In contrast to the enteroviruses, the rhinoviruses are acid labile and transmitted primarily by aerosols or on fomites.
   - More than 100 rhinovirus serotypes cause the "common cold."
2. Pathogenesis
   - Rhinoviruses cannot replicate at temperatures of the lower lung (>33°C)
   - Replication occurs primarily in the nasal mucosa and conjunctiva, causing edema of subepithelial tissue and release of inflammatory mediators responsible for many of the symptoms.
   - Secretory IgA and interferons produced in response to infection limit spread of rhinovirus within the body.
3. Rhinoviral upper respiratory tract infection (common cold)
   - Usual symptoms include sneezing, rhinorrhea (runny nose), headache, sore throat, and malaise.
     a. Fever and chills may occur.
   - Infection peaks in 3 to 4 days, but cough and nasal symptoms may last 7 to 10 days.
   - May be associated with acute sinusitis due to blockage of sinus drainage
4. Incidence
   - Active illness is seen in 50% of those infected.
   - Asymptomatic individuals can spread rhinoviruses.
   - Highest infection rates occur in infants and children.

II. Caliciviridae (Norwalk and Related Viruses)
- This family comprises very small viruses with a naked, icosahedral capsid and single-stranded (+) RNA genome.
- Virus structure and replication resemble picornaviruses.

A. Norwalk virus
1. Pathogenesis
   - Brush border function is compromised by infection, preventing proper absorption of water and nutrients, hence diarrhea.
   - Delayed gastric emptying may also occur, causing vomiting.
2. Gastroenteritis due to Norwalk virus
   - Incubation period of 24 to 60 hours is followed by watery diarrhea with nausea and vomiting for 12 to 60 hours.
   - Fever is present in one third of cases.
   - Illness is self-limited and may be treated with bismuth salicylate to reduce symptoms.
3. Transmission
   - Norwalk virus is spread by the fecal-oral route through contaminated food and water.
   - Outbreaks can be traced to a common source and often occur in contained environments (e.g., cruise ships and schools).

III. Reoviridae
- This family consists of medium-sized viruses with a naked double capsid and segmented double-stranded RNA genome.

A. Rotaviruses
1. Pathogenesis
   - Partial digestion of virions within the GI tract yields infectious particles that directly penetrate the plasma membrane of intestinal epithelial cells.
   - Cholera toxin-like virion protein induces loss of electrolytes, and inability to reabsorb water results from infection of intestinal mucosa.
   - Massive shedding of virions occurs during diarrhea, contributing to transmission of infection.
   - Secretory IgA antibodies in the intestine confer immunity to rotavirus infection.
2. Rotavirus gastroenteritis
   - Incubation period: about 48 hours
   - Symptoms
     a. Watery diarrhea, vomiting, and fever last for 4 or 5 days.
     b. Possible dehydration
   - Severity
     a. Disease is self-limited, and complete recovery usually occurs.
     b. Disease is most severe in infants and may potentially be fatal (due to dehydration) in infants who are malnourished and dehydrated before infection.
     c. Children older than 2 years of age and adults usually develop only mild diarrhea.

Trigger words:
Rhinovirus: heat and pH labile, many serotypes, runny nose, picornavirus

Rhinovirus is the exception to the picornaviruses and acid labile.

Major causes of common colds: rhinovirus, enterovirus, parainfluenza virus, respiratory syncytial virus, coronavirus

Trigger words:
Norwalk virus: cruise ships, nausea, outbreaks of diarrheal disease, schools, watery diarrhea and vomiting

Norwalk virus and other caliciviruses: outbreaks of diarrhea with nausea and vomiting; illness resolves quickly

Reoviruses have a double-stranded segmented RNA genome in a double capsid: *double-double*

Virulence: segmented genome can reassert, fecal-oral transmission, cholera toxin-like induction of diarrhea

Rotaviral infection: most important cause of infant gastroenteritis worldwide

3. Laboratory identification
   - Viral antigens in stool specimens detected by enzyme-linked immunosorbent assay or latex agglutination tests
   - Virions in stool specimens visualized by electron microscopy
4. Transmission
   - Fecal-oral route is primary means of spreading rotaviruses, especially in preschools and day care centers.
5. Prevention and treatment
   - Vaccines include attenuated human virus or hybrid vaccine composed of reassorted components from animal and human rotaviruses.
   - Fluid replacement therapy is needed in severe cases with dehydration.

B. Colorado tick fever virus
1. This reovirus, which is spread by wood ticks, is found in the western and northwestern United States and in Canada.
2. Infection causes a mild clinical syndrome similar to dengue fever, which is usually self-limited.

CHAPTER 24
LARGE ENVELOPED RNA VIRUSES

I. Paramyxoviridae
A. Overview
1. This family consists of large viruses with an enveloped, helical nucleocapsid and (–) RNA genome.
2. Viruses are distinguished by the types of glycoproteins.
   - Parainfluenza and mumps: hemagglutinin-neuraminidase (HN) and F proteins
   - Measles: hemagglutinin (H) and F proteins
   - Respiratory syncytial virus (RSV): nonhemagglutinating glycoprotein (G) and F proteins

B. Shared pathogenic properties
1. Entry into target cells
   - Viral attachment proteins bind to sialic acid or protein receptor.
   - A fusion (F) protein or activity promotes envelope fusion with target cell membrane and release of nucleocapsid into cytoplasm.
2. Target cells
   - Epithelial cells of the upper respiratory tract are the site of initial infection by paramyxoviruses.
   - Viremic spread of measles virus and mumps virus leads to infection in various sites throughout the body.
   - No viremia occurs with parainfluenza virus and RSV, which remain localized to the respiratory tract.
3. Formation of multinucleated cells (syncytia)
   - Infected cells form syncytia, which allow cell-to-cell spread of virions and evasion of antibodies.
4. Host immune responses:
   - Good interferon inducers and highly sensitive to interferon
   - Resolution of infection depends on cell-mediated or inflammatory responses, which are also responsible for most disease manifestations.

C. Measles virus (Box 24-1)
1. Overview
   - Measles virus is a strictly human virus with only one serotype. Infection is usually diagnosed clinically.
   - Viremic spread from upper respiratory tract and local lymph nodes can lead to infection of the conjunctiva, urinary tract, small blood vessels, lymphatic system, and central nervous system (CNS).
2. Measles clinical manifestations
   - This serious febrile illness has an incubation period of 7 to 13 days.
   - Prodromal symptoms include cough, coryza (acute rhinitis), and conjunctivitis (3 Cs).
     a. Photophobia, high fever
   - Koplik's spots (diagnostic) appear on buccal membrane after 2 days and last for 1 or 2 days.
     a. These small lesions have the appearance of a bluish-gray grain of salt surrounded by a red halo.

Paramyxoviruses = parainfluenza (croup), RSV (infant bronchiolitis), measles, and mumps

Paramyxoviruses are sensitive to detergents, replicate in the cytoplasm, and must carry a polymerase into the target cell.

Paramyxoviruses and orthomyxoviruses replicate with a double-stranded RNA intermediate and are excellent inducers of interferon.

Paramyxoviruses, herpes simplex virus, varicella-zoster virus, and human immunodeficiency virus enter by fusion at the cell surface and can cause syncytia.

Trigger words:
Measles: high fever, Koplik spots (blue-gray vesicles in mouth), paramyxovirus, rash, "3 Cs" + photophobia

Mumps and measles: aerosol spread and highly contagious, with most people infected in childhood in the absence of early immunization

Virulence of measles: syncytia formation, neurotropism, immunosuppressive, immunopathogenesis.

BOX 24-1 MEASLES, MUMPS, AND INFLUENZA INFECTIONS: QUICK CASES

Paramyxoviridae

Measles: A 10-year-old boy develops a high fever with cough, conjunctivitis, and coryza and is sensitive to bright lights. After 48 hours, white vesicles are seen in his mouth, followed by a maculopapular rash beginning on the face and spreading over the trunk.

Mumps: One day in late March, a 10-year-old girl experiences a slight fever, headache, and loss of appetite for 24 hours. The next day, her fever increases, and examination shows that the parotid glands have rapidly become swollen. When she tries to chew, she experiences pain.

Orthomyxoviridae

Influenza A: A 70-year-old woman experiences rapid onset of fever with headache, myalgia, sore throat, and nonproductive cough. The disease progresses to pneumonia with bacterial involvement. The woman's history shows no recent immunization with influenza vaccine.

Measles sequelae include secondary bacterial infections, giant cell pneumonia in immunocompromised patients, postinfectious encephalitis, and subacute sclerosing panencephalitis (SSPE).

SSPE is due to accumulation of a defective measles virus in the brain.

- Extensive maculopapular rash, appearing 12 to 24 hours *after* the Koplik spots, starts below the ears and spreads over the body.
    a. Rash results from cytolytic cell-mediated response to infected endothelial cells lining small vessels.
3. Complications of measles infection
    - Secondary bacterial infections can cause pneumonia, which accounts for 60% of deaths from measles infection.
        a. Rare, fatal giant cell pneumonia occurs in children lacking cell-mediated immunity.
    - Acute postinfectious encephalitis, an immune-mediated demyelinating disease, has a mortality rate of 15%.
    - SSPE, a rare, slow viral infection occurring months to years after primary infection, is caused by defective measles virus in the brain.
        a. It is marked by changes in personality, behavior, and memory, followed by myoclonic jerks, blindness, and spasticity.
4. Laboratory identification
    - Diagnosis usually made from symptoms
    - Confirmation by reverse transcriptase–polymerase chain reaction (RT-PCR)
    - Immunofluorescence of cells in urinary sediment or pharyngeal cells
5. Transmission
    - Measles, a highly contagious disease, is spread by virion-containing respiratory droplets both before and after symptoms of infection occur.
6. Prevention and treatment

MMR vaccine contains live attenuated measles, mumps, and rubella viruses.

The MMR vaccine is recommended for children 15 to 24 months of age, after maturation of the child's cell-mediated immunity and dissipation of maternal antibody.

Measles and mumps may be eliminated by effective vaccine programs because only humans can be infected and there is only one serotype of these viruses.

Virulence of mumps: cell-to-cell fusion, immune-mediated disease.

Trigger words:
Mumps: orchitis, pancreatitis and aseptic meningitis or encephalitis (5%), paramyxovirus, parotitis (chipmunk cheeks)

- Live attenuated vaccine is given at 15 to 24 months of age and again before entering elementary or junior high school as part of the MMR triple vaccine.
    a. Use of killed vaccine is associated with more severe, atypical measles infection on exposure to virus.
- Passive immunization with immune serum globulin is effective in protecting unvaccinated immunocompromised children after exposure to measles virus.

D. Mumps virus (see Box 24-1)
1. Overview
    - Mumps virus exists as a single serotype and only infects humans.
    - Initial infection in the upper respiratory tract spreads to parotid glands.
    - Subsequent viremia can spread infection to the testes, ovaries, thyroid, pancreas, and CNS (in 50% of cases).
2. Mumps clinical manifestations
    - Infection with mumps virus often is asymptomatic or accompanied by mild nonspecific symptoms.
    - Fever, sudden onset of bilateral swelling of the parotid glands (parotitis), and redness and swelling of the ostium of Stensen duct mark acute disease.
    - Orchitis, oophoritis, pancreatitis, and CNS infection may occur after a few days.
        a. Unilateral orchitis may result in sterility.
        b. About 5% of cases show aseptic meningitis or encephalitis (meningoencephalitis), which is self-limited.
3. Laboratory identification
    - Histologic detection of syncytia in cultured cells infected by virions isolated from saliva (or from swabs taken from the pharynx and Stensen duct), urine, or cerebrospinal fluid

- Hemagglutination inhibition, RT-PCR for genome, enzyme-linked immunosorbent assay (ELISA) detection of virions, viral antigens, or antibodies to the virus in clinical samples
  4. Transmission
     - Mumps, a highly contagious infection, is spread through respiratory droplets, direct person-to-person contact, and fomites.
     - Contagious period begins before onset of clinical symptoms, and asymptomatic shedding may occur in subclinical cases.
  5. Prevention
     - Live attenuated vaccine is administered as part of the MMR vaccine in early childhood.

E. **Parainfluenza viruses**
  1. Overview
     - Four serotypes of parainfluenza virus infect the upper respiratory tract.
     - Spread of infection to lower respiratory tract (without viremia) occurs in about 25% of cases.
  2. Diseases due to parainfluenza viruses
     - Croup (laryngotracheobronchitis)
        a. Infection of the lower respiratory tract caused by serotypes 1 and 2 (primarily in the fall)
        b. Most common in children 2 to 5 years of age
        c. Characterized by a "seal bark" cough and tracheal swelling that may block the airway
     - Bronchiolitis and pneumonia, caused by serotype 3 (year-round), are most common in infants and elderly patients.
     - Mild cold-like syndrome of the upper respiratory tract is caused by serotype 4.
  3. Transmission
     - Parainfluenza viruses are transmitted through respiratory droplets and direct contact.
     - All serotypes spread quickly in hospitals, causing nosocomial outbreaks in nurseries and pediatric wards.
  4. Treatment
     - Nebulized air or hot-steam therapy, monitoring of the upper airway, and, rarely, intubation can alleviate symptoms.

F. **RSV**
  - A single serotype of RSV causes localized infection of the upper and lower respiratory tract.
  1. RSV diseases
     - Common cold with rhinorrhea (upper respiratory tract infection)
     - Bronchiolitis (lower respiratory tract infection)
        a. Usually self-limited infection of infants
        b. Marked by trapping of air, decreased ventilation, low-grade fever, tachycardia, and expiratory wheezes over all lung fields
        c. It is potentially fatal in immunocompromised or premature infants with lung disease.
  2. Transmission and incidence
     - RSV infection is very contagious, with spread through respiratory droplets and direct contact.
        a. Viral shedding precedes onset of symptoms and may last for many days.
     - Most children are infected by 4 years of age, with clinical manifestations ranging from a mild cold to pneumonia.
        a. Maternal antibody does not protect infants from primary infection.
     - Reinfection of adults causes milder symptoms.
  3. Treatment
     - Ribavirin, a guanosine analogue, may be administered to infants in aerosol form in severe cases.
     - RSV-specific gammaglobulin (RespiGam) or monoclonal antibody (palivizumab [Synergis]) for infants who were born prematurely or have cardiopulmonary disease

G. **Metapneumovirus**
  - Newly discovered, very common, parainfluenza-like disease causing virus

II. **Orthomyxoviridae**
  - This family of large viruses with an enveloped, helical nucleocapsid and segmented (−) RNA genome comprises the influenza viruses.

A. **Key viral proteins (Fig. 24-1)**
  1. Envelope glycoproteins are the major antigens of influenza virus.
     - Hemagglutinin (HA) functions as viral attachment protein and also binds to and aggregates erythrocytes (hemagglutination).

Trigger words:
Parainfluenza virus: barking seal, croup, paramyxovirus, pneumonia, syncytia

Parainfluenza viruses and RSV: infection most common and widespread in infants and young children

Trigger words:
RSV: bronchiolitis, infant, premature birth, paramyxovirus

No antiviral drugs are used in the treatment of paramyxovirus infections, except for aerosol ribavirin in severe RSV infections.

Antibody prophylaxis for RSV in premature infants and those with lung problems

Trigger words:
Orthomyxovirus: antigenic drift (minor mutations) (outbreak/epidemic) versus shift (reassortment = pandemic), hemagglutinin and neuraminidase, influenza, segmented genome = reassortment

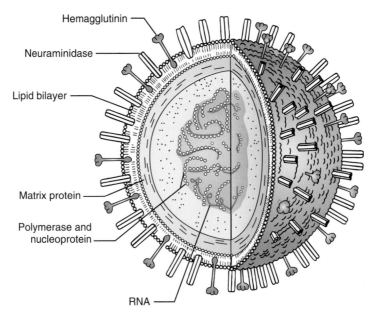

Hemagglutinin

Neuraminidase

Lipid bilayer

Matrix protein

Polymerase and
nucleoprotein

RNA

24-1: General schematic of the influenza virus. The eight (–) RNA genomic segments associate with multiple molecules of nucleoprotein and RNA-dependent RNA polymerase, forming helical nucleocapsid segments. The set of nucleocapsid segments is surrounded by matrix protein, which lines the inside of the membrane envelope. Two glycoproteins, hemagglutinin and neuraminidase, project from the envelope.

- Neuraminidase (NA), an enzyme that removes sialic acid from virion and host glycoproteins and glycolipids, facilitates release of virions from target cells by minimizing clumping.
   2. Nucleoprotein and RNA-dependent RNA polymerase associate with genomic segments to form helical nucleocapsids.
   3. M1 (matrix) protein surrounds the nucleocapsid and is involved in virion assembly.
   4. M2 (membrane) protein, which forms a proton channel that facilitates uncoating and assembly, is a target for amantadine and rimantadine antiviral drugs.
B. **Types and genetic changes in influenza viruses**
   1. Overview
      - Of the three types of influenza virus (A, B, and C), type A is the only one that infects animals (zoonosis) and humans.
      - Influenza A and B are significant human pathogens; influenza C is less important.
   2. Antigenic drift
      - Minor changes due to mutation in the genes encoding HA or NA, which alters viral antigenicity
      - Both influenza A and influenza B exhibit antigenic drift.
   3. Antigenic shift
      - Only influenza A undergoes antigenic shift.
      - Major changes that result from reassortment of genome segments from different human and animal strains
      - Random mixing and packaging of genome segments into virions occurs after coinfection with different strains of viruses, producing new hybrid viruses.
      - For example, reassortment of swine influenza virus (genome segments S1 to S8) and human influenza virus (segments H1 to H8) could create a new, distinct hybrid strain that contains some swine and some human segments and is capable of infecting humans.
C. **Replication**
   1. Attachment and entry
      - After HA binds to sialic acid–containing receptors on epithelial cells, virions enter by endocytosis.
   2. Fusion with endosome and uncoating
      - Release of the nucleocapsid from internalized virion is facilitated by acidification of the endosome and M2 proton channel.
   3. Nucleic acid synthesis
      - As an exception to the rule for RNA viruses, influenza produces its messenger RNAs (transcription) and progeny genome segments (replication) in the nucleus.

Influenza A (but not B or C) is a zoonosis.

New hybrid viruses produced by reassortment of human and animal viral genome segments cause antigenic shift and lead to pandemics.

New vaccines formulated for each year with the projected dominant influenza A and B types.

Influenza A: undergoes both antigenic drift and antigenic shift; most common cause of epidemics and pandemics of influenza

Influenza B: undergoes antigenic drift; causes localized outbreaks

Influenza C: more genetically stable; rarely causes widespread disease

Influenza is the exception to the RNA virus rule and replicates and transcribes its genome in the nucleus.

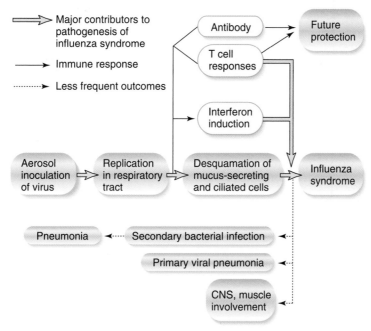

24-2: Pathogenesis of influenza A virus. Viral damage to the respiratory epithelium and host immune responses are responsible for the symptoms of influenza. Infection may also promote secondary bacterial infection. CNS, central nervous system.

4. Envelopment
- After nucleocapsids assemble, they move to the plasma membrane, associate with matrix protein on the viral glycoprotein-modified membrane, and are released by budding.

D. **Pathogenesis and host response** (Fig. 24-2)
1. Killing of ciliated and mucus-secreting epithelial cells results from initial infection of upper respiratory tract.
2. Action of viral NA thins out mucous secretions, compromising airway clearance and promoting viral spread to the lungs, as well as secondary bacterial infection.
   - Virus- or bacteria-induced tissue damage can cause pneumonia.
3. Interferons produced in response to infection help control viral spread but are largely responsible for typical flu-like symptoms.
4. Strain-specific antibody response to HA and NA antigens provides protection against the same but not different strains.
5. Cell-mediated response, which recognizes peptides from less variable proteins (e.g., nucleoprotein), provides more general protection that can help reduce subsequent disease by different strains.

E. **Diseases due to influenza virus**
- Classic acute influenza in adults (Box 24-1)
  a. Time course:
     (1) Incubation period is 1 to 3 days.
     (2) Prodromal period is 3 to 24 hours.
     (3) Disease usually lasts 7 to 10 days.
  b. Clinical manifestations
     (1) Malaise and headache during prodrome are followed by myalgia, fever, and nonproductive cough.
     (2) Secondary bacterial infection (e.g., sore throat) may occur in the second week.
  c. Severity
     (1) Disease may be asymptomatic to severe, depending on the degree of existing immunity to the infecting influenza strain and other factors.
     (2) Severe illness occurs most often in pregnant women and in patients with immunodeficiencies or cardiorespiratory disease.
  d. Childhood influenza
     (1) Disease is similar to that in adults but with higher fever.
     (2) Croup, otitis media, bronchiolitis, abdominal pain, and vomiting are also likely to be present.

Virulence of influenza: cytolytic infection, genetic instability

e. Complications
   (1) Bacterial pneumonia or influenzal pneumonia
   (2) Postinfluenza encephalitis with inflammation may occur 2 to 3 weeks after recovery and is rarely fatal.
   (3) Myositis and aspirin-associated Reye syndrome may occur in children.

F. **Laboratory identification**
   1. ELISA and other immunoassays to detect viral antigens in nasal secretions
   2. Hemadsorption and hemagglutination to detect the influenza virus in infected cultured cells
   3. Hemagglutination inhibition to detect antibodies induced by prior exposure to a specific strain of virus or to identify the virus type, depending on how the assay is set up
   4. RT-PCR to detect and distinguish influenza genomes

G. **Transmission and occurrence**
   1. Respiratory droplets are primary means of spreading influenza virus.
   2. Local outbreaks (epidemics) due to antigenic drift (change in viral antigenicity) occur every few years.
   3. Widespread outbreaks (pandemics) due to antigenic shift (appearance of new strains) occur about every 10 years.
   4. Naming influenza viruses
      • A/Bangkok/1/79 (H3N2): type (A,B,C)/place of origin/date of origin/antigen (HA, NA)

H. **Prevention and treatment**
   1. Vaccines consisting of the predicted endemic strains are produced each year.
      • Inactivated whole virus or detergent-extracted vaccine
         a. Vaccine is produced in embryonated eggs and should not be given to individuals with allergies to eggs.
      • Live attenuated aerosol vaccine for patients aged 2 to 49 years.
         a. Immunization is recommended for everyone, especially at-risk populations, particularly elderly patients, immunodeficient patients, and those with cardiorespiratory disease.
   2. Amantadine and rimantadine, which block uncoating of endocytosed virions, are approved for use against influenza A in unimmunized individuals but are ineffective against influenza B or C.
      • Treatment must start before or within 24 to 48 hours of the appearance of symptoms.
   3. Zanamivir and oseltamivir inhibit neuraminidase and are effective against both influenza A and influenza B.
   4. Acetaminophen (not aspirin) can reduce symptoms of influenza.

III. **Coronaviridae**
   A. **Overview**
      1. This family consists of large, enveloped viruses with a (+) RNA genome.
      2. Virions have a corona-like appearance in electron micrographs.
      3. Transmission occurs through respiratory droplets, with infection localized primarily to the respiratory tract.
   B. **Common cold (most common presentation)**
      1. The disease is similar to that caused by rhinoviruses but with a longer incubation period (3 days).
      2. Infection occurs mainly in infants and children, with sporadic outbreaks in winter and spring.
   C. **Gastrointestinal tract infection (uncommon)**
      • Coronavirus-like particles are occasionally seen in the stools of patients with diarrhea, gastroenteritis, or neonatal necrotizing enterocolitis.
   D. **Severe acute respiratory syndrome (SARS) (uncommon)**
      1. An outbreak of this very lethal disease started in China in 2002, and good public health action limited geographic spread.
      2. First transmitted to humans through contact with masked palm civets (China) and then from human-to-human contact through respiratory secretions (e.g., hospitals, families).
      3. One third of patients improve, and the infection resolves.
         • Others develop severe respiratory infection, and nearly 10% die.
      4. Diagnose with viral detection by PCR or detection of antibodies

---

Margin notes:

Hemagglutination inhibition uses antibodies to type patient virus or with defined virus, can titer patient antibody.

Genetic drift: mutation of the prevalent influenza A or B virus producing a new strain

Genetic shift (only influenza A): coinfection of a cell with a human and an animal influenza A virus can produce a new reassortant hybrid virus with gene segments from both viruses.

Amantadine only for influenza A; neuraminidase inhibitors for both A and B

Aspirin + influenza (or rubella) → Reye syndrome = acute encephalitis with hepatic dysfunction occurring primarily in children; high mortality rate

Trigger words:
Coronaviruses: common cold, fecal-oral and respiratory spread, SARS

Coronaviruses are the enveloped virus exception and are resistant to gastrointestinal conditions.

Microinjection of the coronavirus (+) RNA genome is sufficient to initiate virus replication.

Coronaviruses: responsible for about 15% of upper respiratory tract infections

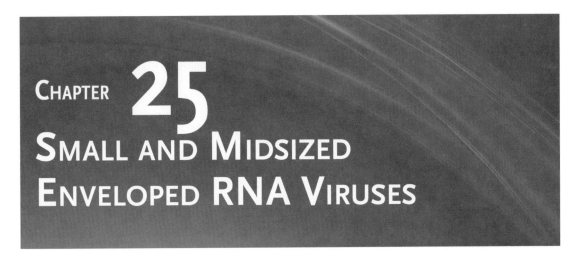

CHAPTER **25**
SMALL AND MIDSIZED ENVELOPED RNA VIRUSES

I. Rhabdoviridae
A. Overview
1. This family comprises medium-sized, bullet-shaped viruses with an enveloped, helical nucleocapsid and single-stranded (–) RNA genome.
2. Only one significant human pathogen, rabies virus, is a rhabdovirus.
B. Pathogenesis and disease progression (Table 25-1)
1. Rabies is a zoonotic disease, with unvaccinated domestic pets (dogs and cats) and wild skunks, raccoons (most common), and bats being the major reservoirs of the rabies virus.
2. The virus is transmitted to humans in saliva from an infected animal (via bite) or in aerosols from infected bats (via inhalation).
3. Inoculation
   - Rabies virions bind to acetylcholine receptors on muscle cells at the site of the bite and enter target cells by endocytosis.
4. Incubation phase
   - The virus replicates within infected muscle cells.
   - The duration of the incubation phase depends on the dose of virus received and the proximity of the bite to the brain.
5. Prodrome phase
   - The virus infects peripheral nerves and travels through retrograde transport to the central nervous system (CNS).
6. Neurologic phase
   - The virus spreads from the CNS through afferent neurons to highly innervated sites (e.g., glands, skin, and eyes).
   - Virions are shed into saliva in the salivary glands.
   - Infection of the brain leads to encephalitis with seizures and hydrophobia.
   - Antibody response occurs only after the virus has infected the CNS and other sites, too late to prevent progression of the disease.

Trigger words:
Rabies: aerosol, bats, bullet-shaped virion, coma, dog bite, hydrophobia, Negri bodies, rhabdovirus, salivation

Rhabdovirus, filovirus, and arenavirus are zoonoses, are sensitive to detergents, and replicate in cytoplasm through a double-stranded RNA intermediate.

Bats, skunks, raccoons are major reservoirs of rabies.

Rabies promotes its own transmission by replicating and shedding from salivary glands when the virus has reached the brain to cause the "mad" phase of the disease.

TABLE 25-1 **Progression of Rabies Disease**

DISEASE PHASE	SYMPTOMS	DURATION	VIRUS AND ANTIBODY STATUS
Incubation phase	Asymptomatic	60-365 days after bite	Low titer; virus in muscle No detectable antibody
Prodrome phase	Fever, nausea, vomiting Loss of appetite Headache, lethargy Pain at site of bite	2-10 days	High titer; virus in peripheral nerves and CNS No detectable antibody
Neurologic phase	Hydrophobia, pharyngeal spasms Hyperactivity, anxiety, depression CNS symptoms: loss of coordination, paralysis, confusion, delirium	2-7 days	High titer; virus in brain and other sites Antibody detectable in serum and CNS
Coma	Cardiac arrest, hypotension, hypoventilation Secondary infections Death	0-14 days	

CNS, central nervous system.

BOX 25-1 RABIES: QUICK CASE

Rhabdoviridae
- **Rabies:** A 10-year-old boy is brought to the pediatrician by his parents because the boy is experiencing a headache, lethargy, vomiting, and fever. He is having difficulty drinking and is suffering from anxiety and confusion. The boy was bitten by a baby raccoon about 4 months before the onset of symptoms.

7. Coma and death are nearly always inevitable, unless prophylactic treatment is administered during incubation phase.

C. Diagnosis of rabies

1. Rabies is diagnosed based on neurologic symptoms and history of an animal bite or contact with bats, with laboratory tests providing confirmation (Box 25-1).
   - Analysis of the brain of the biting animal for rabies antigen can avert need for vaccine therapy.
2. Negri bodies (intracytoplasmic viral inclusions) are found in 70% to 90% of infected brains (animal or human).
3. Viral antigen in the CNS and brain is detectable by immunofluorescence at postmortem.
4. RT-PCR detection of genome

D. Prevention and prophylaxis

1. Preexposure vaccination of pets and high-risk personnel (veterinarians and animal handlers) is recommended.
2. Postexposure prophylaxis can prevent disease in infected people if instituted soon after exposure.
   - Immediate cleansing of the wound reduces viral load.
   - Active immunization with killed rabies vaccine is effective because of the long incubation period (>6 months).
   - Passive immunization with equine antirabies serum or human rabies immune globulin provides protection until antibody is produced in response to vaccine.
     a. Injected close to site of bite as soon as possible
3. Animal immunizations
   - Routine immunization of pets
   - Wild animal (e.g., skunk, raccoon) immunization with bait containing live hybrid vaccinia virus with gene for rabies G protein

II. Other Zoonotic Enveloped (–) RNA Viruses

A. Filoviridae: Ebola and Marburg viruses

1. Long, filamentous, enveloped viruses with a linear (–) RNA genome
2. Transmission and pathogenesis
   - Transmission from monkeys to humans and also among humans by contact with infected body fluids or by accidental injection
   - Viral glycoprotein initiates extensive tissue necrosis in the liver, lymph nodes, spleen, and lungs.
   - Virus initiates potent cytokine release (cytokine storm).
3. African hemorrhagic fever (Ebola fever and Marburg virus disease)
   - Initial flu-like symptoms (headache and myalgia) are followed within a few days by nausea, vomiting, diarrhea, and possibly a maculopapular rash.
   - Extensive hemorrhage, especially from the gastrointestinal tract, results in edema and hypovolemic shock, with death occurring in 50% to 90% of cases depending on strain.

B. Arenaviridae

1. Overview
   - Virions have segmented (–) RNA genome
     a. Virions carry nonfunctional cellular ribosomes, giving them a sandy appearance in electron micrographs.
   - Aerosols, food, or fomites contaminated by feces or urine of infected rodents are routes for spreading virions to humans.
2. Lymphocytic choriomeningitis (LCM)
   - Infection with the LCM virus causes a febrile flu-like illness with CNS involvement in about 25% of cases.
   - Transmission
     a. Food or water contaminated with mouse urine or feces
   - Permanent neurologic damage in more than 25% with encephalitis
3. Lassa fever and other arenaviral hemorrhagic fevers
   - Common clinical features include fever, coagulopathy, petechiae, liver and spleen necrosis, and visceral hemorrhage with no CNS involvement.

Presence of Negri bodies, immunofluorescence assay, or reverse transcriptase–polymerase chain reaction (RT-PCR) is used to diagnose rabies.

Rabies vaccine is inactivated virus grown in diploid fibroblasts.

Rabies vaccine is the only vaccine appropriate for postinfection treatment.

Rabies immunoglobulin G (IgG) and rabies vaccine are administered to a bite victim if animal is not proved uninfected.

Filoviruses and arenaviruses: Ebola virus (filovirus) and Lassa virus (an arenavirus) cause often-fatal hemorrhagic fevers.

Trigger words: Arenaviruses: lymphocytic choriomeningitis virus—flu-like symptoms, ribavirin, rodents, slums; Lassa fever—Africa, hemorrhagic, rodents

4. Treatment
   - Ribavirin, a guanosine analogue, and supportive measures are used in treating infections with arenaviruses.

C. Bunyaviridae

1. Overview
   - Medium-sized, enveloped viruses with a segmented (–) RNA genome
   - Most bunyaviruses are arboviruses, which are transmitted by insect vectors.
   - Hantaviruses are zoonoses carried by rodents.
2. Pathogenesis
   - Initial viremia following exposure causes flu-like symptoms.
   - Secondary viremia spreads virions to target organs (e.g., CNS, liver, lungs, and vascular endothelium).
3. Hantaviral infections
   - Inhalation of infected rodent urine and feces transmits hantaviruses from infected animals to humans.
   - Hantavirus pulmonary syndrome
     a. Acute respiratory distress syndrome, hemorrhage, renal failure
     b. Laboratory
        - Viral RNA in lung tissue (RT-PCR test)
     c. High mortality
4. California encephalitis (e.g., La Crosse virus, California encephalitis virus)
   - This arboviral disease is transmitted by a *Culex* mosquito that inhabits the forests of North America.
   - Illness usually lasts about 1 week with a low fatality rate, although seizures occur in about half of cases.
5. Bunyaviral hemorrhagic fevers (e.g., Rift Valley fever virus, Crimean-Congo hemorrhagic fever virus)
   - High mortality rate (up to 50%) is associated with hemorrhagic manifestations.

III. Togaviridae and Flaviviridae

A. Overview

1. These two families contain small, enveloped viruses with a single-stranded (+) RNA genome.
2. Except for rubella virus, all togaviruses are arboviruses.
3. Except for hepatitis C virus (see Chapter 27), all flaviviruses are arboviruses.

B. Rubella virus

1. Pathogenesis
   - Initial noncytolytic infection is established in the upper respiratory tract and then spreads to local lymph nodes.
   - Viremia spreads virions to the skin and other tissues.
   - Shedding of virions into respiratory droplets occurs during the 2-week prodromal period and for as long as 2 weeks after onset of the rash.
   - Transplacental infection in nonimmune pregnant women leads to viral replication in fetal tissues and possible teratogenic effects due to alterations in fetal growth, mitosis, and chromosome structure.
   - Antiviral antibody appears after viremia and helps limit virion spread.
2. Diseases due to rubella virus
   - Rubella (German measles)
     a. In children, disease is benign, consisting of swollen glands and a pink maculopapular rash that lasts 3 days, starting on the face and spreading downward over the trunk and extremities.
     b. In adults, disease is more severe, with arthralgia, arthritis, thrombocytopenia (rare), and possible postinfectious encephalitis due to the immune response.
   - Congenital rubella
     a. Transplacental infection of fetus until the 20th week of gestation can lead to cataracts, mental retardation, and deafness.
     b. Maternal antirubella antibodies resulting from earlier infection or vaccination prevent viral spread to the placenta and fetus.
3. Laboratory identification
   - Serologic tests demonstrating the presence of antirubella IgM antibodies or a fourfold increase in IgG antibodies confirm diagnosis of rubella infection.
   - RT-PCR for viral genome
4. Transmission
   - Rubella virus is spread by the respiratory route and not by animals or insects.

Trigger words:
Bunyaviruses: arbovirus, California encephalitis viruses: *Culex* mosquito, encephalitis, La Crosse virus, meningitis, forests

Hantaviruses: bleeding tissues, hemorrhagic, ecchymosis, petechiae, rodent feces and urine

Arboviruses infect animal and bird species and are transmitted to humans through insect vectors, causing mild flu-like disease, hemorrhagic fevers, and encephalitis.

Togaviruses and flaviviruses are sensitive to detergents, replicate in cytoplasm through a double-stranded RNA intermediate, and are good inducers of interferon.

Trigger words:
Rubella: rash, arthritis, congenital disease, cataracts, deafness, teratogen, togavirus, vaccine

Rubella virus: togavirus only infects humans, causing German measles and congenital rubella; teratogenic during first trimester of fetal life. Maternal antirubella antibodies prevent spread to fetus.

Congenital diseases include TORCH: *toxo, other, rubella, cytomegalovirus, herpes simplex virus* and *human immunodeficiency virus.*

Antirubella antibodies are commonly assayed in early pregnancy to determine the immune status of the mother.

5. Prevention
   - Routine immunization is done with live attenuated virus as part of the MMR vaccine.

C. Togaviral and flaviviral arboviruses
1. Pathogenesis
   - Bite of insect vector (usually a mosquito) injects virion-containing saliva into blood and initiates viremic spread.
   - Initial infection is established primarily in macrophages and monocytes.
   - Secondary viremia may occur, spreading infection to the brain, liver, vasculature, and skin.
2. Clinical syndromes associated with arboviral infections
   - Most infections start with and may be limited to systemic flu-like symptoms.
   - Tissue tropism of virus determines the nature of subsequent disease.
   - Dengue (breakbone fever)
      a. Caused by a flavivirus that is transmitted by an *Aedes* species mosquito in the Caribbean and Southeast Asia
      b. Initial exposure causes high fever, headache, rash, and back and bone pain lasting 6 or 7 days.
      c. Rechallenge with related strain can result in severe DHF and DSS.
   - Yellow fever
      a. Caused by a flavivirus that is transmitted by an *Aedes* species mosquito found mainly in tropical South America and Africa
      b. Degeneration of the liver, kidneys, and heart can result in high mortality during epidemics.
      c. High fever, jaundice, and "black vomit" due to gastrointestinal tract hemorrhage are common symptoms.
      d. Councilman bodies (apoptotic acidophilic inclusions) are visible in liver.
   - Encephalitis
      a. Caused by numerous arboviruses and flaviviruses, including:
         - Togaviruses such as Eastern and Western equine encephalitis viruses occur in the United States
         - Flaviviruses such as St. Louis encephalitis virus (in the United States) and West Nile encephalitis virus are widely distributed
3. Transmission (Fig. 25-1)
   - *Aedes* species mosquitoes are found near pools of water and transmit dengue and yellow fever to urban populations.
   - *Culex* species mosquitoes breed in forests and cause urban outbreaks of St. Louis encephalitis.
4. Prevention
   - Elimination of mosquitoes or other vectors is primary means for preventing arboviral diseases.
   - Live attenuated vaccine is available for yellow fever and Japanese encephalitis.

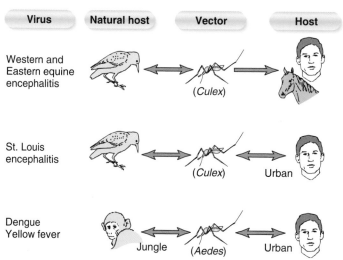

25-1: Patterns of arboviral transmission. Infections in which the host can transmit the virus back to the vector (*double-headed arrow*) maintain and amplify the virus in the environment. Viruses that can be transmitted from humans to vector (e.g., dengue, yellow fever, and St. Louis encephalitis) can cause outbreaks among urban populations. Dead-end infections with no transmission from humans back to the vector (*single-headed arrow*) generally occur as isolated cases in the endemic region of the vector.

CHAPTER 26
RETROVIRUSES

I. Retroviridae: General Features
- Midsized viruses with an enveloped capsid containing two copies of a single-stranded (+) RNA genome, transfer RNA (tRNA), reverse transcriptase, integrase, and protease.
- Two human pathogens—human immunodeficiency virus (HIV) and human T lymphotropic virus (HTLV)—are retroviruses.

A. Retroviral genes
1. All retroviral genomes contain three genes—*gag, pol,* and *env*—and are flanked by long-terminal repeats (Table 26-1).
   - Each gene encodes a polyprotein, which is cleaved to yield the final gene products.
     a. *gag* → nucleocapsid proteins
     b. *pol* → enzymes (reverse transcriptase, integrase, and protease)
     c. *env* → envelope glycoproteins
2. Complex retroviruses, such as HIV, have several other genes encoding auxiliary and regulatory proteins (e.g., *nef, tat,* and *rev*)

B. Key HIV proteins (Fig. 26-1)
1. Major envelope glycoprotein consists of two associated proteins: an attachment protein (HIV gp120) and transmembrane fusion protein (HIV gp41) both cleaved from gp160 precursor.
2. Three enzymes are carried within the nucleocapsid: reverse transcriptase, integrase, and protease.
3. Matrix protein (HIV p17) forms a layer underlying the envelope.
4. Nucleocapsid protein (HIV p24) forms the outer layer of the virion core, and detection in blood indicates infection.

> Retroviruses are enveloped and must carry reverse transcriptase, integrase, and protease enzymes to initiate replication.
>
> Simple retroviruses have three genes (*gag, pol, env*), complex retroviruses (like HIV) have more genes.

TABLE 26-1 **Retrovirus Genes and Their Function**

GENE	VIRUS	FUNCTION
gag	All	Group-specific antigen: core and capsid proteins
int	All	Integrase
pol	All	Polymerase: reverse transcriptase, protease, integrase
pro	All	Protease
env	All	Envelope: glycoproteins
tax	HTLV	Transactivation of viral and cellular genes
tat	HIV-1	Transactivation of viral and cellular genes
rex	HTLV	Regulation of RNA splicing and promotion of export to cytoplasm
rev	HIV-1	Regulation of RNA splicing and promotion of export to cytoplasm
nef	HIV-1	Alteration of cell activation signals; progression to AIDS (essential)
vif	HIV-1	Virus infectivity, promotion of assembly, blocks a cellular antiviral protein
vpu	HIV-1	Facilitates virion assembly and release, decrease of cell surface CD4
vpr (vpx*)	HIV-1	Transport of complementary DNA to nucleus, arresting of cell growth
LTR	All	Promoter, enhancer elements

*In HIV-2.
HIV, human immunodeficiency virus; HTLV, human T lymphotropic virus; LTR, long-terminal repeat (sequence).
From Murray PR, Rosenthal KS, Pfaller MA: Medical Microbiology, 6th ed. Philadelphia, Mosby, 2009, Table 64-2.

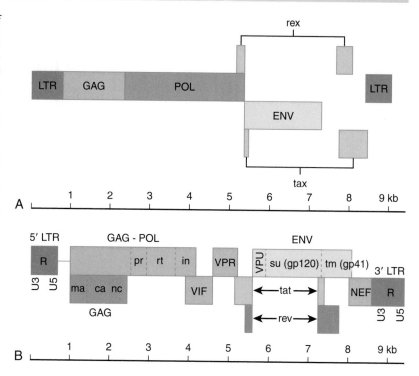

26-1: Genome structure of human retroviruses: (A) HTLV-1 and (B) HIV. The basic retrovirus genome consists of the long terminal repeat (ltr) group–specific antigen (capsid proteins) (gag)-enzymes (polymerase, integrase, protease) (env) and the glycoproteins (env). Complex retroviruses, such as HIV have additional proteins that enhance their virulence. These are described in Table 26-1. *(Redrawn from Belshe RB: Textbook of Human Virology, 2nd ed. St Louis, Mosby, 1991. In Murray PR, Rosenthal KS, Pfaller MA: Medical Microbiology, 6th ed. Philadelphia, Mosby, 2009, Fig. 64-4.)*

C. Replication

- Replication cycle (Fig. 26-2)
1. Attachment and fusion
   - Binding of viral gp120/gp41 to CD4 and a chemokine coreceptor is required for HIV infection of cells.
     a. Preference for chemokine coreceptor genetically switches during disease from:
        - Initial: CCR5—on macrophages, dendritic cells, and T cells
          Later: CXCR4—on T cells
2. Formation of HIV provirus
   - Reverse transcriptase carried in the virion synthesizes a complementary DNA (cDNA) from viral genome, forming an RNA-DNA hybrid. The same enzyme then degrades the RNA strand and synthesizes a complementary DNA strand, forming double-stranded viral DNA.
     a. Reverse transcriptase causes a high mutation rate in newly formed viral DNA.
   - Viral integrase catalyzes integration of viral DNA into host nuclear DNA, forming provirus.
     a. Provirus is part of host chromosome and vertically transmitted with host DNA and passed on to daughter cells.
3. Viral messenger RNA (mRNA) and genome replication
   - Host DNA-dependent RNA polymerase transcribes a full-length (+) RNA copy of the integrated genome and several shorter mRNA copies for individual proteins and polyproteins.
4. Assembly
   - After synthesis of viral proteins, nucleocapsids containing two copies of genome associate with glycoprotein modified plasma membrane and bud off.
   - After budding, protease cleaves gag-pol polyprotein to produce mature (cone-shaped) nucleocapsid and functional integrase and reverse transcriptase enzymes.

D. Genetic variation

1. High rate of mutation in retroviruses results from numerous alterations introduced by reverse transcriptase.
2. Generation of new HIV strains occurs during the course of infection of an individual, leading to changes in tissue tropism, antigenicity, and other properties of the virus.
3. Generation of drug resistance occurs readily, requiring multiple drug therapy (highly active antiretroviral therapy [HAART]).

Initial HIV target cell expresses CD4 and CCR5 chemokine receptor on macrophages, dendritic cell, and T cell; later, HIV mutates and binds to T cells expressing CD4 and CXCR4.

Reverse transcriptase, integrase, and protease are enzymes critical to HIV replication and are major targets of drugs used in the treatment of HIV infection.

HIV polymerase is error prone, and mutations produce new substrains.

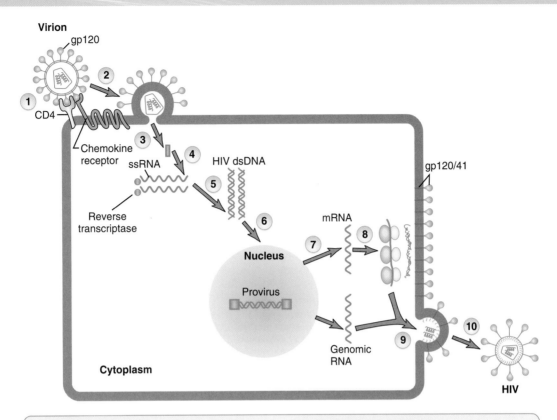

1 Binding of HIV gp120 to CD4 and chemokine coreceptor (early disease: CCR5; late disease: CXCR4)	**6** Transport of HIV dsDNA into nucleus and its integration into host chromosomal DNA by viral integrase forming provirus
2 Fusion of virion with cell membrane mediated by HIV gp41 and a coreceptor on cells	**7** Transcription of proviral DNA into genomic RNA and several mRNAs, which are transported to cytoplasm
3 Release of nucleocapsid into cytoplasm	**8** Synthesis, processing, and assembly of viral proteins in or near cell membrane
4 Uncoating of nucleocapsid and release of 2 copies of single-stranded (ss) RNA genome and reverse transcriptase	**9** Movement of HIV genomic RNA to modified membrane and budding out to form envelope
5 Formation of HIV double-stranded (ds) DNA by viral reverse transcriptase	**10** Release of virion by budding off and subsequent cleavage of polyproteins by viral protease to yield mature virion

26-2: The life cycle of human immunodeficiency virus (HIV). mRNA, messenger RNA.

II. HIV

- HIV is a lentivirus that causes immunosuppression and neurologic disorders.
- HIV has a characteristic morphology with a cone-shaped capsid surrounded by an envelope (see Fig. 26-1).

A. Laboratory diagnosis

1. Serologic and molecular tests
   a. Enzyme-linked immunosorbent assay (ELISA) detects anti-HIV antibodies as the standard screening test.
      1) High false-positive rate requires confirmation.
   b. Western blot for anti-HIV antibodies is used to confirm ELISA test for diagnosis of HIV infection.
      1) Antibody to more than three HIV proteins is required to indicate HIV infection.
   c. Viral RNA and antigens can be detected early in infection (before the appearance of antibody) and late in infection (when antibody titer falls).
      1) Viral RNA (genome load) is detected by reverse transcriptase–polymerase chain reaction (RT-PCR)
      2) Genome load is an early indicator of infection, course of disease, and efficacy of therapy.
      3) Quantitative RT-PCR and other assays are used to evaluate genome load.
   d. HIV p24 antigen is an early marker of infection and active virus replication.

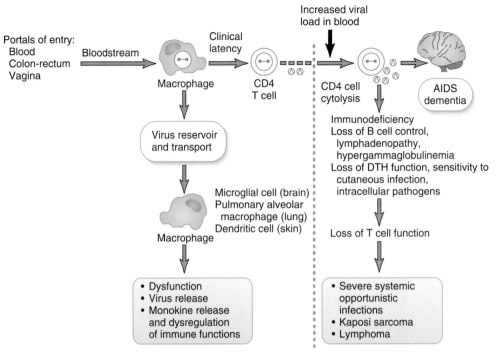

26-3: Pathogenesis of human immunodeficiency virus (HIV). HIV causes lytic and latent infection of CD4 T cells and persistent infection of cells of the monocyte-macrophage family, and it disrupts neurons. The outcomes of these actions are immunodeficiency and acquired immunodeficiency syndrome (AIDS) dementia. DTH, delayed-type hypersensitivity.

2. T cell counts
   - Decreased number of CD4 T cells in peripheral blood and decreased ratio of CD4 to CD8 T cells indicate active HIV disease.
      a. Precipitous decrease in CD8 T cells precedes progression to full-blown AIDS.

Virulence factors of HIV: incapacitation of immune system, rapid mutation, lytic infection, latent infection, syncytia formation, asymptomatic transmission

B. Pathogenesis (Fig. 26-3)
   1. Target cells
      - HIV primarily infects helper T (T_H) cells and myeloid-lineage cells, which express CD4 and a chemokine coreceptor.
         a. Lytic infection and latent infection are established in T cells.
         b. Persistent low-level productive infection is established in macrophages.
   2. Consequences of target cell infection
      - Persistently infected macrophages may act as the major reservoir and distribution vehicle for HIV in the body.
      - Killing of infected CD4 T cells leads to decreased CD4 T cell count and eventually to other immune system abnormalities. Examples include:
         a. Decreased proliferation of CD8 T cells (due to reduced interleukin [IL]-2 production)
            (1) Increased susceptibility to viruses
         b. Decreased macrophage function due to reduced interferon-γ production
            (1) Reduced macrophage function increases susceptibility to fungi, mycobacterial recurrences, and bacterial infections.
         c. Changes in the balance of cytokines
         e. Uncontrolled nonspecific antibody production (hypergammaglobulinemia)
      - Neurologic abnormalities may result from infection of brain macrophages, microglial cells, and neurons.
   3. Factors preventing immune resolution of HIV infection
      - Disruption of immune system by virus
      - Viral replication in inaccessible "privileged sites"
      - Latency of virus
      - Changes in antigenicity of HIV
      - Direct cell-to-cell transmission (e.g., from macrophage or dendritic cell to T cell)

HIV escapes immune control by changing antigenicity, incapacitating CD4 T cells and macrophages, direct cell-cell transmission, and establishment of latency.

C. Clinical course of HIV infection (Fig. 26-4)
   1. Initial acute infection
      - Asymptomatic or resembles mononucleosis and may have aseptic meningitis or a rash; symptoms subside spontaneously.

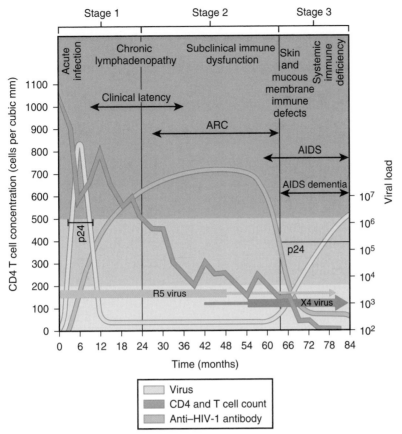

26-4: Time course and stages of human immunodeficiency virus (HIV) disease. A long clinical latency period follows the initial mononucleosis-like symptoms. Initial infection is with the R5-M-tropic virus, and later the X4-T-tropic virus arises. The progressive decrease in the number of CD4 T cells, even during the latency period, allows opportunistic infections to occur. The stages in HIV disease are defined by the CD4 T cell levels and occurrence of opportunistic diseases. AIDS, acquired immunodeficiency syndrome; ARC, AIDS-related complex. *(Data from Redfield RR, Buske DS: Sci Am 1996;259:90-98, updated 1996. In Murray PR, Rosenthal KS, Pfaller MA: Medical Microbiology, 6th ed. Philadelphia, Mosby, 2009, Fig. 64-9.)*

- Viral load increases and then decreases, but HIV persists in the host for months to years with few symptoms.
2. AIDS-related complex
   - Onset is marked by reduction of CD4 T cell count below 500 cells/μL and reduced delayed-type hypersensitivity responses.
   - Symptoms include lymphadenopathy and fever, weight loss, malaise, diarrhea, night sweats, fatigue, and relatively mild opportunistic infections such as oral thrush (oropharyngeal candidiasis), hairy leukoplakia, and listeriosis.
3. Full-blown AIDS
   - AIDS is defined by CD4 T cell count of less than 200 cells/μL and usually is accompanied by the appearance of one or more indicator diseases (Table 26-2).
   - Progression of AIDS is marked by an increase in detectable viral load and further reduction of CD4 T cell count to very low levels.
   - AIDS-related dementia, marked by a slow deterioration of intellect and other neurologic disorders, occurs in some AIDS patients.
     a. AIDS patients are at risk for progressive multifocal leukoencephalopathy, which may be confused with AIDS-related dementia.

D. Transmission
- Blood, semen, breast milk, and vaginal secretions of HIV-infected people contain the virus.
1. Inoculation with infected blood: transfusion of blood or blood products, sharing of needles by intravenous drug abusers, use of infected tattoo needles, accidental needle sticks, and contact with contaminated blood through open wounds and mucous membranes
   - Screening of the blood supply, organ transplants, and clotting factors used by hemophiliacs for the presence of HIV has reduced transmission by these routes.

Primary targets of HIV infection are CD4-expressing cells: T_H cells, macrophages, dendritic cells, and microglial cells in brain.

AIDS diagnosis: based on CD4 T cell count of less than 200 cells/μL and the presence of at least one "indicator" opportunistic infection, neoplasm, or other condition in HIV-infected patients

HIV is transmitted in blood, semen, vaginal secretions, and organ transplants.

TABLE 26-2 **Selected AIDS Indicator Diseases**

TYPE	SPECIFIC DISEASE*
Bacterial infection	*Mycobacterium avium-intracellulare* complex infection, disseminated
	Extrapulmonary tuberculosis (*Mycobacterium tuberculosis*)
	Salmonella septicemia, recurrent
Viral infection	Cytomegalovirus disease
	Herpes simplex virus infection, chronic or disseminated
	Progressive multifocal leukoencephalopathy (JC virus)
Fungal infection	Candidiasis of the esophagus, trachea, or lungs (*Candida albicans*)
	Cryptococcal meningitis (*Cryptococcus neoformans*)
	Histoplasmosis (*Histoplasma capsulatum*)
	Pneumocystis jiroveci pneumonia
Protozoal infection	Cryptosporidiosis, chronic with diarrhea (*Cryptosporidium* species)
	Toxoplasmosis of the brain (*Toxoplasma gondii*)
Neoplasia	Cervical cancer (invasive)
	Kaposi sarcoma
	Primary lymphoma of the brain
	Other non-Hodgkin lymphomas
Other	HIV wasting syndrome

*A diagnosis of AIDS is made for HIV-infected patients who manifest any of these diseases regardless of their T cell count.

Promiscuity is the highest risk factor for HIV infection

HIV therapy: multidrug therapy (HAART) can reduce viral load to near zero.

Treatment is initiated at less than 350 CD4 or AIDS-defining illness. Treatment for CD4 of more than 350 if clinical benefit indicated.

CD4 less than 200, *Pneumocystis pneumoniae*; CD4 less than 100, toxoplasmosis; CD4 less than 50, *Mycobacterium avium-intracellulare* complex

2. Sexual contact: anal or vaginal intercourse
3. Intrauterine or perinatal transmission or through breast milk to the newborn

E. **Treatment (Table 26-3)**
   • Antiviral drug therapy delays the onset and severity of symptoms and decreases virus production and shedding.
   • Targets for therapy are polymerase, protease, integrase, viral binding, and fusion to cell.
   1. Treatment can be initiated when CD4 T cell numbers are less than 500.
   2. Treatment with AZT alone or in combination with lamivudine or other drug treatment of pregnant mother can prevent transmission to fetus.
      • Rapid development of resistance to single drugs by HIV has led to the use of multidrug therapy.
      • Combination therapy: HAART
         a. HAART significantly reduces viral loads and morbidity in most patients.
         b. One or two protease inhibitors and two nucleotide reverse transcriptase inhibitors
         c. Two nucleotide reverse transcriptase inhibitors and a non-nucleoside reverse transcriptase inhibitor

TABLE 26-3 **Anti–Human Immunodeficiency Virus Therapy**

NUCLEOSIDE ANALOGUES (NRTIs)	PROTEASE INHIBITORS*	RECEPTOR OR FUSION INHIBITORS	NNRTIs
Abacavir (ABC)	Amprenavir	Enfuvirtide (T-20)	Delavirdine
Didanosine (ddI)	Atazanavir	Maraviroc (CCR5 antagonist	Nevirapine
Emtricitabine (FTC)	Darunavir		Efavirenz
Lamivudine (3TC)	Indinavir		
Stavudine (d4T)	Lopinavir		**INT inhibitor**
Tenofovir (nucleotide)	Nelfinavir		Raltegravir
Zalcitabine (ddC)	Ritonavir		
Zidovudine (AZT)	Saquinavir		
	Tipranavir		
Examples of Highly Active Antiretroviral Therapy (HAART)			
1-2 Protease inhibitor(s) + 2 NRTIs	Atazanavir, ritonavir, zidovudine, lamivudine		Lopinavir, ritonavir, lamivudine, zidovudine
2 NRTIs + NNRTI	Abacavir, lamivudine, nevirapine		Zidovudine, lamivudine, efavirenz

NNRTI, non-nucleotide reverse transcriptase inhibitor; NRTI, nucleotide reverse transcriptase inhibitor.
*The suffix -*navir* means "no virus."

III. HTLV
- HTLVs are oncoviruses associated with cancer and neurologic disorders.
- Only HTLV-1 has been directly associated with human disease, although infection is usually asymptomatic.

A. Pathogenesis
1. CD4 T cells are the primary targets of HTLV-1 infection, but the virus can also infect neurons.
   - Virus may remain latent in T cells or replicate slowly for years.
2. Viral tax protein stimulates proliferation of infected T cells in the absence of antigen by activating production of IL-2 and the IL-2 receptor.
   - Chromosomal aberrations and rearrangements that arise during continued T cell proliferation may contribute to transformation of infected cells into leukemic cells.

B. Adult T cell leukemia/lymphoma (ATLL)
- This neoplasia of mature CD4 T cells arises many years after infection with HTLV-1.
1. Characteristic signs: circulating malignant cells resembling flowers (pleomorphic cells with lobulated nuclei), bone lesions, lymphadenopathy, hypercalcemia, and skin rash similar to Sézary syndrome
2. Acute disease: usually fatal within 1 year of diagnosis
3. Chronic disease: similar to non-Hodgkin lymphoma

C. Transmission and occurrence
- Spread of HTLV-1 occurs by similar routes as HIV (e.g., blood transfusion, intravenous drug abuse, sexual contact, and breastfeeding).
- HTLV-1 disease is endemic among the black population in the southeastern United States and in southern Japan and the Caribbean.

IV. Endogenous Retroviruses
- Retrovirus genomes have integrated and become part of human chromosomes. They do not produce virus, to our knowledge.

Trigger words:
HTLV: CD4 T cell, flower cell, leukemia, reverse transcriptase

HTLV-1: slow oncogenic retrovirus; infects and promotes CD4 T cell proliferation; ATLL

Like HIV, HTLV-1 infects CD4 T cells and is transmitted by the same routes.

I. General Properties (Table 27-1)

- The hepatitis viruses (types A to E) are a diverse group of viruses that infect the liver, resulting in mild to severe acute disease (all types) and chronic disease (types B, C, and D).

A. Transmission and onset of hepatitis

1. Hepatitis virions are shed and transmissible *before* the onset and during symptomatic and asymptomatic phases of infections.
2. Hepatitis A and E viruses
   - Spread by the fecal-oral route
   - Rapid onset of acute disease
   - No chronic infection
3. Hepatitis B and C viruses
   - Present in body fluids with parenteral and sexual spread
   - Insidious onset of acute disease with potential for chronic infection
4. Hepatitis D virus
   - Transmitted like hepatitis B virus (HBV)
   - Replication only in HBV-infected cells
   - Abrupt onset of acute disease with potential for chronic disease

B. Pathogenesis

1. Host immune response is the primary cause of liver damage resulting from infection by any of the hepatitis viruses.
2. Direct cytopathic effects contribute to pathogenesis in hepatitis A, E, and D infection.

C. Common clinical manifestations of acute hepatitis

1. Acute hepatitis symptoms are similar for all viruses.
2. Severity and duration of acute disease vary among the hepatitis viruses.

Hepatitis A and E have similar structure (capsid) and mode of transmission and cause acute disease.

Hepatitis B, C, and D (enveloped) are transmitted by the same means and can cause chronic disease.

TABLE 27-1 **Comparison of Hepatitis Viral Infections**

PROPERTY	HEPATITIS A	HEPATITIS B	HEPATITIS C	HEPATITIS D	HEPATITIS E
Common name	Infectious	Serum	Posttransfusion non-A, non-B	Delta	Enteric non-A, non-B
Virus structure (family)	Naked, RNA (picornavirus)	Envelope, DNA (hepadnavirus)	Envelope, RNA (flavivirus)	Envelope, RNA	Naked, RNA (calici-like)
Transmission	Fecal-oral	Parenteral, sexual	Parenteral, sexual	Parenteral, sexual	Fecal-oral
Incubation period	Short	Long	Long	Intermediate	Short
Usual onset*	Abrupt	Insidious	Insidious	Abrupt	Abrupt
Severity*	Mild or asymptomatic	Occasionally severe	Usually subclinical	Occasionally to often severe	Mild, but severe in pregnant women
Mortality rate*	Very low	Low	Low	High to very high	Low but high in pregnant women
Chronicity (carrier state)	No	Yes	Yes (common)	Yes	No
Other disease associations	None	HCC, cirrhosis	HCC, cirrhosis	Cirrhosis, fulminant hepatitis	None

*Refers to acute infection. HDV replicates only in HBV-infected cells. Onset of hepatitis D is most rapid, and the prognosis is worst when HDV infects cells already infected with HBV (superinfection).
HCC, hepatocellular cancer.

3. Prodromal symptoms
   - Fever, malaise, anorexia
4. Preicteric symptoms
   - Nausea, vomiting, abdominal pain, fever, chills
5. Icteric signs
   - Jaundice, dark urine, increase in serum levels of liver enzymes due to liver damage

D. **Diagnosis**
   - Hepatitis diagnosis is based on the time course of clinical signs and symptoms and on serologic assays for specific antiviral antibodies or viral antigens.

II. **Hepatitis A Virus (HAV)**

A. **Overview**
   1. HAV is a small, naked (+) RNA virus belonging to the family Picornaviridae (see Chapter 23).
   2. Like other enteroviruses, HAV is acid resistant and can survive in the gastrointestinal tract and sewage systems.

B. **Pathogenesis**
   1. After ingestion, HAV probably replicates in the oropharynx and the intestinal epithelium.
   2. Viremia spreads the virus to the liver, where it replicates within hepatocytes with minimal damage.
   3. Virions are released into the bile and shed into the stool 10 days before symptoms appear.
   4. Disease manifestations result from host immune and inflammatory response.

C. **Hepatitis A disease (infectious hepatitis)**
   1. Acute disease is usually mild, or asymptomatic, and occurs most often in school-aged children and young adults.
   2. Complete recovery occurs in 99% of the cases and confers lifelong immunity.

D. **Laboratory diagnosis**
   - Serologic detection of anti-HAV immunoglobulin M (IgM) antibody provides confirmation of hepatitis A diagnosis.

E. **Prevention and treatment**
   1. Chlorine treatment of water and sewage, good hygienic practices, and avoidance of contaminated food and water (especially uncooked shellfish) reduce HAV transmission.
   2. Inactivated HAV vaccine is recommended for travelers to endemic regions.
   3. Passive immunization with immune globulin before exposure or soon after can protect contacts.

III. **Hepatitis B Virus**

A. **Overview**
   1. HBV is a small, enveloped virus with a circular, partially double-stranded DNA genome.
   2. HBV encodes a reverse transcriptase, which is carried in the virion particle.
   3. Only human virus belonging to the family Hepadnaviridae.
   4. Unlike most enveloped viruses, HBV virion (Dane particle) is resistant to low pH, moderate heating, and detergents.

B. **HBV antigens**
   1. HBcAg (major core antigen) surrounds genome and core enzymes.
   2. HBsAg (surface antigen) is present in the envelope.
   3. HBeAg is shed into blood and indicative of active disease (related to HBc).

C. **Replication of HBV (Fig. 27-1)**
   1. Virions carry a reverse transcriptase similar to the retrovirus enzyme, which is essential to the unique HBV replication mechanism.
   2. Viral genome is transcribed into a longer than genomic length RNA.
      - Viral reverse transcriptase uses the RNA to make double-stranded DNA circles.
      - Circles remain incomplete in virion.
   3. Virions and noninfectious particles composed of HBsAg without genomes are released from infected cells.

D. **Markers of the course and nature of hepatitis B disease (Fig. 27-2; Table 27-2)**
   1. Serum HBeAg and HBV DNA are the best indicators of the presence of infectious virions (transmissibility).
   2. Anti-HBc, IgM antibody to HBcAg, is an indicator of recent acute infection
      - All IgM antibody is converted to IgG antibody by 6 months.

Abdominal pain, anorexia, jaundice, and dark urine indicate hepatitis but does not indicate cause.

Trigger words:
HAV: acute, sudden-onset hepatitis; day care center; fecal-oral spread; food-borne; picornavirus; shellfish

Virulence properties of HAV: fecal-oral spread, asymptomatic transmission, capsid resistant to inactivation

HAV: acute hepatitis with sudden onset; usually self-limited, benign infection

Protection from HAV by passive (immunoglobulin) and active (inactivated vaccine) immunization.

Trigger words:
HBV: contaminated blood and semen and mother's milk, chronic, Dane particle, HBsAg, hepadnavirus, insidious onset, primary hepatocellular carcinoma, serum hepatitis

HBV is a small, enveloped DNA virus that is resistant to detergents but sensitive to reverse transcriptase inhibitors.

HBV: acute hepatitis with slow onset; chronic infection and asymptomatic carriers

Hepatitis B serologic markers: HBsAg and HBe mean virus is present.
- HBeAg = virus shedding (transmissibility)
- HBV DNA = transmissibility
- Antibody (IgM) to HBcAg = recent infection
- Antibody to HBsAg = resolution of infection or vaccination
- Persistent HBsAg = chronic infection

The HBV virion particle contains circular double-stranded DNA with a partially completed strand.

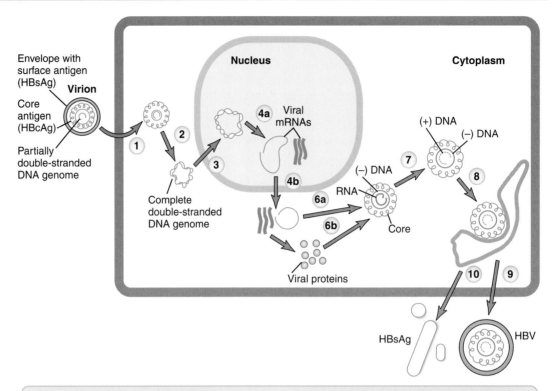

27-1: Proposed pathway for replication of hepatitis B virus (HBV). HBcAg, hepatitis B core antigen; HBsAg, hepatitis B surface antigen; mRNA, messenger RNA.

The figure legend reads:

1. Binding and endocytosis of HBV virion into target cell; and release of nucleocapsid core into cytoplasm

2. Uncoating of core and completion of partially double-stranded DNA genome by viral DNA polymerase

3. Transport of completed genome to nucleus

4. Transcription of viral genome by host enzymes (4a) and transport of mRNAs to cytoplasm (4b)

5. Translation of viral mRNAs into proteins on host ribosomes

6. Synthesis of (−) DNA strand by viral reverse transcriptase using longest mRNA as template (6a) and assembly of core proteins around RNA/DNA hybrid (6b)

7. Degradation of RNA strand and synthesis of (+) DNA strand to replace it

8. Envelopment of nucleocapsid by intracellular membrane before entire (+) DNA strand is completed

9. Exocytosis of HBV virion

10. Exocytosis of noninfectious HBsAg particles

3. Anti-HBs, antibody to HBsAg, indicates resolution of infection or prior vaccination and confers lifelong immunity.
   • IgG anti-HBcAg distinguishes previous infection (positive) from vaccination (negative).
4. The continued presence of HBsAg, presence of IgG anti-HBcAg, and lack of anti-HBsAg are the best indicators of chronic infection.
   • If HBeAg and HBV DNA are negative, the patient is called a *healthy carrier*.
   • If HBeAg and HBV DNA are positive, the patient is called an *infective carrier*.

E. Pathogenesis
1. Viremia spreads HBV virions from the site of entry to the liver.
   • Anti-HBsAg produced by prior infection, vaccination, or gammaglobulin prevents infection by blocking spread to the liver.
2. Viral replication in hepatocytes continues for a long period without damage to the liver.
3. Cell-mediated immune response, responsible for both the symptoms and the resolution of HBV infection, develops during the incubation period.
   • Strong response → acute disease with complete resolution
   • Mild response → mild symptoms (or asymptomatic) with incomplete resolution, leading to chronic infection
     a. Young children have mild disease but become carriers because they mount only a weak cell-mediated response.

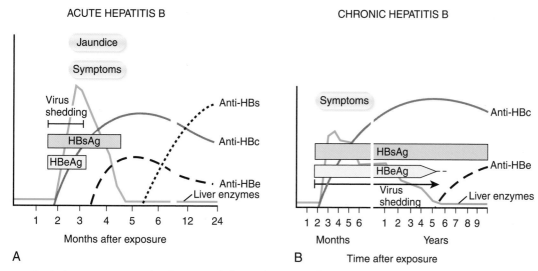

27-2: Serologic events associated with acute and chronic hepatitis B disease. **A,** Acute disease. Hepatitis B early antigen (HBeAg) indicates the presence of infectious virions in the blood. Serum hepatitis B surface antigen (HBsAg) does not correlate well with viral load because of secretion of noninfectious HBsAg particles from infected cells. Antibody to hepatitis B core antigen (HBcAg) indicates recent infection, whereas antibodies to HBsAg or HBeAg become detectable once these antigens cease to be produced as infection resolves. **B,** Chronic disease. Development of the chronic hepatitis B carrier state is characterized by the continued presence of HBsAg and HBeAg, high serum levels of liver enzymes, and the absence of detectable anti-HBsAg antibody.

TABLE 27-2 **Serology of Hepatitis A and B Viruses**

DISEASE	HAV IgM	HAV IgG	HBsAg	HBeAG/HBV DNA	ANTI-HBc IgM	ANTI-HBc IgG	ANTI-HBs
Acute hepatitis A virus (HAV)	+	+/−					
Previous HAV	−	+					
Acute hepatitis B virus (HBV)			+	+	−/+	−	−
"Window"*			−	−	+	−	−
Chronic HBV healthy carrier			+	−	−	+	−
Chronic HBV infective carrier			+	+		+	
Previous HBV			−	−	−	+	+
Vaccinated			−	−	−	−	+

*The window period of HBV disease occurs after infection has been resolved but before anti-HBs can be detected.

4. HBsAg secreted by infected liver cells forms immune complexes with serum antibody that can trigger type III hypersensitivity reactions (e.g., glomerulonephritis, polyarthritis, rash, and itching).
5. Permanent liver damage and cirrhosis can result from fulminant infection, activation of a chronic infection, or coinfection with hepatitis D virus.
6. Long-term chronic infection predisposes patient to primary hepatocellular carcinoma.

F. Hepatitis B disease (serum hepatitis)
1. Acute hepatitis
   - About 25% of HBV infections manifest acute symptoms, primarily in adults.
2. Chronic hepatitis
   - About 5% to 10% of HBV infections become chronic, usually after a mild or asymptomatic initial infection.
   - Prolonged elevation of serum liver enzymes and the continued presence of HBsAg in the blood mark the chronic state (see Fig. 27-2B).
   - Up to 10% of patients with chronic hepatitis B develop cirrhosis and permanent liver damage.
   - After about a 30-year period, chronic infection can lead to primary hepatocellular carcinoma (PHC).

Anti-HBV immune response causes symptoms and resolution of disease: no pain, no gain. No pain, chronic disease, as in children.

HBV, HCV, and HDV are transmitted in blood, semen, vaginal secretions, saliva, and mother's milk by transfusions, needle stick, sexual contact, and breastfeeding.

Blood supply is routinely screened for HBV, HCV and HIV.

HBV vaccine is a virus-like particle formed by HBsAg.

Immunization for HBV prevents HDV disease and PHC.

HBV reverse transcriptase is a target for lamivudine and other nucleotide and nucleoside analogue antiviral drugs.

Trigger words:
HCV: chronic; cirrhosis; flavivirus; non-A, non-B hepatitis

HCV: causes 90% of the cases of non-A, non-B hepatitis; major cause of posttransfusion hepatitis. Slow onset of usually subclinical acute disease; usually causes chronic infection.

Virulence factors of HCV: chronic infection, immune escape, rapid mutation, asymptomatic transmission

HCV is most likely to cause chronic disease and then lead to liver failure.

Trigger words:
HDV: fulminant hepatitis, HBV required as helper virus

HDV: major cause of fulminant hepatitis; infection of an HBV carrier causes more severe disease than simultaneous coinfection.

G. Transmission
1. Asymptomatic and chronic carriers shed HBV and are major sources for spread of the virus.
2. Virion-containing body fluids (blood, semen, vaginal secretions, saliva, and mother's milk) can be acquired through transfusions, needle stick, sexual contact, and breastfeeding.

H. Prevention
1. Screening of blood supply with enzyme-linked immunosorbent assay (ELISA) for HBsAg and antibody to HBcAg
2. HBsAg subunit vaccine is recommended for newborns, health care workers, and other at-risk groups (e.g., individuals with multiple sex partners and patients requiring numerous blood and blood product treatments).
   - Vaccine prevention of chronic HBV will also prevent PHC.

I. Treatment
1. Nucleotide analogue inhibitors of reverse transcriptase polymerase: lamivudine, entecavir, emtricitabine, adefovir, dipivoxil, famciclovir
   - Passive immunization with anti-HBV gammaglobulin.

IV. Hepatitis C Virus (HCV)

A. Overview
1. HCV is a small, enveloped (+) RNA virus belonging to the family Flaviviridae (see Chapter 25).
2. It is transmitted by the same routes as HBV.

B. Hepatitis C (non-A, non-B hepatitis)
1. Antibody is *not* protective.
2. Acute infection
   - Clinical course and symptoms are similar to those of HBV infection, but the symptoms are milder.
3. Chronic infection
   - About 75% of HCV infections become chronic with viremia (virus shedding) lasting more than 10 years.
   - Can lead to cirrhosis liver failure and hepatocellular carcinoma

C. Prevention
- Blood supply and transplant organs are screened by ELISA.

D. Laboratory diagnosis
1. ELISA does not distinguish IgG from IgM antibodies or whether the disease is acute, chronic, or resolved.
2. Recombinant immunoblot assay (RIBA) is ordered if ELISA test is positive.
3. Positive RIBA
   - Order polymerase chain reaction to detect viral RNA

E. Treatment
- Recombinant interferon-α and ribavirin with supportive therapy are used for treatment of hepatitis C.

V. Hepatitis D Virus (HDV, Delta Agent)

A. Overview
1. HDV replicates only in HBV-infected cells.
2. Virion comprises circular, single-stranded (–) RNA genome and delta antigen surrounded by an HBsAg-containing envelope.

B. Pathogenesis
1. HDV is acquired by the same routes as HBV.
2. Coinfection occurs when hepatocytes are infected simultaneously (or nearly so) with HBV and HDV.
3. Superinfection occurs when HDV infects cells that are already infected with HBV → most rapid and severe disease progression.
4. Cytotoxicity and liver damage result from replication of HDV.
5. Persistent HDV infection may occur in HBV carriers.

C. Hepatitis D disease
1. Clinical manifestations are similar to but occur more rapidly and are more severe than those associated with HBV infection alone.
2. Fulminant hepatitis is more likely with HDV than with other hepatitis viruses.
   - Is associated with severe liver damage accompanied by ascites fluid and bleeding; may be fatal
   - Occurs in 1% of HBV-infected patients due to coinfection or superinfection with HDV

D. Prevention
- Immunization with HBV vaccine (preventing infection with the cofactor) reduces the incidence of HDV infection.

VI. Hepatitis E Virus (HEV)
  A. Overview
- HEV is a small, naked (+) RNA virus that resembles Norwalk virus (see Chapter 23).

  B. HEV disease
- Epidemiologically and clinically, HEV infection resembles HAV infection, except the mortality rate is higher, especially in pregnant women (see Table 27-1).

VII. Hepatocellular Carcinoma (HCC)
- Postnecrotic cirrhosis from chronic HBV and HCV infections is the most important risk factor.

Trigger words:

HEV: acute, sudden-onset hepatitis; calicivirus, fecal-oral spread, pregnant women

HEV: abrupt onset of acute disease; high mortality rate in expectant mothers

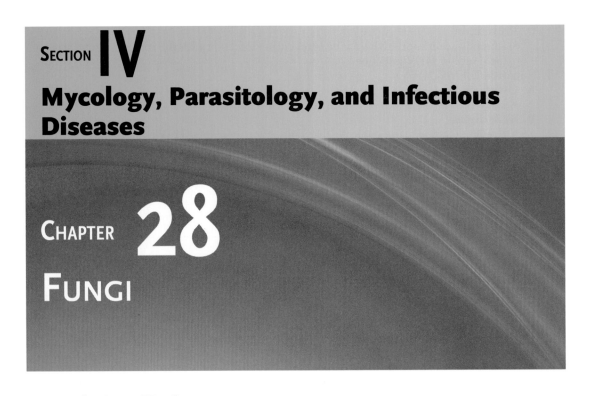

I. Introduction to Mycology

A. Overview

1. Fungi are eukaryotic organisms.
2. Fungal membranes contain ergosterol rather than cholesterol found in other eukaryotic membranes.
3. The cell wall surrounding fungal cells, which differs in composition from bacterial cell walls, contains chitin, glucans, and protein.

B. Morphologic forms

1. Molds, or filamentous fungi, are composed of a mass of branching, thread-like tubular filaments (hyphae) that elongate at their tips.
   - Septate hyphae are divided into individual walled-off cells, each containing a nucleus.
   - Aseptate (coenocytic) hyphae are hollow and multinucleate.
2. Yeasts are unicellular, usually round fungi.
   - Some yeasts develop pseudohyphae, which are strings of elongated cells linked like sausages.
3. Dimorphic fungi exist as molds or yeasts depending on temperature or other environmental factors.
4. Dematiaceous fungi are dark colored and usually from soil.

C. Asexual reproduction

1. All fungi can reproduce asexually, and asexually reproducing forms are most commonly encountered in clinical situations.
2. Some fungi can also reproduce sexually.
3. Molds
   - Aerial hyphae release spores, which germinate on suitable substrates, leading to growth of new hyphae.
4. Yeasts
   - Budding or binary fission of a yeast cell produces two daughter cells.

D. Conditions conducive to fungal infections

- Although fungi are ubiquitous in the environment, they generally colonize tissues and cause infection only when the body's normal defenses or the normal flora are disrupted.
1. Disruption of the body's physical, chemical, or physiologic barriers
   - Intact skin, pH, fatty acids in the skin, normal bacterial flora, and various humoral factors normally prevent fungal infection.
2. Immunosuppression, particularly loss of CD4 T_H1 responses
   - Opportunistic infections by normal flora (e.g., *Candida albicans*) or increased susceptibility to environmental fungi (e.g., *Aspergillus* species) may result.

Ergosterol is unique to fungal membranes.

Ergosterol and cell wall metabolism are antifungal drug targets.

Dimorphic fungi are yeasts at 37°C and molds at lower temperatures.

Many fungi cause opportunistic infections of immunosuppressed individuals with hereditary or acquired T cell deficiencies.

3. Disruption of normal bacterial flora
   - Use of antibacterial drugs sometimes allows colonization by fungi that otherwise would not establish infection.

E. **Types of fungal infections (mycoses)**
   - Fungal infections and the agents causing them are commonly classified based on the site of disease or the immune status of the host.
   1. Superficial mycoses involve the keratinized outermost layers of skin, hair, and nails.
   2. Cutaneous mycoses involve the keratin-containing epidermis and deeper layers of the hair, skin, and nails.
   3. Subcutaneous mycoses involve the dermis, subcutaneous tissues, muscles, and fascia.
   4. Systemic mycoses often originate in the lungs but disseminate to other organs (especially in immunocompromised individuals).
   5. Opportunistic mycoses generally occur only in patients with compromised immune systems (e.g., cancer patients receiving immunosuppressive therapy and human immunodeficiency virus [HIV]-infected individuals).

F. **Diagnosis of fungal infections**
   - Fungal infections mimic other diseases and therefore must be distinguished through careful differential diagnosis (Table 28-1).
   1. Culture and microscopic examination
      - Isolation of fungi from specimens may require culturing for up to 30 days at 25°C and 35°C on appropriate media.
        a. Sabouraud agar, Mycosel agar
        b. Antibacterial antibiotics are often included in the medium to inhibit bacterial overgrowth.
      - Specific histologic stains can be used for direct visualization of fungi in tissue specimens.
        a. Skin scrapings are treated with 10% to 15% potassium hydroxide (KOH) to destroy tissue elements.
        b. Mucicarmine stain is used for cryptosporidia.
      - Sugar utilization tests (similar to the fermentation tests for Enterobacteriaceae) are useful in identifying yeasts.
   2. Detection of fungal antigens in blood or cerebrospinal fluid (CSF) by Ouchterlony (double-immunodiffusion) test or enzyme-linked immunosorbent assay

G. **Antifungal agents**
   - Table 28-2 lists common drugs used in treating mycoses and their mode of action.

Fungi are great mimickers and resemble other diseases, such as tumor growths.

KOH preparation discloses fungal structures in sample.

Mucicarmine stains cryptosporidia.

TABLE 28-1 Differential Diagnosis of Fungal Infections

INFECTION	ETIOLOGIC AGENT	OTHER CONDITIONS TO EXCLUDE
Aspergillosis	*Aspergillus* species	Zygomycoses and other mold infections
Blastomycosis	*Blastomyces dermatitidis*	Bacterial and viral pneumonia, atypical mycobacterial infection, other systemic mycoses, bacterial or mycobacterial skin infections
Candidiasis	*Candida albicans*	Bacterial and other fungal infections
Chromoblastomycosis	Dematiaceous soil fungi	Sporotrichosis, tularemia, plague, gangrene, actinomycosis, atypical mycobacterial infection
Coccidioidomycosis	*Coccidioides immitis*	Bacterial and viral pneumonia; skin infections caused by bacteria, viruses, or other fungi
Cryptococcosis	*Cryptococcus neoformans*	Meningitis caused by bacteria (e.g., *Mycobacterium tuberculosis*) and viruses, lung cancer, other systemic mycoses (especially histoplasmosis)
Histoplasmosis	*Histoplasma capsulatum*	Other systemic mycoses, bacterial and viral pneumonia, tuberculosis
Mycetoma, eumycotic	Dematiaceous soil	Mycetoma caused by soil bacteria fungi
Paracoccidioidomycosis	*Paracoccidioides brasiliensis*	Bacterial and viral pneumonia; skin infections caused by bacteria, viruses, or other fungi
Ringworm (tinea)	*Trichophyton, Microsporum,* and *Epidermophyton* species	Candidal infections; bacterial and viral skin infections
Sporotrichosis	*Sporothrix schenckii*	Tularemia, plague, gangrene, nocardiosis, chronic staphylococcal skin infections, atypical mycobacterial infection, other mycoses
Zygomycosis	*Rhizopus* and *Mucor* species	Aspergillosis and other mold infections

TABLE 28-2 Antifungal Drugs

CLASS AND EXAMPLES	MECHANISM	PRIMARY USES
Polyenes		
Amphotericin B	Disrupt fungal membranes by binding to ergosterol in the membrane	Broad spectrum, for systemic and opportunistic mycoses Amphotericin B can cause renal toxicity
Liposomal amphotericin		Less toxic, more useful form
Nystatin	Topical	
Azole Derivatives (Imidazole and Triazole)		
Miconazole Ketoconazole Fluconazole Itraconazole Posaconazole Voriconazole	Depress biosynthesis of lanosterol and ergosterol by inhibiting cytochrome P-450 enzymes	Systemic and opportunistic mycoses Broader spectrum of activity Broader spectrum of activity Broader spectrum of activity and *Aspergillus* species infections
Nucleoside Analogues		
5-Fluorocytosine (in combinations)	Inhibits DNA and RNA synthesis	Cryptococcosis Chromoblastomycosis
Allylamines and Thiocarbamates		
Naftifine Terbinafine Tolnaftate Tolciclate	Depress ergosterol biosynthesis by inhibiting squalene oxidase	Topical treatment of cutaneous mycoses caused by dermatophytes
Grisans		
Griseofulvin	Inhibits fungal mitosis by interacting with microtubules	Cutaneous mycoses that are unresponsive to topical agents
Candins (echinocandins)		
Micafungin Caspofungin Anidulafungin	Depress cell wall formation by inhibiting glucan synthesis	Candidiasis, aspergillosis

II. Superficial and Cutaneous Mycoses

A. Superficial mycoses
- Occur in outer cornified tissues, elicit no immune response, and pose only cosmetic problems
1. Pityriasis versicolor and pityriasis nigra involve the outer layer of the skin.
   - Treated with keratin-removing agents or with topical miconazole
2. White piedra and black piedra involve the hair shaft.
   - Treated by cutting hair below the nodular lesions

B. Cutaneous mycoses
1. Caused by various *Trichophyton*, *Microsporum*, and *Epidermophyton* species, collectively referred to as *dermatophytes*.
2. These infections are generally restricted to keratin-containing tissues and may elicit cellular immune responses, leading to inflamed, outward-spreading lesions. They may also contribute to seborrhea and dandruff.
3. Clinical manifestations
   - *Ringworm*, the common name for these infections, describes the lesions, which are in the form of a ring and resemble a worm burrowing in the skin.
   - Tinea plus modifier specifically indicates the site involved. For example:
     a. Tinea capitis = scalp (Fig. 28-1)
     b. Tinea cruris = groin (jock itch)
     c. Tinea pedis = feet (athlete's foot)
     d. Tinea unguium = nails
4. Laboratory diagnosis
   - Branching, septate hyphae are seen in KOH preparations of skin scrapings.
   - Spores and fragmented hyphae are seen in KOH preparations of hair.
5. Treatment
   - Skin infections
     a. Topical azole antifungal such as ketoconazole, miconazole, or clotrimazole
   - Hair infections
     a. Ketoconazole or sulfur-containing shampoos; griseofulvin
   - Nails
     a. Azole antibiotics (topical or systemic); surgical or chemical removal of the infected nail

Malassezia furfur causes pityriasis versicolor and looks like spaghetti (short septate hyphae) and meatballs (small yeasts).

Trichophyton infects all three: hair, nails, and skin. Dermatophyte infections causing ringworm (tinea) are often mixed with bacteria.

Microsporum fluoresce when exposed to ultraviolet light (Wood lamp)

Trigger words:
Tinea: azoles; circular, scaling lesion with central clearing and hair loss; crumbling nails; discoloring; keratin; ringworm

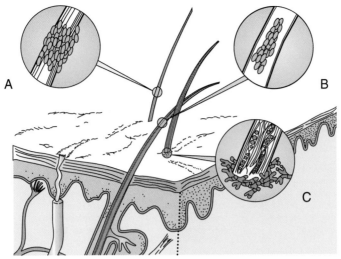

28-1: Schematic illustration of ringworm of the scalp, which involves the hairs and takes various forms. In an ectothrix infection, fungal spores form a sheath around the hair shafts (**A**), whereas in an endothrix infection, spores invade the hair shafts (**B**). **C**, In a favic hair infection, honeycomb-appearing masses usually form at the base of scalp hairs.

III. Subcutaneous, Opportunistic, and Systemic Mycoses
- Pertinent information about common mycoses and the fungi causing them are summarized in Table 28-3.
A. Subcutaneous mycoses
1. Overview
   - These infections are often caused by melanin-containing (dematiaceous) fungi present in the soil or decaying vegetation.
   - Organisms usually enter through cuts, punctures, or stabs caused by contaminated thorns or sharp tools.
2. Sporotrichosis
   - Caused by *Sporothrix schenckii*, a dimorphic fungus
   - Chronic nodular and ulcerative nodular lymphocutaneous lesions along lymphatics (e.g., rose gardener's disease)
3. Chromoblastomycosis
   - Caused by various dematiaceous soil fungi
   - Verrucoid (warty) nodules with cauliflower-like appearance; pseudoepitheliomatous hyperplasia
4. Eumycotic mycetoma
   - Caused by numerous dematiaceous fungi
   - Swollen, deforming lesions that contain numerous draining sinus tracts
     a. Grains or granules composed of fungal tissue in exudate
     b. Commonly on hand or foot

TABLE 28-3 Summary of Common Fungal Pathogens

ORGANISM	DISEASE FEATURES	IDENTIFICATION	PATHOGENESIS	TRANSMISSION	TREATMENT
Aspergillus fumigatus	Lung infection with hemoptysis. Invasive form: blood vessels often involved. Allergic form: respiratory distress increasing with age.	Mold with septate, branched hyphae; spherical mass of hyphae ("fungus ball") visible in lung radiograph	Opportunistic; growth in preexisting lung cavity; tissue invasion in immunocompromised; host allergic reactions	Inhalation of airborne spores	Surgery to remove infected tissue; amphotericin B, itraconazole, voriconazole, posaconazole, echinocandins
Blastomyces dermatitidis	Suppurative and tuberculosis-like lung infections. Possible involvement of skin and bones	Dimorphic; large yeast cells with **broad-based** buds in tissue samples; exoantigen	Invasion of respiratory tract inducing cell-mediated response and granuloma formation; possible spread	Inhalation of airborne spores; endemic in areas of midwestern United States (Mississippi River Valley)	Azole derivatives; amphotericin B for serious cases

TABLE 28-3 **Summary of Common Fungal Pathogens—Cont'd**

ORGANISM	DISEASE FEATURES	IDENTIFICATION	PATHOGENESIS	TRANSMISSION	TREATMENT
Candida albicans	Oral thrush (neonates, diabetic patients, AIDS patients) Vulvovaginitis (high pH, antibiotic use, diabetes) Mucocutaneous lesions in those with T cell or endocrine defects	Budding yeasts, pseudohyphae, septate hyphae in tissues; germ-tube formation at 37°C; pasty, cream-colored colonies on agar	Opportunistic; infection associated with trauma, immunosuppression, use of broad-spectrum antibiotics or oral contraceptives	Part of normal mucosal flora	Ketoconazole, fluconazole, voriconazole, echinocandin
Coccidioides immitis	San Joaquin Valley fever: self-limited respiratory infection with fever and cough Involvement of meninges and/or skin in immu-nosuppressed	Dimorphic; spore-containing spherules in tissue; skin test for fungal antigen (similar to PPD test)	Invasion of respiratory tract inducing inflammatory response and granuloma formation	Inhalation of arthrospores; endemic to desert areas of **southwestern United States**	Amphotericin B, ketoconazole, fluconazole, itraconazole
Cryptococcus neoformans	Primary lung infection often asymptomatic with a solitary nodule Meningitis similar to that due to *Mycobacterium tuberculosis* Disseminated skin and bone lesions	Not dimorphic; encapsulated yeast in soil and tissue; capsule detected by India ink staining of cerebrospinal fluid; capsular antigens	Capsule protects against phagocytosis in respiratory tract; spread via bloodstream mostly in immunosuppressed	Inhalation of yeast cells; often in pigeon droppings	Amphotericin B plus flucytosine for meningitis; long-term fluconazole in AIDS patients
Histoplasma capsulatum	Progressive respiratory infection with granulomas in lung tissue Disseminated disease with fever, weight loss, and splenomegaly in immunosuppressed	Dimorphic; small yeasts visible in tissue macrophages; exoantigen in serum or urine	Growth in pulmonary macrophages with granuloma formation; spread via monocytes to lymphoid and other tissues	Inhalation of airborne spores; endemic in **Ohio and Mississippi River valleys**; found in bird droppings	Amphotericin B for acute disease; long-term itraconazole in AIDS patients
Mucor and *Rhizopus* species	Rhinocerebral infection originating in paranasal sinuses and ocular orbit; possible extension to brain; usually in acidotic diabetic patients Involvement of lungs in neutropenic patients and of gastrointestinal tract in malnourished children	Mold with broad, aseptate hyphae and wide-angle branching	Opportunistic; invasion of blood vessels and formation of hyphal emboli causing ischemia and necrosis of adjacent tissue	Inhalation of airborne spores	Surgery to remove necrotic tissue; amphotericin B
Paracoccidioides brasiliensis	Primary lung infection often asymptomatic Ulcerative lesions of oral and nasal mucosa	Dimorphic; yeasts with multiple buds ("captain's wheel") in tissue	Initial infection of respiratory tract with dissemination and granuloma formation	Inhalation of spores; endemic in Central and South America	Long-term azole derivatives
Pneumocystis jiroveci (carinii)	Interstitial pneumonia with plasma cell infiltrates; common in AIDS patients	Cup-shaped organisms seen in lung tissue with silver stain	Opportunistic; alveolar inflammation with pulmonary exudate and fibrosis; cyst formation	Inhalation	TMP-SMX, pentamidine Clindamycin
Sporothrix schenckii	Nodular and ulcerative lesions along lymphatic vessels; lesions initially pink, then turn purple or black	Dimorphic; moist, white mold with thin, branching hyphae at 25°C; small budding yeast at 35°C	Chronic subcutaneous infection; swelling and inflammation of lymph nodes and vessels draining inoculation site	Thorn prick most common route (rose gardener's disease)	Potassium iodide (oral), amphotericin B, itraconazole

PPD, purified protein derivative; TMP-SMX, trimethoprim-sulfamethoxazole.

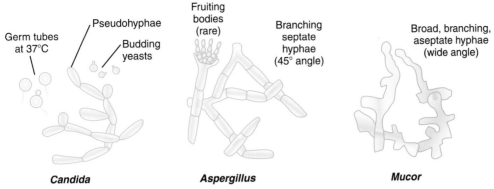

28-2: Morphology of common opportunistic fungal agents in tissues.

- May require total excision of lesion or amputation of the affected limb because antifungal drugs are generally ineffective against causative fungi

B. **Agents of opportunistic mycoses (Fig. 28-2)**

- Major characteristics distinguishing fungi that cause opportunistic and systemic mycoses are outlined in Box 28-1.

1. *Candida albicans*
   - Part of the normal flora in mucous membranes
   - Dimorphic, germ tubes at 37°C
   - Cutaneous candidiasis
     a. Oral thrush is most common in neonates, diabetics, AIDS patients, and those receiving antibiotics or steroids.
     b. Vulvovaginitis is promoted by antibiotic use, higher pH, and diabetes mellitus.
   - Chronic mucocutaneous candidiasis (rarely disseminates but is resistant to treatment)
     a. T cell deficiency or endocrine defects (e.g., hypoparathyroidism, hypothyroidism, hypoadrenalism, or thymoma) are predisposing factors.
   - Disseminated disease
     a. In immunosuppressed cancer and transplant recipients, candidal infection commonly presents as disseminated disease (bloodstream infections).

2. Other candida:
   - *Candida glabrata* causes bloodstream infections and is azole drug resistant

3. *Aspergillus fumigatus* and other *Aspergillus* species
   - Filamentous with septate, branched hyphae; "fungus ball" in lungs seen on radiograph; induces allergic reactions
   - Pulmonary infection established in preexisting cavitary lesion (fungus ball)
   - Becomes invasive in immunocompromised patients, especially neutropenic patients
   - Produces a severe extrinsic type of bronchial asthma

4. *Rhizopus* and *Mucor* species
   - Filamentous with broad, aseptate hyphae; hyphal emboli
   - Rhinocerebral zygomycosis (most common presentation) originates in paranasal sinuses and ocular orbit with possible spread to palate and frontal lobes.
     a. Usually seen in diabetic ketoacidosis

Acquired immunodeficiency syndrome (AIDS) patients are prone to develop severe candidal infections of the oropharynx and the upper gastrointestinal tract (thrush) but only rarely exhibit disseminated disease.

Trigger words:
Candida albicans: "cobblestones"; immunocompromised (AIDS patients, chemotherapy patients, diabetic patients, infants, transplant recipients); thrush; vaginal yeast; white, curd-like, adhesive plaques that bleed when removed for culture, prolonged use of antibiotics

Trigger words:
Aspergillus species: allergic bronchopulmonary, angioinvasive, fruiting bodies, fungus ball, hypersensitivity pneumonitis (allergic alveolitis), malt (grain) workers, septate branching hyphae

Trigger words:
Rhizopus and *Mucor* species: acidotic diabetic, black nasal discharge, bread mold, coenocyte (aseptate) hyphae, paranasal sinus and ocular orbit involvement

BOX 28-1 SYSTEMIC VERSUS OPPORTUNISTIC FUNGAL AGENTS	
Agents of Systemic Infection	**Agents of Opportunistic Infection**
Disease often is asymptomatic or resolves quickly in both normal and compromised hosts	Disease often is serious primarily in compromised hosts
Endemic in limited geographic area	Found worldwide
Usually not part of normal flora	Usually part of normal flora
Dimorphic (except *Cryptococcus*)	Not dimorphic (except *Candida*)

5. *Pneumocystis jiroveci (carinii)*
   - A fungus, but used to be classified as a protozoan
   - Interstitial pneumonia occurs only in severely immunocompromised individuals, especially AIDS patients.
   - Gomori silver stain of lung tissue reveals diagnostic rounded, cup-shaped organisms.

C. Agents of systemic mycoses (Fig. 28-3)
   1. Overview
      - Most agents of systemic mycoses are dimorphic, existing as filamentous fungi in soil (saprobic phase) and as yeasts or spherules in tissue at 37°C (parasitic phase)
      - In healthy individuals, many systemic mycoses are asymptomatic or manifest as a relatively mild, self-limited pulmonary infection.
      - In immunocompromised individuals, systemic mycoses generally exhibit more serious lung involvement and often disseminate to other organs.
   2. *Blastomyces dermatitidis*
      - Dimorphic
      - Large yeasts with broad-based buds seen in tissue samples
      - Endemic in portions of the midwestern United States
      - Blastomycosis is marked by tuberculosis-like pneumonia with possible skin, bone, or prostate involvement.
   3. *Coccidioides immitis*
      - Dimorphic
      - Spherules with endospores seen in tissue specimens
      - Contracted by inhaling arthrospores in dust
      - Endemic in desert areas of the southwestern United States
      - Primary coccidioidomycosis (San Joaquin Valley fever)
        a. Acute, self-limited, flu-like illness with fever, cough, joint pain, and sometimes erythema nodosum (painful nodules on the shins)
   4. *Cryptococcus neoformans*
      - Nondimorphic encapsulated yeast visible in India ink preparations of CSF
      - Found worldwide, commonly in pigeon droppings and nests
      - Primary cryptococcosis is often discovered accidentally as a solitary pulmonary nodule that may mimic carcinoma.
      - Granulomatous meningitis is the most common form of systemic disease.
   5. *Histoplasma capsulatum*
      - Dimorphic
      - Small budding yeast seen within macrophages

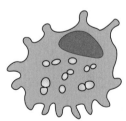

Histoplasma capsulatum
(intracellular budding yeasts)

Blastomyces dermatitidis
(broad-based budding yeasts)

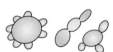

Paracoccidioides brasiliensis
(multiple-budded yeasts; captain's wheel)

Coccidioides immitis
(spherule of spores)

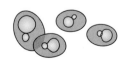

Cryptococcus neoformans
(encapsulated yeasts with narrow-based, unequal buds)

28-3: Morphology of tissue forms of common systemic fungal agents. Except for *Cryptococcus neoformans,* all are dimorphic, exhibiting a mold-to-yeast (or spherule) transition when infecting susceptible species.

- Endemic in the Ohio and Mississippi River valleys
- Especially abundant in bird (chickens, starlings) and bat droppings
- Histoplasmosis is marked by pulmonary granulomas, which may be seen on radiograph.

6. *Paracoccidioides brasiliensis*
   - Dimorphic
   - Captain's wheel morphology of yeast cells in tissues due to multiple budding
   - Endemic in Central and South America
     a. Paracoccidioidomycosis is marked by ulcerative lesions of oral and nasal mucosa.

IV. Case Presentations: Fungal Infections (Box 28-2)

Trigger words:
H. capsulatum: bird and bat droppings, "Cincinnati spleen," granulomas, lung and spleen, Ohio and Mississippi River Valleys, yeasts inside macrophages

Histoplasma are small yeasts often seen within macrophages.

BOX 28-2   CLASSIC FUNGAL INFECTIONS: QUICK CASES

Aspergillus species
Pulmonary aspergillosis: A 35-year-old man has a respiratory infection. His sputum is blood stained. A chest radiograph shows a ball-like mass of fungal hyphae (aspergilloma) in an apical cavity.

Blastomyces dermatitidis
Systemic blastomycosis: An otherwise healthy man who had successfully recovered from a respiratory illness marked by fever, cough, and chest pain 3 months ago now develops several chronic suppurative skin lesions. A chest radiograph shows pulmonary infiltrates.

Candida albicans
Oral thrush: An HIV-positive man has white patches on the tongue.
Candidal vaginitis: A 39-year-old woman who has diabetes is being treated with antibiotics for a bacterial infection. She develops vaginal pruritus, erythema, and a thick, creamy vaginal discharge.

Coccidioides immitis
San Joaquin Valley fever (primary coccidioidomycosis): After vacationing in the desert areas of New Mexico, a 40-year-old woman develops a respiratory infection with pulmonary infiltrates and has red, nodular, painful lesions (erythema nodosum) on both shins.

Cryptococcus neoformans
Cryptococcal meningitis: An immunosuppressed woman has a chronic headache and stiff neck. India ink preparation of cerebrospinal fluid shows encapsulated yeast cells.

Histoplasma capsulatum
Primary histoplasmosis: A chicken farmer living in southern Ohio has a mild respiratory infection with flu-like symptoms that resolve within 10 days. Two months later, numerous diffuse, small calcific densities are seen on a chest radiograph.

Mucor species
Rhinocerebral zygomycosis: A diabetic patient in ketoacidosis has a frontal lobe abscess.

Pneumocystis jiroveci (carinii)
***Pneumocystis* pneumonia:** An AIDS patient with a low CD4 T cell count has a respiratory infection with fever, cough, shortness of breath, and pulmonary infiltrates.

Sporothrix schenckii
Sporotrichosis: A woman develops suppurating, nodular skin lesions on the lower arm after pruning rose bushes in her garden.

29 PARASITES

I. Introduction to Parasitology

A. Overview

1. Two groups of parasitic organisms cause human disease: the single-celled protozoa and the multicellular helminths (worms).
2. Like fungi, parasites are eukaryotes, but they lack the plant-like cell wall present in fungi.
   - Humans are usually not the primary host for parasites.
   - Humans acquire infection when they encounter the primary host (vector) or its environment.

B. Pathogenesis

1. Entry of organisms occurs primarily by ingestion or direct penetration of the skin (sometimes by bite of insect vector).
   - Not part of normal flora
2. Replication of parasites takes place in specific cell types or organs.
   - A characteristic route of entry leads to infection.
   - Site and route of entry and release are determined by the life cycle of the organism.
   - Life cycle may differ in different hosts, for example, human versus snail or mosquito.
3. Cell and tissue damage result from four general mechanisms.
   - Toxic substances produced by parasites
   - Mechanical damage due to the size and movement of parasites
   - Cell-mediated immune response elicited in the host
   - Degradation of tissue to feed parasite
4. Immune escape
   - Variation of surface antigens: trypanosomes, plasmodia
   - Molecular mimicry of host antigens: plasmodia
   - Coating by host proteins: schistosomes, trypanosomes, hydatid cyst
   - Intracellular growth
   - Immunosuppression: trypanosomes, plasmodia, schistosomes

C. Disease manifestations

1. Disease determined by affected tissue and nature of disruption
2. Periodicity of symptoms due to life cycle of parasite
   - For malaria, rupturing of erythrocytes on maturation of merozoites
   - Pinworm females come out of anus at night to lay eggs.

D. Diagnosis

1. Definitive diagnosis of most parasitic diseases depends on microscopic identification of parasitic forms (e.g., larvae, eggs, and adults) in clinical specimens (Fig. 29-1).
2. Serologic testing is useful in diagnosis of *Entamoeba* and *Strongyloides* species infection.

E. Prevention

- No vaccines are available for parasitic infections.
1. Effective sanitation for organisms spread by fecal-oral route
2. Thorough cooking for organisms transmitted in meat or fish
3. Elimination of vectors and protection from their bites for organisms transmitted by insects

F. Treatment (Table 29-1)

1. Antiparasite drug targets are differentially sensitive to the drug compared with humans.
2. No vaccines are available.

For parasites, make sure to know your trigger words, diagnostic features, and epidemiology (means of spread, vectors, hosts, seasons, risk factors).

PROTOZOA

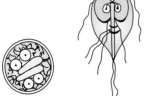 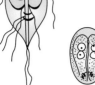 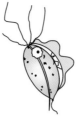

Cyst	Troph	Cyst	Adult	Troph	Oocyst
Entamoeba histolytica	*Giardia*	*lamblia*	*Trypanosoma and Leishmania* spp.	*Trichomonas vaginalis*	*Cryptosporidium* spp.

HELMINTHS

Sucker

Egg

Unfertilized egg

   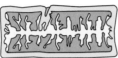 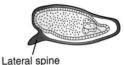

Lateral spine on egg

Fertilized egg

Larva in muscle	Gravid proglottid	Ascaris lumbricoides	Schistosoma mansoni
Trichinella spiralis	**Taenia solium**	***Ascaris lumbricoides***	***Schistosoma mansoni***

29-1: Diagnostic or characteristic morphology of selected parasites. Troph, trophozoite.

TABLE 29-1 Antiparasitic Drugs

PARASITE	DRUG	TARGET	EXAMPLES
Protozoa	Sulfonamides	Folate pathway	Toxoplasma, malaria
	Doxycycline, clindamycin	Protein synthesis	Malaria, amebiasis, babesia, cryptosporidia
	Diamidines	Bind to DNA	Pneumocystis, leishmania
	Arsenic, antimony compounds	Sulfhydryl groups	Trypanosomes, leishmania
Antimalarial	Aminoquinoline analogues (e.g., chloroquine, primaquine)	DNA replication, heme digestion	
	Doxycycline	Protein synthesis	
	Artemisinin	Reacts with heme	
	Halofantrine	Reacts with heme	
Antihelminth and antiworm	Mebendazole, thiabendazole, albendazole	Fumarate reductase, glucose metabolism, microtubules	Broad-spectrum antihelminth, antinematode, anticestode
	Pyrantel pamoate	Blocks neuromuscular action: fumarate reductase	Ascariasis, pinworm, hookworm
	Ivermectin	Blocks neuromuscular action, reproduction	Filaria
	Praziquantel	Calcium agonist	Antihelminth, antinematode, anticestode
	Niclosamide	Uncouples ox phos	Intestinal tapeworm
	Suramin	Blocks G proteins	Trypanosomes

II. Protozoan Parasites (Table 29-2)
A. Intestinal and urogenital protozoa
1. *Cryptosporidium* species
   - Self-limited watery diarrhea and flu-like symptoms in normal individuals
   - Severe, prolonged diarrhea in AIDS patients
2. *Entamoeba histolytica*
   - Watery diarrhea with blood and mucus in stools (amebic dysentery)
   - Cecal ulcers
   - Liver abscesses
   - Trophozoites phagocytose red blood cells

Cyst is resistant to inactivation and is transmitted. Trophozoite is the replicative form.

Trigger words:
Cryptosporidium species: immune suppression, water supply

Entamoeba histolytica: amebic dysentery, cyst with one to four nuclei, liver abscesses

TABLE 29-2 Parasites: Protozoa

NAME	DISEASE FEATURES	IDENTIFICATION	PATHOGENESIS	TRANSMISSION	TREATMENT
Cryptosporidium species	Watery diarrhea; severe in AIDS patients	Acid-fast stain of oocysts in stools	Invasion of gastrointestinal tract mucosa	Fecal-oral spread of oocysts	Rehydration, nitazoxanide
Entamoeba histolytica	Amebic dysentery, right upper quadrant pain, urn-shaped intestinal ulcers; Liver abscess	Cysts or trophozoites in stools or biopsy	Invasion of intestinal mucosa, cell destruction	Fecal-oral spread of cysts	Metronidazole, iodoquinol, paromomycin
Giardia lamblia	Mild to severe watery foul-smelling diarrhea; nausea, anorexia, cramps	Cysts or flagellated trophozoites (less common) in stools; stool antigen	Adherence to villi, perhaps causing malabsorption and irritation	Fecal-oral spread of cysts	Metronidazole, tinidazole,
Leishmania donovani	Visceral disease (kala-azar): blackening of skin, anemia, fever, hepatosplenomegaly	Intracellular organisms seen in tissue biopsy	Multiplication in macrophages; spread to liver and spleen	Bite of sandfly (*Phlebotomus* species)	Stibogluconate (antimony)
Naegleria species	Meningoencephalitis	Amebae in CSF or other sterile tissue	Colonization of nasal passages; invades nasal mucosa and travels to brain	Swimming in contaminated water	Amphotericin B plus miconazole and rifampin
Plasmodium species	Malaria: cyclical fever and chills; anemia, liver and spleen enlarged; Cerebral involvement and blackwater fever (*P. falciparum*)	Blood smear showing ring forms and signet-like trophozoites within RBCs and crescent-shaped gametophytes	Sporozoites invade hepatocytes and form merozoites, which infect and reproduce asexually in RBCs causing hemolysis	Bite of female *Anopheles* species mosquito	Chloroquine, primaquine, artemisinin, quinine, mefloquine, pyrimethamine, doxycycline, artesunate as single drug or combinations
Toxoplasma gondii	Mononucleosis-like illness: fever, enlarged lymph nodes; Lesions in brain, eyes, and liver possible in AIDS patients and neonates	ELISA for increased antibody titer; cysts or trophozoites in biopsy	Proliferation of organisms within cells; induced cellular immune response	Ingestion of cysts in meat; cat feces; transplacental	Sulfonamides plus pyrimethamine; clindamycin plus dapsone
Trichomonas vaginalis	Vaginitis with frothy discharge, itching, and burning; Asymptomatic in men	Trophozoites in vaginal secretions or Papanicolaou smear	Adherence to vaginal wall; erosion of surface cells	Sexual contact	Metronidazole, tinidazole
Trypanosoma brucei (African)	Sleeping sickness: fever, Winterbottom sign, CNS involvement (headache, blank look, lethargy)	Trypanosomes visible in blood, CSF, or lymph node aspirates	Invasion of brain; antigenic shift	Bite of tsetse fly	Suramin for acute disease; melarsoprol for chronic disease involving CNS
Trypanosoma cruzi (American)	Chagas disease: fever, enlarged liver and spleen, Romaña sign (orbital edema) Chronic form: cardiac involvement common, cardiomegaly; megacolon, megaesophagus	Trypanosomes visible in blood	Proliferation within cells (especially muscle and neuroglial cells); induced cellular immune response	Contact with cysts in feces of reduviid bugs at bite site	Nifurtimox

AIDS, acquired immunodeficiency syndrome; CNS, central nervous system; CSF, cerebrospinal fluid; ELISA, enzyme-linked immunosorbent assay; RBCs, red blood cells.

Trigger words:
Giardia species: contaminated creek water (beavers and bears), foul-smelling diarrhea, hikers, old man looking over his shoulder (troph)

Trichomonas species: flagella, hanging drop test for motility, STD

Trigger words:
Leishmania species: blackening of skin, sandflies, soldiers returning from Persian Gulf, trip to Asia or South America

3. *Giardia lamblia*
   • Watery, foul-smelling diarrhea with malabsorption, flatulence, and cramps
   • Often acquired from drinking contaminated creek water (campers, hikers)
   • Common in immunodeficiency conditions with absent immunoglobulin A (IgA)
4. *Trichomonas vaginalis*
   • Vaginitis with frothy discharge (due to flagella motion)
   • Sexually transmitted
B. **Blood and tissue protozoa**
   1. *Leishmania* species
      • Endemic to tropical and subtropical regions
      • Transmitted by sandfly (*Phlebotomus* species)
      • Infection of macrophages leading to cutaneous, mucocutaneous, or visceral disease
   2. *Plasmodium* species
      • Endemic to tropical regions

- Transmitted by female *Anopheles* species mosquito
- Malaria
  a. Characterized by episodic paroxysms of high fever and severe chills followed by sweats
  b. Life cycle of plasmodia within humans includes an exoerythrocytic phase within hepatocytes and a series of erythrocytic cycles within red blood cells (RBCs) (Fig. 29-2).
  c. Malarial paroxysms are due to simultaneous hemolysis of large numbers of infected RBCs and release of motile merozoites.
  d. Asexual ring forms and signet-like trophozoites within RBCs and crescent-shaped gametocytes in blood are diagnostic.
- *Plasmodium vivax* and *Plasmodium ovale* infect only young erythrocytes.
  a. Paroxysms at 48-hour intervals.
  b. These species can establish a dormant stage (hypnozoite) in the liver.
  c. Reactivation of hypnozoites leads to relapse of clinical manifestations months to years after the initial disease.
- *Plasmodium malariae* infects only old erythrocytes.
  a. Paroxysms at 72-hour intervals.
- *Plasmodium falciparum*
  a. Infects all erythrocytes and causes the most serious disease
  b. Has shortest incubation period (7 to 10 days)
  c. Only species that involves the central nervous system
  d. Only species with only ring forms and gametocytes in the peripheral blood
  e. Typical paroxysms, if present, initially occur daily, then every 36 to 48 hours.
  f. Malignant tertian malaria
     - Blackwater fever with kidney failure
     - Cerebral malaria
3. *Toxoplasma gondii*
   - Acquired from cat litter, ingestion of undercooked meat, or in utero
   - Mononucleosis-like syndrome in healthy individuals
   - Potentially fatal encephalitis in immunocompromised patients

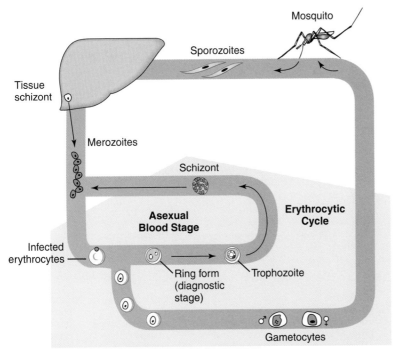
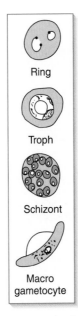

29-2: Life cycle of plasmodia in humans. The bite of an infected female *Anopheles* species mosquito injects **sporozoites** into the blood. These infect the liver and develop into **merozoites** (motile, infective stage), which are released and invade erythrocytes. Asexual reproduction within erythrocytes proceeds through several stages (ring form, trophozoite, and schizont), culminating in rupture of the cell and release of more merozoites. Some **gametocytes** are also produced within erythrocytes. Ingestion of male and female gametocytes by a mosquito during a blood meal initiates sexual reproduction of plasmodia within the mosquito, leading to production of more sporozoites that can infect humans.

4. *Trypanosoma cruzi*
   - Endemic to South America
   - Transmitted by reduviid bug
   - Chagas disease
     a. Myocarditis with heart failure
     b. Acquired achalasia (megaesophagus)
     c. Acquired Hirschsprung disease (megacolon)
     d. Orbital edema (Romaña sign)
5. *T. brucei* (gambiense and rhodesiense)
   - Endemic to West Africa
   - Transmitted by tsetse fly
   - Sleeping sickness
     a. Early enlargement of posterior cervical lymph nodes
     b. Later development of encephalitis
     c. Death by starvation

III. **Helminthic Parasites (Table 29-3)**
   A. **Roundworms**
      1. *Ascaris lumbricoides* (roundworm)
         - Accumulation of large worms that may cause small intestinal obstruction
           a. No eosinophilia
         - Pneumonitis with eosinophilia associated with larval migration
      2. *Enterobius vermicularis* (pinworm)
         - Perianal pruritus and itching
         - Self-reinfection by scratching anal area and transmitting eggs to mouth

TABLE 29-3 Parasites: Helminths

NAME	DISEASE FEATURES	IDENTIFICATION	PATHOGENESIS	TRANSMISSION	TREATMENT
Ascaris lumbricoides (roundworm)	Abdominal pain, diarrhea, intestinal obstruction, asthma-like pneumonitis	Oval-shaped eggs in stools	Larval migration; obstruction due to large numbers in gastrointestinal tract; induced allergic reactions	Ingestion of food or soil containing larvae	Mebendazole, albendazole
Enterobius vermicularis (pinworm)	Perianal itching, vaginal irritation	Scotch tape test for eggs in perianal region	Invasion of colon by adult worms; host allergic reactions	Fecal-oral spread of eggs; self-reinfection	Albendazole, mebendazole, pyrantel pamoate
Necator americanus (hookworm)	Diarrhea, cramps, nausea; microcytic, hypochromic anemia	Eggs in stools	Larval migration; blood ingested by adult worms attached to intestinal villi; host allergic reactions	Penetration of skin by larvae in soil	Mebendazole, albendazole, pyrantel pamoate, iron replacement therapy
Strongyloides stercoralis (threadworm)	Dermatitis, pneumonitis, eosinophilia	Larval worms	Larval migration; induced allergic reactions	From soil; autoinfection	Ivermectin, albendazole
Schistosoma species (blood and bladder flukes)	Initial urticarial skin rash at exposure site; Pipestem fibrosis of liver and ascites (*S. mansoni, S. japonicum*); Bladder granulomas and hematuria (*S. haematobium*)	Eggs with characteristic spines in stools or urine	Inflammation, fibrosis, and granuloma formation due to host reaction to eggs	Skin penetration by motile larvae (cercariae); snails are intermediate hosts	Praziquantel
Taenia species (tapeworms)	Taeniasis: abdominal pain, diarrhea, weight loss; Cysticercosis (*T. solium*): cysts and inflammation in brain, eyes, and muscle; potentially fatal	Suckers and circle of hooks on larvae; eggs or gravid proglottids in stools	Attachment of adult worms to intestinal mucosa; encystment of larvae within tissues	Ingestion of larvae in beef (*T. saginata*) or pork (*T. solium*); fecal-oral spread of eggs	Niclosamide or praziquantel (especially for cysticercosis), albendazole
Trichinella spiralis	Trichinosis: fever, diarrhea, eye edema, acute muscle pain, hemorrhages under nails	Spiral-shaped encysted larvae in muscle biopsy; eosinophilia	Larval migration; immune reaction to encysted larvae	Ingestion of larvae in raw or undercooked meat	Albendazole, mebendazole

- Other conditions: acute appendicitis, urethritis in girls
- Scotch tape test for eggs in perianal folds
  a. Tape applied to perianal area and then viewed under microscope to detect adhered eggs
- No eosinophilia

3. *Necator* and *Ancylostoma* species (hookworm)
   - Microcytic hypochromic anemia
   - Pneumonitis with eosinophilia associated with larval migration
4. *Strongyloides stercoralis* (threadworm)
   - Dermatitis, pneumonitis with eosinophilia
   - Disseminated hyperinfection in immunocompromised
   - Autoinfection due to maturation of larvae in intestine
   - Larva, *not* eggs, in stool
5. *Trichinella spiralis*
   - Undercooked meat, especially pork
   - Encysted larvae in muscle
   - Periorbital edema
   - Exquisite muscle pain
   - Marked eosinophilia
6. *Wuchereria bancrofti*
   - Elephantiasis due to clogging of lymphatics
   - Spread by mosquitoes
   - Microfilariae in blood is diagnostic

B. Flukes and flatworms
1. *Schistosoma* species (blood and bladder flukes)
   - Spines on eggs
   - Snails first intermediate host in tropical regions
   - *Schistosoma mansonii*
     a. Ascites, pipestem fibrosis of liver, portal hypertension with splenomegaly
   - *Schistosoma hematobium*
     a. Hematuria, squamous cell carcinoma of urinary bladder
2. *Taenia* species (beef and pork tapeworms)
   - Suckers and hooks on larvae
   - *Taenia solium* (pork tapeworm)
     a. Human eats undercooked pork with larva
       - Human has adult worms in intestine (definitive host)
     b. Human eats eggs from adult worms (human is intermediate host); develops cysticercosis
       - Cysts in brain
       - Blindness
       - Muscle involvement
3. Diphyllobothrium latum (fish tapeworm)
   - Contracted by eating raw and undercooked fish
   - Vitamin B_{12} deficiency with megaloblastic anemia
4. *Echinococcus granulosus* (dog tapeworm)
   - Dog eats sheep liver with hydatid cysts.
     a. Sheep is intermediate host; dog is definitive host with adult worms.
   - Sheepherder eats eggs and develops hydatid cysts in liver.
     a. Sheepherder is intermediate host.

C. Disease manifestations caused by infection with representative helminthic parasites
1. Creeping eruption or serpent-like lesions caused by migrating larva in the skin (cutaneous larva migrans)
   - *Ancylostoma braziliense* and *Necator americanus* (dog hookworm) cutaneous larva migrans
   - *Strongyloides stercoralis* (threadworm)
2. Subcutaneous swelling or nodules due to infections of subcutaneous tissue (*not* commonly seen in the United States)
   - *Loa loa* (worm native to West Africa)
   - *Dracunculus medinensis* (worm native to India, Africa, Arabian peninsula)
   - Maggots (larvae) of various fly species
3. Pulmonary infiltrates with eosinophilia caused by passage of migrating larva through the lungs
   - *Necator americanus, Ancylostoma duodenale* (hookworm)

Scotch tape test detects pinworm eggs

Trigger words:
Necator americanus: anemia, hookworm, pneumonitis

Strongyloides stercoralis: autoinfection life cycle, dermatitis, eosinophilia, pneumonitis, threadworm

Trigger words:
Schistosoma species: fluke, injection, Mansoni (spine on egg), snails

Haematobium species: bladder cancer

Trigger words:
T. solium: cysticercosis, tapeworm, undercooked pig

Cysticercosis due to pork tapeworm (*T. solium*)

Trigger words:
Diphyllobothrium latum: raw fish (fish tapeworm), tapeworm, vitamin B_{12} deficiency

- *Ascaris lumbricoides* (intestinal roundworm)
- *Strongyloides stercoralis* (threadworm)
4. Central nervous system involvement
    - *Toxoplasma gondii* (especially in patients with acquired immunodeficiency syndrome [AIDS])
    - *P. falciparum* (cerebral malaria)
    - *T. brucei* (African sleeping sickness)
    - *T. spiralis* (worm causing trichinosis)
    - *T. solium* larvae (cysticercosis)
5. Lesions in the liver and the lungs
    - *Clonorchis sinensis, Fasciola hepatica* (liver flukes)
    - *Schistosoma* species (blood fluke)
    - *Paragonimus westermani* (lung fluke)
    - *Entamoeba histolytica* (amebic dysentery)
    - *Echinococcus granulosus* (hydatid cyst)
6. Bladder lesions with hematuria
    - *Schistosoma haematobium* (bladder fluke)
7. Eye lesions
    - *T. solium* (pork tapeworm)
    - *Toxoplasma* species (especially in immunocompromised)

IV. Case Presentations: Parasitic Infections (Box 29-1)

BOX 29-1 PARASITIC INFECTIONS: QUICK CASES

Ascaris lumbricoides
Ascariasis: An 18-year-old immigrant from Cambodia complains of severe abdominal cramping. He reports having seen a 10-inch long, pearl white-colored worm in his stool a few months ago.

Trypanosoma species
Sleeping sickness (African trypanosomiasis): A 50-year-old man who had been camping for several weeks along a river in Africa began experiencing intermittent high fevers, headaches, and joint pains about 2 weeks after returning from the trip. He reports being bitten by many insects while camping.
Chagas disease (South American trypanosomiasis): A Latin American immigrant child has nonspecific findings of fever, malaise, and tachycardia. Physical examination shows unilateral conjunctivitis and unilateral periorbital edema. A family member had similar symptoms several months ago and subsequently experienced congestive heart failure.

Entamoeba histolytica
Amebic dysentery: Soon after returning from a visit to rural villages in India, a 40-year-old woman develops severe abdominal pain, cramping, and fever accompanied by bouts of diarrhea with blood and mucus in her stools about 8 times per day. Two weeks later, she seeks medical care because her condition has not improved.

Cryptosporidium species
Cryptosporidiosis: A 25-year-old man has profuse watery, nonbloody diarrhea but has no fever. He tests positive for human immunodeficiency virus (HIV), and his current CD4 T cell count is 50 cell/mm^3.

Giardia lamblia
Giardiasis: For the past 10 days, a 27-year-old man has been experiencing profuse, foul-smelling diarrhea with stools that float in the toilet. He has abdominal cramping and severe flatus. He had returned from a camping trip in the Rocky Mountains a few weeks before onset of these symptoms.

Plasmodium species
Malaria: An immigrant from tropical Africa complains of having a fever every other day that is accompanied by shaking chills followed by heavy sweating. He comments that his urine is darker than usual. Physical examination shows jaundice and splenomegaly.

Toxoplasma gondii
Acute toxoplasmosis: An otherwise healthy woman develops a fever, painful cervical lymphadenopathy, sore throat, muscle pains, and a rash. She has an outdoor cat.
Chronic toxoplasmosis: An AIDS patient who owns a cat begins to experience seizures. A computed tomography (CT) scan of the brain shows ring-enhancing lesions.

BOX 29-1 PARASITIC INFECTIONS: QUICK CASES—Cont'd

Schistosoma mansoni, Schistosoma japonicum (Blood Flukes)
Hepatic schistosomiasis: A businessman who has traveled frequently to northern Africa for many years has ascites, hepatosplenomegaly, and other signs of portal hypertension.

Taenia solium (Pork Tapeworm)
Taeniasis: A recent Mexican immigrant to the United States experiences diarrhea, abdominal pain, and weight loss. Before leaving Mexico, the patient had often eaten pork dishes in neighborhood restaurants.
Cysticercosis: A patient has right-sided weakness and seizures of recent onset. A CT scan of the head shows a cystic lesion.

Diphyllobothrium latum (Fish Tapeworm)
Diphyllobothriasis: A Jewish woman from Minnesota complains of abdominal pain and recent weight loss. Laboratory studies indicate that she has megaloblastic anemia. She is known for her homemade gefilte fish and usually tastes the seasoned minced fish before cooking it.

Echinococcus granulosus (Dog Tapeworm)
Hydatid cyst: A worker in a dog kennel has right upper quadrant pain. A CT scans show a cystic lesion in the liver.

CHAPTER 30
INFECTIOUS DISEASES: CLINICAL CORRELATIONS

I. Sexually Transmitted Diseases (STDs)
A. Overview
1. Usually spread during asymptomatic period when partners are unaware of problem
2. *Chlamydia trachomatis* and human papillomavirus (HPV) infections are the most common STDs worldwide.
   - *C. trachomatis* is often masked by coinfection with *Neisseria gonorrhoeae*.

When treating for *N. gonorrhoeae*, also treat for *C. trachomatis*.

B. Table 30-1 summarizes diseases spread primarily by sexual contact.
II. Urinary Tract Infections (UTIs) (Table 30-2)
- Most common causes of nosocomial UTIs are *Escherichia coli*, *Enterococcus* species, and *Pseudomonas aeruginosa*.

TABLE 30-1 **Sexually Transmitted Diseases**

DISEASE	ORGANISMS	CLINICAL FEATURES
HIV/AIDS	Human immunodeficiency virus	Opportunistic infections and neoplasms
Anogenital warts	Human papillomavirus	Koilocytotic cells and possible progression to **squamous cell carcinoma** (types 16, 18) Condylomata acuminata (types 6, 11)
Chancroid	*Haemophilus ducreyi*	**Painful** ulcers on external genitalia
Genital herpes	Herpes simplex virus 2	**Painful** ulcerative lesions on genitalia
		Fever and swelling of regional lymph nodes
Granuloma inguinale	*Calymmatobacterium granulomatis*	Multiple ulcerating granulomatous lesions in inguinal region and genitalia
		Donovan bodies (intracellular bacteria) seen in biopsy or smear
Hepatitis	Hepatitis virus (types B, C)	Acute: jaundice, rash, arthritis, nausea, right upper quadrant pain
Lymphogranuloma venereum	*Chlamydia trachomatis* (types L1 to L3)	**Painful** genital lesions; draining lymph nodes
		Rectal strictures in women
Syphilis	*Treponema pallidum*	Hard, **painless** chancres on genitalia (primary)
		Gray wart-like, **painless** lesions (condylomata lata), fever, lymphadenopathy, skin rash (secondary), gummas, neurologic manifestations (tabes dorsalis, dementia), ascending aortic aneurysm (tertiary)
Trichomoniasis	*Trichomonas vaginalis*	Vulvovaginitis with frothy discharge; usually asymptomatic in men
Urethritis, cervicitis	*C. trachomatis* (types D to K), *Neisseria gonorrhoeae*	**Coinfection common** **Acute pelvic inflammatory disease** associated with both diseases
		Conjunctivitis and Reiter syndrome (chlamydia)
		Arthritis and pharyngitis (gonorrhea)

AIDS, acquired immunodeficiency syndrome.

TABLE 30-2 **Bacteria Causing Urinary Tract Infections**

ORGANISM	DISTINGUISHING FEATURES	NOTES
Escherichia coli	Gram negative, no capsule, red-black colonies on EMB agar	Most common cause of UTIs (50% to 80%)
Staphylococcus saprophyticus	Gram positive, coagulase negative, resistant to novobiocin	Second most common cause of UTIs in young women (10% to 30%)
Proteus mirabilis	Gram negative, urease positive, swarming growth on agar	Associated with struvite urinary stones
Klebsiella pneumoniae	Gram negative, nonmotile, prominent capsule, large mucoid colonies	Usually in catheterized patients
Enterobacter species	Gram negative, motile, capsule, moist colonies, often drug resistant	Usually in immunocompromised patients
Pseudomonas aeruginosa	Gram negative, oxidase positive, fruity odor, blue-green pigment	Usually in patients with kidney stones, chronic prostatitis, or a catheter
Enterococcus faecalis	Gram positive, variable hemolysis, salt tolerant (6.5% NaCl)	Usually in immunocompromised or catheterized patients

UTI, urinary tract infection.

A. **Cystitis (lower UTI)**
   1. Most commonly caused by *E. coli*.
   2. Higher incidence in women
   3. Dysuria, frequency, urgency, suprapubic pain
   4. Not accompanied by bacteremia
B. **Pyelonephritis (upper UTI): flank pain, fever, chills, dysuria**
   1. Results from ascension of bacteria from infected bladder
   2. May be accompanied by bacteremia
C. **Genitourinary tract pathogens that are not sexually transmitted**
   • *Candida albicans* (vulvovaginitis), *Staphylococcus aureus* (toxic shock syndrome), and various organisms that infect the urinary tract.

III. **Infectious Diarrheas (Tables 30-3 and 30-4)**
   A. **Distinguishing features of three types**
      1. Noninflammatory diarrhea is watery
         • Site of pathology: **small intestine**
         • Fever rare
         • Bacteremia and fecal leukocytes not present
         • Mediated by bacterial toxins and viruses

E. coli is the most common UTI.

TABLE 30-3 **Major Infectious Agents of Diarrhea**

ORGANISM	TYPE OF DIARRHEA	TOXIN RELATED	NOTES AND KEY WORDS
Bacteria			
Vibrio cholerae	Watery (NI)	Cholera toxin ($\uparrow$ cAMP)	**Rice-water stools**, vomiting, dehydration
Bacillus cereus	Watery (NI)	Enterotoxins (preformed)	**Reheated rice** and beans rapid onset
Campylobacter jejuni	Watery or bloody (I)		Undercooked meats and poultry, unpasteurized milk; fever, cramps; may last 3 to 4 weeks
Clostridium difficile	Watery or bloody (I)	Toxin A (cholera-like); toxin B (cytotoxic)	**Antibiotic use**; pseudomembrane
Clostridium perfringens (type A)	Watery (NI)	Heat-labile enterotoxin (disrupts ion transport)	Leftover meat and poultry dishes
Escherichia coli (EHEC)	Bloody (I-I)	Shigatoxin (Vero-toxin)	**Undercooked hamburger**; hemorrhagic colitis, hemolytic uremic syndrome (**strain O157:H7**)
Escherichia coli (ETEC)	Watery (NI)	Cholera-like enterotoxin Heat-labile ($\uparrow$ cAMP); heat-stable enterotoxin ($\uparrow$ cGMP)	**Traveler's diarrhea**; fever and vomiting sometimes
Salmonella species	Watery or bloody (I and I-I)	None	Often food-borne (eggs or poultry); **typhoid fever** (invasive *Salmonella typhi*)

TABLE 30-3   **Major Infectious Agents of Diarrhea—Cont'd**

ORGANISM	TYPE OF DIARRHEA	TOXIN RELATED	NOTES AND KEY WORDS
Shigella species	Watery, then bloody (I)	Shiga toxin inhibits protein synthesis	Mild disease *(Shigella sonnei)* common in day care centers; severe invasive disease *(Shigella flexneri, Shigella dysenteriae)*
Staphylococcus aureus	Watery (NI)	Enterotoxins (preformed)	**Picnic foods** (cold cuts, potato salad), custards; nausea, vomiting; rapid onset
Vibrio parahaemolyticus	Watery (I and I-I)	None	**Shellfish**
Yersinia enterocolitica	Watery (I-I)	None	Cabbage, other raw vegetables, cheese
Viruses			
Norovirus	Watery (NI)	None	Often in **outbreaks** (schools, ships); nausea, vomiting, fever sometimes
Rotavirus	Watery (NI)	None	**Infants,** winter months; fever, vomiting, dehydration
Protozoa			
Cryptosporidium species	Watery (NI)	None	Large fluid loss; most common in **immunocompromised patients**
Entamoeba histolytica	Bloody (I)	None	**Amebic dysentery;** lower abdominal pain, **mucus and blood in stools**
Giardia lamblia	Watery (NI)	None	Contaminated stream water (campers, hikers); fatty, **foul-smelling stools**

cAMP, cyclic adenosine monophosphate; cGMP, cyclic guanosine monophosphate; I, inflammatory; I-I, inflammatory, invasive; NI, noninflammatory.

TABLE 30-4   **Food Sources of Bacterial Infections**

FOOD	BACTERIA
Poultry	*Salmonella enteritidis, Campylobacter* species
Raw eggs	*Salmonella enteritidis*
Dairy products	*Listeria monocytogenes, Brucella* species, *Mycobacterium bovis*
Shellfish	*Vibrio* species
Reheated rice	*Bacillus cereus*
Undercooked beef	*Escherichia coli* O157:H7, *B. cereus*, *Brucella* species, *C. perfringens*
Picnic foods (mayonnaise, custard, salted meats)	*S. aureus* toxin mediated

2. Inflammatory diarrhea is watery or bloody
   - Lesion in **colon**
   - Fever and fecal leukocytes common
   - Bacteremia uncommon
3. Inflammatory, invasive diarrhea is bloody
   - Lesion in Peyer patches
   - Fever prolonged
   - Bacteremia and fecal leukocytes common

B. **Typical time of onset after infection by various agents**
   1. 1 to 6 hours
      - *S. aureus* and *Bacillus cereus* (preformed toxin)
   2. 8 to 16 hours
      - *Clostridium perfringens* and *B. cereus* (toxin produced after infection)
   3. 24 to 48 hours
      - Norwalk virus and rotavirus
   4. 48 hours
      - *E. coli* (ETEC) and *Vibrio cholerae* (toxin produced after infection)
   5. More than 24 hours
      - *E. coli* (EHEC); *Shigella, Salmonella,* and *Campylobacter* species; *Yersinia enterocolitica, Entamoeba histolytica,* and *Giardia lamblia* (adherence, growth, invasion)

TABLE 30-5 **Primary Causes of Pneumonia by Age Group**

CHILDREN (6 WK TO 19 YR)	ADULTS (20-60 YR)	OLDER ADULTS (>60 YR)
RSV, parainfluenza virus, and influenza virus	M. pneumoniae	Strep pneumoniae
	C. pneumoniae	RSV, parainfluenza virus, influenza virus
Mycoplasma pneumoniae	Strep pneumoniae	
Chlamydophila pneumoniae	Haemophilus influenzae anaerobes	
Streptococcus pneumoniae		H. influenzae

Streptococcus pneumoniae and Haemophilus influenzae cause typical pneumonia; other organisms may cause atypical pneumonia.
RSV, respiratory syncytial virus.

IV. Pneumonia (Table 30-5)
A. Clinical presentation
1. Typical
   - Abrupt onset, high fever (>39°C), productive cough with blood-tinged sputum, chest pain, consolidated "whited-out" infiltrate throughout lower lobe on chest radiograph
   - *Streptococcus pneumoniae, Haemophilus influenzae,* and *S. aureus*
2. Atypical
   - Slow onset of nonproductive cough, moderate fever (<39°C), headache, sore throat, gastrointestinal symptoms, patchy infiltrates on chest radiograph
   - *Mycoplasma pneumoniae, Chlamydophila* species, *Legionella* species, viruses, and fungi
B. Bacterial pneumonia
1. Community acquired
   - *Streptococcus pneumoniae, H. influenzae, M. pneumoniae, Chlamydophila pneumoniae, Legionella* species, *S. aureus*
2. Nosocomial
   - *S. aureus* and gram-negative rods including *E. coli, Klebsiella pneumoniae,* and *P. aeruginosa*
C. Viral pneumonia
1. Respiratory syncytial virus (RSV), parainfluenza virus, and influenza virus are most common causes.
2. **Bacterial superinfection,** usually by *S. aureus,* often complicates these infections.
D. Fungal pneumonia
   - **Immunocompromised patients** are most at risk for atypical, chronic pneumonia due to fungi.
1. ***Pneumocystis jiroveci (carinii)*** causes potentially fatal pneumonia, in acquired immunodeficiency syndrome (AIDS) patients.
2. *Histoplasma capsulatum, Coccidioides immitis,* and *Blastomyces dermatitidis* can cause pneumonia in both immunocompetent and immunocompromised individuals.
V. Meningitis and Encephalitis (Table 30-6)
   - **Analysis of cerebrospinal fluid** usually can distinguish bacterial, viral, and fungal causes of meningitis (Table 30-7).
A. Acute bacterial meningitis
1. In adults: *Streptococcus pneumoniae* and *Neisseria meningitidis* are most common causes in immunocompetent individuals.
   - Terminal complement deficiency (C5 -C9) predisposes to *N. meningitidis* infection.
   - Meningitis due to **Listeria monocytogenes** is seen in **immunocompromised patients** and the **elderly.**
2. In neonates
   - Group B streptococci, *E. coli,* and *Listeria* species are major causes.
3. In children
   - **H. influenzae** B is a common cause, as well as *Strep pneumoniae* and *N. meningitidis.*
   - **Hib vaccine** has almost eliminated **H. influenzae** meningitis cases.
B. Viral (aseptic) meningitis
1. Enteroviruses (especially Coxsackie viruses) and herpes simplex virus are the most common causes.
2. Mumps virus and lymphocytic choriomeningitis virus (LCMV) are less common causes.
3. LCMV in immunocompromised patients
C. Chronic meningitis
   - *Mycobacterium tuberculosis* and fungi (e.g., *Cryptococcus neoformans* and *C. immitis*) are common causes.

TABLE 30-6 **Central Nervous System Disease**

DISEASE	ORGANISMS	COMMENTS
Bacterial meningitis	*Neisseria meningitidis**	Accompanied by petechiae, capsule
	Streptococcus pneumoniae*	Capsule
	Haemophilus influenzae	Capsule
	Listeria monocytogenes	
	Mycobacterium tuberculosis	
Neonatal meningitis	Group B streptococci*	
	Escherichia coli*	
	Listeria monocytogenes*	
	Echovirus	
Fungal meningitis	*Cryptococcus neoformans*	India ink test, capsule
Viral (aseptic) meningitis	Enteroviruses: Coxsackie, echo, polio	
	Lymphocytic choriomeningitis (LCMV)	
	Mumps	
	Arboviruses	
	HSV (especially HSV-2)	
Encephalitis	HSV*	Frontal lobe, nonseasonal, sequelae
	Arboviruses: flavivirus (Japanese, West Nile, St. Louis), togavirus (equine encephalitis), bunyavirus (California)*	Seasonal, minimal sequelae
	Measles	
	Mumps	
	Rabies	Treatable after infection
Tropical spastic paraparesis	HTLV-1	
SSPE	Defective measles virus	Vaccine preventable
PML	JC polyoma virus	In immunocompromised (e.g., AIDS)
Cerebral malaria	*Plasmodium falciparum*	
Neurologic syphilis	*Treponema pallidum*	
Lyme disease	*Borrelia burgdorferi*	
Brain abscess	Various bacteria, *Toxoplasma gondii*	Toxoplasma: especially neonates and AIDS
Cysticercosis	*Taenia solium*	
Spongiform encephalopathies	Prions: Creutzfeldt-Jakob disease agent	

*Most common cause of disease.
AIDS, acquired immunodeficiency disease; HSV, herpes simplex virus; HTLV-1, human T lymphotropic virus type 1; PML, progressive multifocal leukoencephalopathy; SSPE, subacute sclerosing panencephalitis.

TABLE 30-7 **Analysis of Cerebrospinal Fluid in Meningitis**

PROBABLE CAUSE	CEREBROSPINAL FLUID FINDINGS				
	PRESSURE	PROTEIN	SUGAR	LYMPHOCYTES	PMNs
Bacterial	↑	↑	↓↓	N	↑
Viral	N	N or ↑	N	↑	N
Fungal, *Mycobacterium tuberculosis*	↑↑	↑	↓	↑	N

N, normal values; PMNs, polymorphonuclear leukocytes; single arrow, increase (↑) or decrease (↓); double arrows, marked increase or decrease.

D. Encephalitis
1. Nonseasonal
   - Herpes simplex virus
2. Seasonal
   - Arboviruses (arthropod borne)
3. Other
   - Measles, mumps, rabies
E. Other diseases
1. Progressive multifocal leukoencephalopathy—JC virus in immunocompromised patients

2. Subacute sclerosing panencephalitis—defective measles virus
3. Spongiform encephalopathy (Creutzfeldt-Jakob disease)—prions
4. Cysticercosis—*Taenia solium*
5. Brain abscess
   - Anaerobic streptococci, staphylococci, bacteroides, and other bacteria; *Aspergillus* species, *Toxoplasma gondii* (immunosuppressed)

VI. **Arthropod-Associated Diseases (Table 30-8)**
   - Arthropods may act as simple **vectors** and, in some cases, also as **intermediate hosts** in the transmission of human pathogens.
   - Humans are most likely to contract these diseases when they enter the native habitat of the vectors.

VII. **Common Infectious Causes of Other Conditions**
   A. **Ear infections**
      1. Otitis media, sinusitis in children
         - *Strep pneumoniae, H. influenzae, Moraxella catarrhalis*, anaerobes
      2. Otitis externa (swimmer's ear)—*P. aeruginosa*
   B. **Osteomyelitis**
      1. *S. aureus* in most individuals (especially children)
      2. *Salmonella* in individuals with sickle cell disease
   C. **Congenital, neonatal complications**
      - **TORCHES**—*to*xoplasma, *r*ubella virus, *c*ytomegalovirus, *he*rpes simplex virus, *s*yphilis

TABLE 30-8 **Arthropod-Associated Diseases**

DISEASE	ETIOLOGIC AGENT	VECTOR	DISTRIBUTION*
Bacterial			
Lyme disease	*Borrelia burgdorferi*	Tick (*Ixodes* species)	New England, West Coast
Epidemic relapsing fever	*Borrelia recurrentis*	Louse	Europe, North Africa, India
Endemic relapsing fever	*Borrelia* species	Tick	North and South America, Africa, Asia
Tularemia	*Francisella tularensis*	Tick	Worldwide
Rocky Mountain spotted fever	*Rickettsia rickettsii*	Deer tick	Southeastern and (*Dermacentor* species) south-central United States
Epidemic typhus	*Rickettsia prowazekii*	Louse	Worldwide
Murine typhus	*Rickettsia typhi*	Flea	Southeastern United States, near Gulf of Mexico
Ehrlichia	*Ehrlichia* species	Tick	Southeastern and south-central United States
Anaplasmosis	*Anaplasma phagocytophilum*	Tick	Worldwide
Plague	*Yersinia pestis*	Flea	Asia, Africa
Protozoan			
Visceral leishmaniasis	*Leishmania donovani*	Sandfly (*Phlebotomus* species)	Tropical and subtropical areas
Malaria	*Plasmodium* species	Mosquito (*Anopheles* species)	Worldwide
African sleeping sickness	*Trypanosoma brucei*	Tsetse fly	Africa
Chagas disease	*Trypanosoma cruzi*	Reduviid bug	Latin America
Viral			
Equine encephalitis (Eastern, Western, and Venezuelan)	Alphavirus (togavirus)	Mosquito (different species)	North and South America
California encephalitis	Bunyavirus	Mosquito (*Culex* species)	North America
Yellow fever	Flavivirus	Mosquito (*Aedes* species)	South America, Africa
Dengue fever	Flavivirus	Mosquito (*Aedes* species)	Tropics
St. Louis encephalitis	Flavivirus	Mosquito (*Culex* species)	North America
West Nile encephalitis	Flavivirus	Mosquito	Eastern United States, Africa, Asia
Colorado tick fever	Reovirus	Wood tick	North America

*Outbreaks and spread of the vector may go beyond the indicated regions.

    D. Endocarditis
      1. Acute
- Rapid onset; usually involves previously **normal valves**
- *S. aureus* (most common cause) and *Strep pneumoniae*

      2. Subacute
- Slow onset over months; usually involves **diseased, abnormal,** or **prosthetic valves**
- **Viridans streptococci** (most common) and *Enterococcus* species
- *Staphylococcus epidermidis* and *S. aureus* (particularly involving prosthetic valves)
- **HACEK** organisms—*H*aemophilus, *A*ctinobacillus, *c*ardiobacterium, *E*ikenella, *K*ingella

    E. Toxic shock and septic shock
      1. Toxic shock is caused by superantigen activation of T cells and massive cytokine release.
- *S. aureus* TSST, *Streptococcus pyogenes* erythrogenic toxin A or C

      2. Sepsis induces systemic release of acute phase cytokines
- Toll-like receptor–mediated response of leukocytes to presence of bacterial cell wall components in blood
- Usually gram-negative bacteria

APPENDIX 1

BACTERIOLOGY SUMMARY TABLES AND TRIGGER WORDS

Summary: Gram-Positive Bacteria

ORGANISM	DISEASE FEATURES	IDENTIFICATION	PATHOGENIC FACTORS	TRANSMISSION	PREVENTION/TREATMENT*
Actinomyces spp.	Abscesses with draining sinus tracts, especially in cervicofacial region Mycetoma	Gm(+); filamentous; anaerobic Seen as macroscopic "sulfur" granules in clinical specimens	Unknown (normal colonizer of upper respiratory and GI tracts)	Endogenous spread across mucosal barriers after trauma or disease	Débridement and penicillin
Bacillus anthracis	Cutaneous anthrax: ulcerated lesions and septicemia Pulmonary anthrax: often fatal Gastrointestinal anthrax (developing countries)	Gm(+) rod; spore-former; nonmotile; aerobic Medusa-head colonies on blood agar	Exotoxin consisting of a protective factor, edema factor, and lethal factor; antiphagocytic polypeptide capsule	Spores from animal products or soil through skin or by inhalation	Attenuated vaccine for at-risk groups Penicillin, ciprofloxacin, doxycycline
Bacillus cereus	Food poisoning: emetic disease (early vomiting); diarrheal disease (later onset) Traumatic eye infections	Gm(+) rod; spore-former; motile Aerobic	Heat-stable exotoxin (emetic disease); heat-labile exotoxin (diarrheal disease)	Preformed toxin in reheated rice (emetic form); spores in meat and vegetables	Refrigeration of foods Supportive therapy
Clostridium botulinum	Classic botulism: weakness, bilateral descending paralysis Infant form: floppy baby syndrome, constipation Wound form: similar to classic but longer onset	Gm(+) rod; spore-former; anaerobic	Heat-resistant spores; A-B type toxin inhibits release of acetylcholine	Preformed toxin in canned foods (classic); spores, often in honey (infant)	Discard bulging cans of food; no honey for infants Trivalent antitoxin IgG; Trivalent antitoxin Respiratory support Penicillin (infant and wound)
Clostridium difficile	Pseudomembranous colitis with bloody diarrhea: associated with antibiotic use	Gm(+) rod; spore-former; anaerobic; ELISA detection of toxin in stool culture, antigen in stool	Growth after antibiotic depletion of competing intestinal flora; enterotoxin A (fluid loss); cytotoxin B (mucosal damage)	Opportunistic intestinal flora; nosocomial spread	Cessation of causative antibiotic Metronidazole or vancomycin
Clostridium perfringens	Myonecrosis (gas gangrene), Cellulitis Food poisoning (watery diarrhea)	Gm(+) large, boxcar-shaped rod; spore-former; aerotolerant anaerobe Double zone of hemolysis	Cytolytic alpha toxin; heat-labile enterotoxin (fluid loss); other toxins (increased vascular permeability, tissue necrosis)	Spores in food and soil; endogenous spread from GI tract to sterile sites	Proper cooking and refrigeration of foods Wound cleaning and débridement Penicillin
Clostridium tetani	Tetanus: lockjaw (trismus), spastic paralysis (opisthotonos), grinning expression (risus sardonicus)	Gm(+) small rod (tennis racket); terminal spore; strict anaerobe	A-B type exotoxin (tetanospasmin) blocks release of inhibitory neurotransmitters (e.g., GABA, glycine)	Spores via cut or stab wound	Toxoid vaccine (childhood DPT vaccine); booster every 10 years; Antitoxin immunoglobulin to neutralize toxin Penicillin

Continued

Summary: Gram-Positive Bacteria—Cont'd

ORGANISM	DISEASE FEATURES	IDENTIFICATION	PATHOGENIC FACTORS	TRANSMISSION	PREVENTION/TREATMENT*
Corynebacterium diphtheriae	Respiratory diphtheria: pseudomembrane on throat ("bull neck"), sore throat Cutaneous diphtheria Systemic toxemia	Gm(+) club-shaped rod Black colonies on tellurite agar (Löffler medium)	A-B type exotoxin inhibits protein synthesis by ADP ribosylation of EF-2; toxin encoded by gene on phage	Aerosol droplets (asymptomatic carriage); contact with skin of infected person (cutaneous)	Toxoid vaccine (childhood DPT vaccine); booster every 10 years Antitoxin immunoglobulin to neutralize toxin Penicillin, erythromycin
Enterococcus faecalis	UTI Endocarditis (especially in those with genitourinary manipulation)	Gm(+) cocci in pairs or chains Variable hemolysis; growth in bile-esculin; salt tolerant	Widespread antibiotic resistance	Endogenous spread from normal flora of GI tract	Ampicillin (UTI) Aminoglycoside + ampicillin for systemic disease Vancomycin for ampicillin resistant strains
Listeria monocytogenes	Meningitis and sepsis in immunocompromised and neonates (early onset) Late-onset neonatal disease (granulomatosis infantisepticum) Multiple-organ abscesses and granulomas	Gm(+) rod; tumbling motility β Hemolysis	Intracellular growth in macrophages; listeriolysin O; cold enrichment	Food-borne (unpasteurized dairy products, raw vegetables); transplacentally or during birth to infected mother	Ampicillin ± gentamicin
Staphylococcus aureus	Toxin mediated: food poisoning; toxic shock syndrome; scalded skin syndrome Pyogenic infections: skin lesions, endocarditis, osteomyelitis, nosocomial pneumonia	Gm(+) cocci in clusters Salt tolerant; coagulase(+); catalase(+)	Antiphagocytic capsule; protein A; enterotoxins; TSST (superantigen); cytolytic toxins and enzymes; coagulase; catalase; penicillinase (β-lactamase) in many strains; Panton-Valentine leukocidin (PVL) toxin CA-MRSA	Preformed toxin in lunch meats, creamy foods, custards; normal skin and nasal flora; endogenous spread	Methicillin, cephalosporins MRSA: vancomycin, linezolid daptomycin, tigecycline
Staphylococcus epidermidis	Infection around catheters and other implants Wound infections	Gm(+) cocci in clusters Coagulase(−); catalase(+); sensitive to novobiocin	Colonizes implanted devices; tissue-degrading enzymes	Endogenous spread of normal skin flora; IV drug use	Vancomycin, linezolid, daptomycin
Staphylococcus saprophyticus	UTI in young women	Gm(+) cocci in clusters Coagulase(−); catalase(+); resistant to novobiocin	Adheres to transitional epithelium	Sexual contact	Quinolones
Streptococcus agalactiae (group B)	Neonatal meningitis, pneumonia, sepsis Postpartum sepsis	Gm(+) cocci in chains β Hemolysis; catalase(−); + cAMP test	Antiphagocytic capsule; hemolysins and other degradative enzymes	Colonization of GI and vaginal tract in some women	Third-trimester screening and ampicillin before delivery
Streptococcus pneumoniae	Pneumonia Sinusitis, otitis media Bronchitis Meningitis	Gm(+) football-shaped cocci in chains α Hemolysis; catalase(−); quellung reaction; sensitive to Optochin (P disk)	Antiphagocytic capsule; IgA protease; pneumolysin	Normal throat and nasal flora; person-to-person spread via contact and aerosol droplets	Capsular vaccine for high-risk groups (children, elderly) Penicillin, amoxicillin, ceftriaxone, fluoroquinolones, macrolides
Streptococcus pyogenes (group A)	Pharyngitis Skin lesions, necrotizing fasciitis Toxin mediated: scarlet fever, toxic shock syndrome Sequelae: rheumatic fever, glomerulonephritis	Gm(+) cocci in chains β Hemolysis; catalase(−); sensitive to bacitracin (A disk)	M protein and hyaluronic acid capsule (antiphagocytic); F protein (adherence); streptolysins O and S; exotoxins	Aerosol droplets, person-to-person	Penicillin G, cephalosporins

*Drugs other than those listed may also be effective.
ADP, adenosine diphosphate; BL-BLI, β-lactam antibiotic with β-lactamase inhibitor; cAMP, cyclic adenosine monophosphate; ELISA, enzyme-linked immunosorbent assay; GABA, γ-aminobutyric acid; GI, gastrointestinal; Gm(+), gram positive; IV, intravenous; MRSA, methicillin-resistant *Staphylococcus aureus*; CA-MRSA, community acquired MRSA; UTI, urinary tract infection.

Summary: Gram-Negative Bacteria

ORGANISM	DISEASE FEATURES	IDENTIFICATION	PATHOGENIC FACTORS	TRANSMISSION	PREVENTION/TREATMENT*
Bacteroides fragilis	Intra-abdominal abscesses; pelvic infections; peritonitis Bacteremia Wound infection	Gm(−) rod; anaerobic, produce foul-smelling fatty acids	Antiphagocytic capsule; cytolytic enzymes; weak endotoxin; mixed infections common	Endogenous spread of normal colonic flora promoted by surgery or trauma	Surgical intervention Metronidazole, imipenem, clindamycin, BL-BLI
Bordetella pertussis	Whooping cough	Gm(−) coccobacillus; capsule Oxidase(+); growth on Bordet-Gengou agar	A-B type exotoxin increases cAMP by inhibiting "off" G protein; hemagglutinin; tracheal cytotoxin	Respiratory droplets from cough of infected person	Acellular or inactive whole cell vaccine (childhood DPT vaccine) Azithromycin
Brucella spp.	Undulant fever: malaise, chills, sweats, weight loss, fever in waves	Gm(−) coccobacillus; facultative intracellular	Growth in phagocytes and spread to spleen, liver, lymph nodes, bone marrow; granuloma formation	Zoonotic spread via contaminated milk and cheese or contact with animal hosts	Pasteurization of dairy products Tetracycline + streptomycin, or TMP-SMX
Campylobacter jejuni	Gastroenteritis: profuse watery or bloody diarrhea, pus in stool, fever, cramps	Gm(−) comma-shaped rod; motile Growth on Campy plate; oxidase(+); catalase(+)	Ulceration of mucosal surfaces of jejunum and colon; very infective (low ID_{50})	Zoonotic spread via contaminated milk, water, poultry, meat	Symptomatic treatment Fluoroquinolones
Escherichia coli	Watery diarrhea in infants and travelers (ETEC, EPEC, EAggEC) Dysentery (EIEC) Hemorrhagic colitis (EHEC); hemolytic uremic syndrome (strain O157:H7) Urinary tract infection (UPEC) Septicemia, neonatal meningitis	Gm(−) rod; Oxidase(−); lactose(+)	Endotoxin in all strains; enterotoxins in ETEC (increases cAMP or cGMP); verotoxin in EHEC (inhibits 28S rRNA); pili in UPEC (adherence)	Fecal-oral spread of normal GI tract flora (nosocomial, contaminated food and water, self-inoculation)	Ampicillin or sulfonamides (UTI) TMP-SMX and rehydration (diarrhea, not EHEC) Cephalosporins (septicemia) quinolones
Francisella tularensis	Tularemia: skin ulcers, lymphadenopathy, eye ulcers (ocular form)	Gm(−) coccobacillus; facultative intracellular Growth on cysteine media	Antiphagocytic capsule; growth in macrophages; very infective (low ID_{50})	Zoonotic spread from animal reservoirs (rabbits, ticks)	Attenuated vaccine for at-risk individuals Streptomycin
Haemophilus ducreyi	Chancroid: painful genital ulcer; inguinal buboes with purulent exudate	Gm(−) coccobacillus Catalase(−); factor X (heme) but not factor V (NAD) needed for growth	Pili that adhere to genital and perianal mucosa	Sexual contact	Ceftriaxone, azithromycin
Haemophilus influenzae	Infantile meningitis, pediatric epiglottitis, otitis media (children and adults) Pneumonia (elderly, those with chronic pulmonary disease)	Gm(−) coccobacillus Catalase(+); factor X (heme) and factor V (NAD) needed for growth	Colonization of upper respiratory tract; endotoxin; systemic infection only by encapsulated strains (e.g., Hib)	Endogenous spread from upper respiratory tract; respiratory droplets	Hib vaccine at 2, 4, 6, and 15 mo Ceftriaxone BL-BLI
Helicobacter pylori	Type B gastritis Gastric and duodenal ulcers	Gm(−) curved rod; highly motile Urease(+); oxidase(+); catalase(+)	Motility; epithelial damage mediated by urease products, mucinase, and cytotoxin	Ingestion	Triple-drug therapy: bismuth + metronidazole + tetracycline + H_2 blocker Omeprazole + amoxicillin+ clarithromycin
Klebsiella pneumoniae	Pneumonia (especially in alcoholics and those with poor lung function) UTI (especially in catheterized patients) Bacteremia	Gm(−) rod Oxidase(−); mucoid-appearing colonies in culture	Large antiphagocytic capsule	Aspiration of respiratory droplets	Cephalosporins, BL-BLI

Continued

Summary: Gram-Negative Bacteria—Cont'd

ORGANISM	DISEASE FEATURES	IDENTIFICATION	PATHOGENIC FACTORS	TRANSMISSION	PREVENTION/TREATMENT*
Legionella pneumophila	Legionnaires disease: atypical pneumonia Pontiac fever: self-limited, febrile illness	Gm(–) coccobacillus; silver stain; facultative intracellular BCYE agar (need cysteine and iron) Urine antigen	Growth in macrophages; degradative enzymes kill parasitized cells	Aerosols from contaminated water sources (no person-to-person spread)	Chlorination of water sources Erythromycin, new macrolides, fluoroquinolones
Neisseria gonorrhoeae (gonococcus)	Acute gonorrhea: urethral or vaginal discharge PID and salpingitis Septic arthritis Neonatal conjunctivitis Dermatitis-arthritis syndrome	Gm(–) diplococcus; no capsule Ferments glucose (not maltose); growth on Thayer-Martin or chocolate agar	Pili; strong endotoxin effect; protein I (intracellular survival); protein II (adhesin); IgA protease; β-lactamase	Sexual contact; during birth from infected mother	Condoms Prophylaxis with silver nitrate or erythromycin for neonates (for eyes) Ceftriaxone + antichlamydial drug
Neisseria meningitidis (meningococcus)	Meningitis Meningococcemia: generalized petechial/purpura rash, septicemia	Gm(–) diplococcus; capsule Ferments glucose and maltose; growth on Thayer-Martin or chocolate agar High protein and low glucose in CSF	Antiphagocytic capsule; strong endotoxin effect	Respiratory droplets	Anticapsular vaccine Penicillin, chloramphenicol, ceftriaxone Fluoroquinolones for contacts
Proteus mirabilis	UTI often with renal stone formation	Gm(–) rod; swarming growth on agar Urease(+); oxidase(–); lactose(–)	Increased urine pH due to urease activity promotes renal stones and is toxic to uroepithelium	Endogenous spread of normal GI tract flora	Ampicillin, TMP-SMX Cephalosporins
Pseudomonas aeruginosa	Nosocomial infections Burn infections with bacteremia UTI (catheters) Pulmonary infections (cystic fibrosis) Keratitis, "swimmer's ear," "hot-tub folliculitis" Malignant external otitis in diabetics	Gm(–) rods; motile Oxidase(+); flat colonies; fruity odor; blue-green pigment	Pili; capsule; A-B type exotoxin inhibits protein synthesis by ribosylation of EF-2; leukocidin; degradative enzymes	Ubiquitous in environment and water; nosocomial spread via water reservoirs	Fluoroquinolones, ceftazidime, polymyxin, aztreonam, aminoglycoside, special β-lactams
Salmonella enteritidis	Gastroenteritis with vomiting, nonbloody diarrhea	Gm(–) rod Oxidase(–); Lactose(–); colonies with black center (H₂S) on SS agar	Antiphagocytic capsule; exotoxin; intracellular growth	Fecal-oral via water or food (raw eggs, poultry, dairy products)	Rehydration No antibiotics used
Salmonella typhi	Typhoid fever: increasing fever, necrosis and hemorrhage of GI tract, bacteremia	Same as *S. enteritidis* but is motile	Antiphagocytic capsule; invasion of Peyer patches	Same as *S. enteritidis*	Chloramphenicol, cephalosporins, quinolones
Shigella spp.	Shigellosis (bacterial dysentery): fever, cramps, tenesmus, and bloody stools *S. sonnei*: mild disease (day care centers) *S. flexneri*, *S. dysenteriae*: more severe disease (less common)	Gm(–) rod Oxidase(–); lactose(–), colorless colonies (no H₂S) on SS agar	Invades and replicates within colonic mucosa; A-B type exotoxin (Shiga toxin) that inhibits 28S rRNA *(S. dysenteriae)*	Fecal-oral usually via hands	Rehydration in mild cases Ampicillin in severe cases
Vibrio cholerae	Cholera: rice-water stools, profuse watery diarrhea	Gm(–) comma-shaped rod; motile Salt tolerant; oxidase(+)	Adherence to gut mucosa; A-B type exotoxin increases cAMP by stimulating "on" G_s protein, causing loss of water and ions from cells	Fecal-oral via water, fish, and shellfish; shedding by asymptomatic carriers	Rehydration Tetracycline
Vibrio parahaemolyticus	Gastroenteritis with explosive, watery diarrhea, cramps, nausea	Same as *V. cholerae*	Invasion and destruction of colonic epithelium	Ingestion of contaminated shellfish	Usually self-limited

Summary: Gram-Negative Bacteria—Cont'd

ORGANISM	DISEASE FEATURES	IDENTIFICATION	PATHOGENIC FACTORS	TRANSMISSION	PREVENTION/TREATMENT*
Yersinia enterocolitica	Enterocolitis with bloody diarrhea, fever, abdominal pain	Gm(−) rod; motile Oxidase(−); lactose(−); cold tolerant	Antiphagocytic capsule; intracellular growth; endotoxin; cold tolerant	Zoonotic via contaminated food, water, or blood products	Aminoglycosides, TMP-SMX
Yersinia pestis	Bubonic plague: high fever, painful buboes, conjunctivitis	Gm(−) rod Oxidase(−); lactose(−)	Antiphagocytic capsule; intracellular growth; exotoxin; fibrinolysin	Zoonotic via flea vectors	Killed vaccine Streptomycin, chloramphenicol

*Drugs other than those listed may also be effective.
BL-BLI, β-lactam antibiotic with β-lactamase inhibitor; cAMP, cyclic adenosine monophosphate; cGMP, cyclic guanosine monophosphate; CSF, cerebrospinal fluid; GI, gastrointestinal; Gm(−), gram negative; PID, pelvic inflammatory disease; rRNA, ribosomal RNA; TMP-SMX, trimethoprim-sulfamethoxazole; UTI, urinary tract infection.

Summary: Other Bacteria

ORGANISM	DISEASE FEATURES	IDENTIFICATION	PATHOGENIC FACTORS	TRANSMISSION	PREVENTION/TREATMENT*
Borrelia burgdorferi	Lyme disease: rash (erythema chronicum migrans); severe fatigue; involvement of heart, CNS, and joints	Large spirochetes; microaerophilic; numerous flagella Serologic tests for antibodies	Induced cell-mediated and inflammatory responses; weak endotoxin effect	Zoonotic via ticks (*Ixodes* spp.); Northeast, upper Midwest, and Pacific Northwest	Doxycycline and amoxicillin (early) Ceftriaxone (late)
Chlamydophila pneumoniae	Atypical pneumonia: children and young adults at greatest risk; association with coronary artery disease	Obligate intracellular No peptidoglycan in cell wall	Similar to *C. trachomatis*	Respiratory droplets	Same as *C. trachomatis*
Chlamydophila psittaci	Psittacosis (parrot fever): dry cough, pneumonitis, splenomegaly, CNS involvement	Obligate intracellular No peptidoglycan in cell wall	Similar to *C. trachomatis*	Aerosols from dried bird feces	Same as *C. trachomatis*
Chlamydia trachomatis	Strains A-C: trachoma (conjunctivitis) leading to blindness if untreated Strains D-K: urogenital infections, neonatal conjunctivitis Strains L1-L3: lymphogranuloma venereum	Obligate intracellular No peptidoglycan in cell wall; iodine-staining inclusion body; serologic tests	Extracellular inert form (elementary body) enters target cells; active form (reticulate body) replicates within cells leading to cell lysis and host inflammatory response	Sexual contact or via birth canal; contact with tears (strains A-C)	Tetracycline, erythromycin, new macrolides, fluoroquinolones (respiratory)
Coxiella burnetii	Q fever: usual symptoms of rickettsial disease but no rash Atypical pneumonia, endocarditis, liver involvement	Obligate intracellular		Aerosols of urine or feces and contact with birth products from infected animals (no insect vector)	Tetracycline
Mycobacterium leprae	Tuberculoid leprosy: few skin lesions with few bacilli Lepromatous leprosy: numerous skin lesions with many bacilli, tissue damage, loss of sensation	Acid-fast rod; obligate intracellular Positive lepromin skin test; infects cool tissues	Cell wall phenolic glycolipids; host T$_H$1 response → tuberculoid form; host T$_H$2 response → lepromatous form	Direct contact with lesions; inhalation of infectious droplets	Tuberculoid form: dapsone + rifampin (6 mo) Lepromatous form: dapsone + rifampin + clofazimine (2 yr)
Mycobacterium tuberculosis	Tuberculosis: young children, elderly, and immunocompromised at greatest risk	Acid-fast rod; facultative intracellular Slow growth on Löwenstein-Jensen medium; + PPD skin test, IFN-γ tests	Cord factor, mycolic acid; intracellular growth; granuloma formation and caseation due to induced DTH response	Respiratory droplets from coughing by infected person	Prophylactic isoniazid BCG vaccine (rare in United States) Multidrug therapy for 6-9 mo

Continued

Summary: Other Bacteria—Cont'd

ORGANISM	DISEASE FEATURES	IDENTIFICATION	PATHOGENIC FACTORS	TRANSMISSION	PREVENTION/TREATMENT*
Mycobacterium avium-intracellulare complex (MAC)	Disseminated infections of AIDS and other immunocompromised	Mycobacterial characteristics	Like *M. tuberculosis* but even more of an opportunistic infection	Respiratory droplets	Azithromycin or clarithromycin + ethambutol + rifabutin, *NOT* isoniazid
Mycoplasma pneumoniae	Atypical ("walking") pneumonia Pharyngitis, tracheobronchitis	No cell wall; sterols in cell membrane; obligate aerobe Granular colonies on Eaton agar	Adherence to respiratory epithelium; damage to epithelium due to H_2O_2 and lytic enzymes	Respiratory droplets	Erythromycin, tetracycline, quinolones
Nocardia spp.	Cutaneous infections (mycetoma) Pneumonia with cavitation and spread to CNS or skin (abscesses) in immunocompromised	Acid-fast (weakly), filamentous, aerobic	Colonization of oropharynx or wounds with subsequent necrosis and abscess formation	Ubiquitous soil organisms; inhaled and aspirated to lower airways or enter via wounds	Sulfonamides Surgical intervention
Rickettsia spp.	Rocky Mountain spotted fever (*R. rickettsii*): inward-spreading rash Endemic typhus (*R. typhi*): rash on trunk Epidemic typhus (*R. prowazekii*): outward-spreading rash	Obligate intracellular Weil-Felix reaction to distinguish rickettsial species; serology	Invasion and destruction of endothelial cells	*R. rickettsii*, deer tick vector; *R. typhi*, flea vector; *R. prowazekii*, person-to-person via body lice	Tetracycline, chloramphenicol
Treponema pallidum	First-degree syphilis: painless skin ulcers (chancres), buboes Second-degree syphilis: flu-like syndrome, disseminated rash Third-degree syphilis (rare): gummas, aortitis, CNS involvement Congenital: triad—unusual teeth, deafness, interstitial keratitis, + other	Thin spirochetes visualized by dark field microscopy VDRL or RPR test for cardiolipin FTA-ABS test for treponemal antibodies	Hyaluronidase (tissue invasion); protective outer coat; induced host response	Sexual contact, transplacental, transfusion with contaminated blood	Penicillin

*Drugs other than those listed may also be effective.
AIDS, acquired immunodeficiency syndrome; CNS, central nervous system.

Trigger Words: Bacteria

Actinomyces spp.	Sulfur granules in draining sinuses
	Anaerobic
	Filamentous
Bacillus anthracis	Sheep, goat, goat hair
	Fur, spore
	Bioterror
	Malignant pustule
	Wool-sorters' disease
Bacillus cereus	Rice, preformed toxin
	Heat-stable toxin—vomiting
	Heat-labile toxin—diarrhea
Bacteroides fragilis	Foul smelling
	Mixed infection
	Abscess

Trigger Words: Bacteria—Cont'd

Bordetella pertussis	Bordet-Gengou agar
	Lymphotoxin (lymphoid leukocytosis)
	Whooping cough
	DPT vaccine
Borrelia burgdorferi	Deer tick
	High grass
	Lyme disease
	White-tail deer reservoir of spirochete
	Erythema chronicum migrans (bite site)
	Disabling arthritis; bilateral Bell palsy
Brucella spp.	Undulant fever
	Unpasteurized milk and cheese
	Intracellular growth
	Goats and sheep
Campylobacter jejuni	Bloody diarrhea
	Undercooked poultry
	Puppies
	Thin, curved gram negative
	Association with Guillain-Barré syndrome
Chlamydia trachomatis	Sexually transmitted disease, urinary tract infection
	Pelvic inflammatory disease, lymphogranuloma venereum
	Trachoma
	Iodine stain
	Intracellular inclusion bodies
	Elementary bodies (infective particle)
	Reticulate bodies
Chlamydia psittaci	Birds, parrots
Clostridium perfringens	Boxcar shaped
	Double zone of hemolysis
	Lecithinase
	Toxins
	Gas gangrene (myonecrosis)
	Diarrhea
	Anaerobe
Clostridium difficile	Spores
	Pseudomembranous colitis
	Toxin A + B
	Antibiotic associated
Clostridium botulinum	Botulism
	Floppy baby
	Honey (spores; infant)
	Food-borne (adults; preformed toxin)
	A-B toxin
	Anaerobe

Continued

Trigger Words: Bacteria—Cont'd

Clostridium tetani	A-B toxin
	Anaerobe
	Lockjaw
	DPT
	Twitching spasms, sardonic grin
	No protective antibodies
Corynebacterium diphtheriae	Pseudomembrane
	DPT vaccine
	A-B toxin
	Schick test
	Toxic myocarditis (cause of death)
Enterococcus spp.	Entero-feces-gut bug
	Nosocomial
	Vancomycin resistant (VRE)
Escherichia coli	Diarrhea
	Neonatal meningitis
	EIEC, EHEC, ETEC, EAEC, EPEC
	Lactose positive
	O157:H7
	Urinary tract infection
	Acute cholecystitis, diverticulitis, appendicitis
	Septic shock in hospital
Francisella tularensis	Intracellular
	Rabbit
	Ulcer
	Tularemia
Haemophilus spp.	X and V factors
	Hib
	Capsule
	Meningitis uncommon due to vaccine
	Epiglottitis
	Otitis media; sinusitis
Helicobacter pylori	Gastric or duodenal ulcer
	Urease
	Urease breath test
	Stool antigen test (active versus inactive disease)
	Stomach cancer (adenocarcinoma, lymphoma)
Klebsiella pneumoniae	Currant jelly (blood) sputum
	Alcoholic
	Pneumonia, aspiration
	Capsule
Legionella pneumophila	Air-conditioning, warm mist (rain forest)
	Shower and other lukewarm water sources
	Charcoal yeast agar (BCYE agar)

Trigger Words: Bacteria—Cont'd

	Atypical pneumonia
	Urine antigen test
Listeria spp.	Meningitis
	Intracellular growth
	Baby
	Cold enrichment
	Milk products
	Motility
	Undercooked meat, soft cheese
Mycoplasma spp.	Walking pneumonia
	No cell wall
	Atypical pneumonia, crowded conditions
	Association with Guillain-Barré syndrome
	Cold agglutinins
Neisseria meningitidis	Gram-negative diplococci in cerebrospinal fluid
	Meningitis
	Lipooligosaccharide
	Endotoxin
	Septic shock
	Petechiae, purpura
	Waterhouse-Friderichsen syndrome
Neisseria gonorrhoeae	Gram-negative diplococci
	Urethritis
	Sexually transmitted disease
	Thayer-Martin medium
	Chocolate agar
Mycobacterium leprae	Nerve damage, anesthetic skin lesion
	Lepromatous leprosy—T_H2
	Tuberculoid leprosy—T_H1
Mycobacterium tuberculosis	Mantoux reaction
	PPD
	Acid-fast
	Granuloma
	Caseation
	Opportunistic disease
	Ghon complexes (primary disease)
	Intestinal tuberculosis (swallowed organisms in primary lung disease)
	Isoniazid
Proteus mirabilis	Urinary tract infection
	Swarmer
	Urease
	Alkaline urine pH
	Ammonia smell

Continued

Trigger Words: Bacteria—Cont'd

Pseudomonas aeruginosa	Nosocomial infection
	Cystic fibrosis
	Opportunistic
	Green pigment in sputum
	Fruity smell
	Burn patient
	Hot tub folliculitis
	Malignant external otitis in diabetic
	Osteomyelitis in punctured rubber foot wear
Rickettsia spp.	Tick
	Southeastern Atlantic and south central states
	Palmar petechia
	Weil-Felix reaction
	Obligate intracellular growth
Staphylococcus aureus	Grapelike clusters
	Coagulase
	Catalase
	Toxins, TSST
	Methicillin-resistant *Staphylococcus aureus*
	Pus
	Impetigo
Staphylococcus epidermidis	Catalase
	Coagulase negative
	Catheters, shunts, prosthetic devices
Salmonella spp.	Dairy foods
	Motile
	Animal reservoirs
	Raw eggs and chicken
	Nonlactose fermenter
	Nonbloody diarrhea
	Osteomyelitis in sickle cell disease
Shigella spp.	Watery, bloody diarrhea
	Gram-negative bacillus
	Lactose negative
	No hydrogen sulfide
	Shiga toxin
Streptococcus pneumoniae	Gram-positive diplos
	α Hemolysis
	Capsule
	P disk (Optochin) sensitive
	Polysaccharide vaccine
	Pneumonia
	Meningitis
	Otitis media

Trigger Words: Bacteria—Cont'd

	Sinusitis
	Spontaneous peritonitis
Streptococcus pyogenes	β Hemolysis
	Streptolysin O and S
	A disk (group A) bacitracin sensitivity
	Gram-positive cocci in chains
	Necrotizing fasciitis
	Pus
	Erysipelas, scarlet fever
	Rheumatic fever, poststreptococcal glomerulonephritis
Treponema pallidum	Syphilis
	FTA-ABS
	Painless ulcer (chancre)
	Palm and sole rash
	Spirochete
	Gumma
	Unculturable
	VDRL, RPR tests
	FTA-ABS confirm disease
	Sexually transmitted disease
Vibrio cholerae	Comma (S) shaped
	Rice-water secretory diarrhea
	Shellfish
	A-B toxin
Yersinia pestis	Plague, fleas, rodent and other animal host, buboes

APPENDIX 2

VIROLOGY SUMMARY TABLES AND TRIGGER WORDS

Summary: DNA Viruses

FAMILY/ORGANISM	DISEASE FEATURES	IDENTIFICATION	TARGET TISSUE	TRANSMISSION	PREVENTION/TREATMENT
Adenoviridae					
Adenovirus Appendicitis	Pharyngitis Atypical pneumonia Acute respiratory disease (military recruits) Conjunctivitis Gastroenteritis	Nonenveloped; dsDNA genome; midsize Dense intranuclear inclusion body in infected cells	Respiratory tract and eyes	Aerosols, fecal-oral, fomites, close contact, hand-to-eye	Supportive No antiviral
Hepadnaviridae					
Hepatitis B virus	Acute hepatitis: arthritis, rash, jaundice Chronic hepatitis (about 15%-20%): cirrhosis; may progress to primary hepatocellular carcinoma	Enveloped; partially double-stranded circular DNA genome; small Serology: IgM for core antigen (HBcAg) = recent infection; surface antigen (HBsAg) = acute or chronic infection; HBeAg = virus shedding	Hepatocytes; acute or chronic infection	Body fluids via sexual contact, transfusion, needle stick, breastfeeding	HBsAg subunit vaccine for children and at-risk groups Lamivudine, tenofovir, entecavir, emtricitabine, adefovir, dipivoxil
Herpesviridae					
Cytomegalovirus	Mild mononucleosis Neonatal disease Pneumonia, hepatitis, retinitis (AIDS and transplant recipients)	Enveloped; dsDNA genome; large Owl's-eye nuclear inclusions in infected cells	Oral epithelium; latency in lymphocytes, CNS, eyes, salivary glands, GI tract	Body fluids, organ transplants, transplacental	Screening of blood and transplants Valganciclovir, ganciclovir, foscarnet
Epstein-Barr virus	Infectious mononucleosis (mostly in adolescents, young adults) Hairy oral leukoplakia (AIDS patients) Associated with Burkitts lymphoma	Structure same as above Downey cells (atypical T cells); heterophile antibody (monospot test), serology for antiviral antigens	B cells	Saliva	No antiviral
Herpes simplex virus (HSV), types 1 and 2	Oral herpes: fever blisters, cold sores (usually HSV-1) Genital herpes: painful ulcers (usually HSV-2) Encephalitis, meningitis, keratoconjunctivitis, neonatal disease	Structure same as above Syncytia and Cowdry type A nuclear inclusion bodies syncytia, Tzanck smear; PCR for genome	Mucoepithelium of skin, oropharynx, mouth, genitalia, eyes, elsewhere latency in neurons	Mixing and matching of mucous membranes via kissing, sharing utensils, sexual contact, passage through birth canal	Acyclovir, valacyclovir, famciclovir, penciclovir
Human herpesvirus (HHV), types 6 and 8	Roseola (HHV-6): high fever and rash (children) Kaposi sarcoma (HHV-8): mostly in AIDS patients	Structure same as above PCR for viral DNA	Lymphocytes	Respiratory droplets; saliva	No antiviral

Summary: DNA Viruses—Cont'd

FAMILY/ORGANISM	DISEASE FEATURES	IDENTIFICATION	TARGET TISSUE	TRANSMISSION	PREVENTION/TREATMENT
Varicella-zoster virus	Chickenpox: primary infection (usually in children) Shingles: recurrent infection along a single dermatome	Structure same as above Syncytia and Cowdry Type A nuclear inclusion bodies in smears of infected cells; immunofluorescence; ELISA; PCR	Skin and liver; latency in neurons	Respiratory droplets	Attenuated live vaccine VZIG (immune globulin) Famciclovir, valacyclovir, acyclovir
Papillomaviridae					
Human papillomaviruses	Skin warts (types 1-4) Condylomata acuminata (types 6, 11) Cervical intraepithelial neoplasia (types 16, 18)	Nonenveloped; circular dsDNA genome; small Koilocytotic cells (vacuoles and enlarged nuclei) on Papanicolaou smear in CIN; PCR for viral DNA	Skin and epithelia; inactivation of host growth suppressors p53 and RB by early viral proteins E6 and E7	Direct contact with lesions	Interferon-α Nonsurgical removal of warts Vaccine
Polyomaviridae					
JC virus	Progressive multifocal leukoencephalopathy (PML) with demyelination in CNS (pregnant women and those with poor T cell immunity)	Structure same as above	Respiratory tract, kidney; reactivation of latent infection and spread to CNS	Respiratory droplets	No antiviral
Parvoviridae					
Parvovirus B19	Erythema infectiosum (fifth disease): slapped-cheek rash Aplastic crisis in sickle cell disease Polyarthritis	Nonenveloped; ssDNA genome; small	Erythroid precursor cells	Respiratory droplets, transplacental	No antiviral
Poxviridae					
Poxviruses	Smallpox, vaccinia, molluscum contagiosum	Large, enveloped, complex brick-shaped dsDNA genome	Skin and organs	Respiratory droplets and contact	Smallpox: live vaccinia vaccine, quarantine

CNS, central nervous system; ds, double-stranded; ELISA, enzyme-linked immunosorbent assay; GI, gastrointestinal; PCR, polymerase chain reaction; ss, single-stranded.

Summary: RNA Viruses

FAMILY/ORGANISM	DISEASE FEATURES	IDENTIFICATION	TARGET TISSUE	TRANSMISSION	PREVENTION/TREATMENT
Arenaviridae					
Lymphocytic choriomeningitis virus	Febrile flu-like illness Meningitis (immune compromised)	Enveloped; segmented (−) ssRNA genome; midsize	Lungs, CNS	Aerosols, fomites, or food contaminated by infected rodents urine or feces	Ribavirin, supportive measures
Lassa fever virus	Hemorrhagic fever (similar to Ebola fever)	Structure same as above	Blood vessels and numerous organs	Same as above	Same as above
Bunyaviridae					
La Crosse virus and California encephalitis virus	Flu-like syndrome Encephalitis	Enveloped; segmented (−) ssRNA genome; midsize	CNS	Bite of *Culex* spp. mosquito	No antiviral
Hantavirus	Pulmonary syndrome: flu-like prodrome, interstitial pulmonary edema, respiratory failure	Structure same as above	Lungs	Inhalation of aerosols of infected rodent urine or feces	No antiviral
Calicivirus					
Hepatitis E	Hepatitis E: abrupt onset similar to hepatitis A but more severe, especially in pregnant women, not common in United States	Nonenveloped; small (+) ssRNA genome	Liver	Fecal-oral	No antiviral
Norwalk virus	Gastroenteritis: watery diarrhea with nausea and vomiting	Nonenveloped; small (+) ssRNA genome Detection of virions in stools	GI tract	Fecal-oral	Bismuth salicylate to reduce symptoms, fluids

Continued

Summary: RNA Viruses—Cont'd

FAMILY/ORGANISM	DISEASE FEATURES	IDENTIFICATION	TARGET TISSUE	TRANSMISSION	PREVENTION/TREATMENT
Coronaviridae					
Coronavirus	Common cold: 15% of cases, mostly in infants and children	Enveloped; (+) ssRNA genome; large	Upper and lower respiratory tract	Respiratory droplets	No antiviral
SARS	Severe acute respiratory syndrome	Structure same as above	Lung	Aerosols	No antiviral
Filoviridae					
Ebola virus and Marburg virus	African hemorrhagic fever: initial flu-like symptoms, widespread hemorrhage, hypovolemic shock (often rapidly fatal)	Enveloped; (−) ssRNA genome; midsize	Numerous organs	Zoonotic (monkeys are natural hosts); contact with body fluids	No antiviral
Flaviviridae					
Hepatitis C virus	Acute disease: gradual onset; usually subclinical Chronic infection (common): predisposes to primary hepatocellular cancer	Enveloped; (+) ssRNA genome; small	Liver	Body fluids via sexual contact, transfusion, needle stick, breastfeeding	Pegylated interferon-α and ribavirin
Yellow fever virus	Yellow fever: high fever, jaundice, black vomit	Structure same as above	Liver	Bite of *Aedes* spp. mosquito; tropical South America, Africa	Attenuated vaccine, control vector
Dengue virus	Dengue fever, Dengue hemorrhagic fever, dengue shock syndrome	Structure same as above	Vascular endothelium, macrophage, liver	*Aedes* spp. mosquito	No antiviral, control vector
West Nile or St. Louis encephalitis virus	Encephalitis, febrile illness	Structure same as above	CNS and brain	*Culex* spp. mosquito	No antiviral, control vector
Orthomyxoviridae					
Influenza virus	Influenza; complications include pneumonia, myositis, and Reye syndrome (in children)	Enveloped; segmented (−) ssRNA genome; large Types A, B, C; ELISA; hemagglutination; RT-PCR	Upper and lower respiratory tract	Respiratory droplets; antigenic drift (types A and B) promotes epidemics; antigenic shift (type A) promotes pandemics	Killed and live vaccines Type A: amantadine or rimantadine Types A and B: oseltamivir, or zanamivir for prophylaxis and treatment
Paramyxoviridae					
Measles virus	Measles: 3Cs + K (cough, conjunctivitis, coryza, Koplik spots); maculopapular rash Subacute sclerosing panencephalitis (SSPE)	Enveloped; (−) ssRNA genome; large Single serotype; syncytia in infected cells	Lung, skin, CNS	Respiratory droplets	Live attenuated vaccine (childhood MMR vaccine)
Mumps virus	Mumps: bilateral parotitis; spread to testes (unilateral orchitis) may lead to sterility	Structure same as above Single serotype; syncytia in infected cells; ELISA; hemagglutination inhibition	Parotid glands, ovaries, testes, thyroid gland	Respiratory droplets	Live attenuated vaccine (childhood MMR vaccine)
Parainfluenza virus	Croup (types 1, 2): young children Atypical pneumonia (type 3): infants and elderly Common cold (type 4)	Structure same as above Four common serotypes; syncytia in infected cells	Upper and lower respiratory tract	Respiratory droplets, nosocomial spread common	Hot moist air for symptoms
Respiratory syncytial virus (RSV)	Common cold Bronchiolitis and atypical pneumonia (immunocompromised, infants)	Structure same as above Syncytia in infected cells	Upper and lower respiratory tract	Respiratory droplets, direct contact	Anti-RSV immune globulin Ribavirin
Coxsackie A virus	Hand-foot-and-mouth disease and herpangina (young children) Aseptic meningitis with possible skin rash Hemorrhagic conjunctivitis	Unenveloped; (+) ssRNA genome; small	Oral mucosa, skin, CNS	Fecal-oral; respiratory droplets	Pleconaril for serious disease

Summary: RNA Viruses—Cont'd

FAMILY/ORGANISM	DISEASE FEATURES	IDENTIFICATION	TARGET TISSUE	TRANSMISSION	PREVENTION/TREATMENT
Coxsackie B virus	Neonatal myocarditis and pericarditis Pleurodynia (young adults)	Structure same as above	Muscle, skin	Fecal-oral; respiratory droplets	Pleconaril for serious disease
Hepatitis A virus	Hepatitis A: abrupt onset; usually mild disease	Structure same as above	Liver	Fecal-oral (uncooked shellfish)	Inactivated vaccine Immune globulin before or soon after exposure
Poliovirus	Aseptic meningitis Paralytic poliomyelitis	Structure same as above Isolation from CSF or feces	Oropharynx, CNS, muscle	Fecal-oral	Salk vaccine (inactivated; injected) Sabin vaccine (attenuated; oral)
Rhinovirus	Common cold	Structure same as above Numerous serotypes	Nasal mucosa, conjunctiva	Respiratory droplets; fomites; hand-to-nose contact	No antiviral
Reoviridae					
Rotavirus	Gastroenteritis: watery diarrhea, fever, vomiting (most severe in infants and children)	Nonenveloped; segmented (+/−) dsRNA genome; midsize Detection of virions or viral antigens in stools	GI tract	Fecal-oral	Rehydration Vaccine for infants
Retroviridae					
Human immunodeficiency virus (HIV)	AIDS: marked decrease in T cell count, increase in opportunistic infections and neoplasms (e.g., Kaposi sarcoma)	Enveloped; (+) ssRNA genome; midsize; reverse transcriptase in virion ELISA screening for antibodies; Western blot to confirm; RT-PCR to quantitate viral load	CD4 T lymphocytes, macrophages, neurons	Vaginal and anal intercourse, blood transfusion, needle sharing, transplacental blood exposure	Screening of blood supply HAART
Human T cell lymphotropic virus	Acute T cell leukemia Tropical spastic paraparesis	Structure same as above	CD4 T lymphocytes, neurons	Same as above	No antiviral
Rhabdoviridae					
Rabies virus	Rabies: lethal encephalitis with seizures and hydrophobia	Enveloped; (−) ssRNA genome; bullet-shaped; midsize Negri bodies in infected neurons; RT-PCR; immunofluorescence	Muscle and nerve cells	Zoonotic via bite of infected animal (skunks, raccoons) or aerosols (bats)	Pet vaccination Killed rabies vaccine before or soon after human exposure to animal with Antirabies immune serum
Togaviridae					
Rubella virus	Rubella (German measles): swollen glands, rash spreading downward from face Complications in adults: encephalitis, arthritis Teratogenic for fetus, especially with infection during first trimester	Enveloped; (+) ssRNA genome; small IgM antibodies or fourfold increase in IgG antibodies to confirm recent infection	Viremia, lymph nodes, skin, CNS	Respiratory droplets; transplacental	Live attenuated vaccine (childhood MMR vaccine) Maternal antibodies prevent spread to fetus
Equine encephalitis viruses (WEE, EEE, VEE)	Encephalitis	Structure same as above	CNS, brain	*Aedes, Culex* spp. and other mosquitoes	Control vector
Other					
Hepatitis D	Acute disease: similar to hepatitis B but more severe; most common cause of fulminant hepatitis	Enveloped; (−) ssRNA genome; defective virion; HBsAg in envelope; Serology for delta antigen	Hepatocytes; can replicate only in cells also infected with hepatitis B virus	Body fluids via sexual contact, transfusion, needle stick, breastfeeding	HBsAg subunit vaccine Interferon-α

AIDS, acquired immunodeficiency syndrome; CNS, central nervous system; CSF, cerebrospinal fluid; ds, double-stranded; ELISA, enzyme-linked immunosorbent assay; GI, gastrointestinal; HAART, highly active antiretroviral therapy; RT-PCR, reverse transcriptase–polymerase chain reaction; ss, single-stranded; (+), sequence same as mRNA; (−), sequence complementary to mRNA.

Virology Trigger Words

Adenovirus	Conjunctivitis, pharyngitis, hemorrhagic cystitis
	Dense basophilic intranuclear inclusion bodies
	Diarrhea in infant
	Appendicitis in kids
	Infectious genome
	Icosadeltahedral capsid with fibers
	Poorly chlorinated swimming pools
Bunyaviruses	California encephalitis viruses: *Culex* spp. mosquito, arbovirus, woods, La Crosse virus, encephalitis, meningitis
	Hantaviruses: hemorrhagic, petechiae, ecchymosis, bleeding tissues, rodent feces and urine
Arenaviruses	Lymphocytic choriomeningitis virus: rodents, flu-like symptoms, slums, ribavirin
	Lassa fever: hemorrhagic, rodents
Coronaviruses	Common cold
	SARS
	Fecal-oral and respiratory spread
Herpes simplex virus	Enveloped, large, DNA, Cowdry type A inclusion bodies, vesicular lesion, neurotropic, Tzanck smear (multinucleated squamous cells), stress-induced recurrence, encephalitis, destruction of temporal lobe, blindness, neonatal HSV
Cytomegalovirus	Large owl's-eye nuclear inclusion body
	Hypertrophied *(megalo)* cells
	Opportunistic disease
	Mononucleosis-like syndrome
	Blindness, diarrhea, pancreatitis in AIDS
	Congenital CMV (intracerebral calcifications)
	Microcephaly
Epstein-Barr virus	Mononucleosis, fatigue, pharyngitis, heterophile antibody, atypical lymphocytes, rash, monospot test, ampicillin-induced rash, B cell, lymphocytosis
	Burkitt lymphoma
Varicella-zoster virus	Crops of vesicular lesions
	All stages of lesions at once
	Vesicles, latency
	Multinucleated giant cells (syncytia)
	Cowdry type A nuclear inclusion bodies
	Neurotropic
	Thymidine kinase
	Shingles, dermatome distribution of vesicles
	Chickenpox (association with Reye syndrome)
Hepatitis A	Fecal-oral spread
	Acute, sudden-onset hepatitis
	Day care center
	Food-borne
	Shellfish
	Protective antibodies
	Picornavirus
Hepatitis E	Fecal-oral spread
	Acute, sudden-onset hepatitis
	Pregnant women
	Calicivirus
Hepatitis B	Serum hepatitis, chronic, contaminated blood and semen and mother's milk, Dane particle, insidious onset, HBsAg, primary hepatocellular carcinoma, hepadnavirus
Hepatitis C	Non-A, non-B hepatitis, chronic, flavivirus
	Posttransfusion hepatitis
	No protective antibodies
	Hepatocellular carcinoma
Hepatitis D	Fulminant hepatitis, HBV helper virus
HIV	AIDS (most common acquired immunodeficiency)
	Cytolytic to CD4

Virology Trigger Words—Cont'd

	Chemokine coreceptor
	Opportunistic diseases: PCP, Kaposi sarcoma, *Candida albicans* thrush, CMV retinitis, pneumonitis, reverse transcriptase
HTLV	Leukemia, flower cell, CD4 T cell, reverse transcriptase
Parainfluenza virus	Croup, barking seal, pneumonia, syncytia, paramyxovirus
Respiratory syncytial virus	Infant, bronchiolitis, paramyxovirus
Measles	Koplik spots (blue-gray spots in mouth; precede rash)
	3 Cs + photophobia, high fever, rash
	Paramyxovirus
Mumps	Parotitis: chipmunk cheeks
	Orchitis
	Pancreatitis and aseptic meningitis or encephalitis (5%),
	Paramyxovirus
Norovirus	Norwalk virus
	Outbreaks of diarrheal disease
	Nausea
	Watery diarrhea and vomiting
	Schools
	Cruise ships
Orthomyxovirus	Influenza, flu
	Segmented genome = reassortment
	Hemagglutinin and neuraminidase
	Antigenic drift (minor mutations) (outbreak/epidemic) versus shift (reassortment = pandemic)
Papillomavirus	Warts, koilocytes, CIN, cervical cancer, STD
Polyomaviruses	JC, demyelination, abnormal oligodendrocytes opportunistic disease, PML
Parvovirus B19	Fifth disease
	Slapped cheeks
	Lacy pattern rash
	Aplastic anemia, sickle crisis, spontaneous abortions
Coxsackie virus and echovirus	Fecal-oral
	Vesicular lesions; hand, foot, and mouth
	Coxsackie B for body
	Meningitis, myocarditis, pericarditis
	Picornavirus
Poliovirus	Asymmetric flaccid paralysis
	Major disease
	Minor disease
	Fecal-oral
	Postpolio syndrome
	Picornavirus
Rhinovirus	Runny nose, many serotypes, heat and pH labile, picornavirus
Poxviruses	Large, brick-shaped virus
	Replicates in cytoplasm
	Vesicular lesion
	Zoonosis
	Molluscum contagiosum: skin-colored papules
	Smallpox: synchronized crop of vesicular lesions (smallpox), vaccinia vaccine
Prions	Spongiform encephalopathy, CJD, vCJD, beef, no inflammation, presenile dementia, shakes, resistant to inactivation, mad cow
Rabies	Raccoon, skunk bite
	Bats (aerosol)
	Hydrophobia
	Coma
	Salivation
	Negri bodies
	Bullet-shaped virion
	Rhabdovirus

Continued

Virology Trigger Words—Cont'd

Rotavirus	Watery (secretory) diarrhea in young child
	Oral vaccine (risk for intussusception)
	Double capsid and double-stranded segmented RNA (remember: double-double)
Rubella	Rash, vaccine, congenital disease, arthritis, teratogen, cataracts, togavirus
Togavirus	Arbovirus
	Encephalitis viruses: mosquito, seasonal encephalitis, swamp
	Hemorrhagic viruses: blood everywhere, petechiae
Flavivirus	Arbovirus
	Encephalitis viruses: mosquito, seasonal encephalitis, swamp
	Hemorrhagic viruses: blood everywhere, petechiae

APPENDIX 3

MYCOLOGY AND PARASITOLOGY TRIGGER WORDS

Mycology Trigger Words

Aspergillus spp.	"Fungus ball"
	Septate branching hyphae
	Fruiting bodies
	Hypersensitivity pneumonitis (allergic alveolitis)
	Angioinvasive
	Malt (grain) workers
	Allergic bronchopulmonary
Black piedra	Black nodules along hair shaft, ascospores
White piedra	Sleeve or collar around the hair shaft
	Found on mustache, beard, and scalp
Blastomyces dermatitidis	Mississippi River Valley, rotting wood (beaver dams); broad-based budding yeast
	Healthy and immunocompromised
	Granuloma
Candida albicans	White, curd-like, adhesive plaques that bleed when removed for culture
	"Cobblestones"
	Prolonged use of antibiotics
	Immunocompromised: AIDS, diabetic people, transplant recipients, chemotherapy patients, infants
	Vaginal yeast
	Yeast and pseudohyphae (sign of infection)
	Thrush
Chromoblastomycosis	Dematiaceous (brown or black, melanin-producing) sclerotic bodies, skin disease
	Cauliflower-like verrucous (warty) nodules
Eumycotic mycetoma	Dematiaceous fungus
	Many draining sinus tracts
	"Grains" of microcolonies in the deep layer of skin
	Localized infection
Coccidioides immitis	San Joaquin River Valley
	American Southwest deserts
	Inhale arthrospores in dust
	Spherules with endospores
	Skin test for antigen exposure
Cryptococcus neoformans	Pigeon droppings
	Capsule
	India ink preparations
	Capsular antigens
	AIDS patients
	Meningitis in immunocompromised host
	The *crypt* of *Cryptococcus* is the *capsule* that houses the *round* yeast (coccus).

Continued

Mycology Trigger Words—Cont'd

Histoplasma capsulatum	Ohio and Mississippi River Valleys
	Lung and spleen
	Granulomas
	Yeasts inside macrophages
	Bird and bat droppings (spelunker)
	"Cincinnati spleen"
Pneumocystis jiroveci (carinii)	Most common initial AIDS-defining disease
	Diffuse interstitial pneumonia
	Gomori silver stain
	AIDS patient, intravenous drug abuser
	Fluffy, foamy alveolar exudate
	Cup-shaped (flying saucer)
	Ground-glass appearance on radiograph
	Organisms in bronchoalveolar lavage
Pityriasis versicolor	Hypopigmented/hyperpigmented patches
	"Spaghetti and meatballs" KOH preparation
	Seborrheic dermatitis; cradle cap in newborn
Rhizopus and *Mucor* spp.	Acidotic diabetic
	Paranasal sinus and orbit involvement
	Frontal lobe abscess in diabetic ketoacidosis
	Coenocytic (aseptate) hyphae
	Black nasal discharge
	Bread mold
Sporothrix schenckii	Roses
	Thorn prick
	Sphagnum moss
	Splinter
	Gardener
	Lymphocutaneous nodules
Tinea	Infect stratum corneum; KOH preparation
	Ring worm
	Circular, scaling lesion with central clearing and hair loss
	Discoloring
	Crumbling nails
	Azoles

Parasitology Trigger Words

Schistosoma spp.	Snails
	Injection
	Fluke
	Mansoni (lateral spine on egg)
	Haematobium (nipple on egg; squamous bladder cancer)
Taenia solium	Undercooked pig (intermediate host)
	Tapeworm
	Cysticercosis (human intermediate host)
Echinococcus granulosus (dog tapeworm)	Dog (definitive host)
	Hydatid cyst (human intermediate host)
	Tapeworm
Diphyllobothrium latum (fish tapeworm)	Raw fish
	Tapeworm
	Vitamin B_{12} deficiency

Parasitology Trigger Words—Cont'd

Plasmodium spp.	Malaria
	Paroxysms of fever and chills correspond with RBC hemolysis
	Falciparum: multiple ring forms
	Cyclic disease
	Anopheles spp. female mosquito
	Falciparum: blackwater fever
	Thick smears
Giardia spp.	Old man looking over his shoulder (troph)
	Hikers
	Contaminated creek water (beavers and bears)
	Foul-smelling diarrhea
	IgA deficiency
	Stool antigen test
Cryptosporidium spp.	Immune suppression
	Water supply contaminant
	Partially acid-fast oocyst
	AIDS diarrhea
Entamoeba histolytica	Amebic dysentery
	Cyst with one to four nuclei
	Intracellular RBCs
	Hepatic abscess
	Flask-shaped ulcers in cecum
Trichomonas spp.	STD
	Hanging drop test for motility
	Flagella
Toxoplasma spp.	Cats and cat litter
	TORCHS (*toxoplasma, other, rubella, cytomegalovirus, HIV, syphilis*)
	Mononucleosis-like syndrome
	Space-occupying lesion brain in AIDS
Leishmania spp.	Sandflies
	Soldiers returning from Persian Gulf
	Blackening of skin
	Trip to Asia or South America
Trypanosoma brucei	Tsetse fly
	Sleeping sickness
	Trip to Asia or South America
	Death by starvation
	Winterbottom sign
Trypanosoma cruzi	Chagas disease
	Reduviid bug
	Mega organs (e.g., colon)
	Romaña sign
	Acquired achalasia, Hirschsprung disease
	Myocarditis leading to heart failure
Enterobius vermicularis	Pinworm
	Scotch tape test
	Anal itching (itchy butt)
	Appendicitis; urethritis in girls
	No eosinophilia
Ascaris lumbricoides	Roundworm
	Large, pearl-white worm
	Adults: intestinal obstruction
	No eosinophilia *except* in lung transmigration phase

Continued

Parasitology Trigger Words—Cont'd

Trichinella spiralis	Hunter
	Undercooked pig or game meat
	Splinter hemorrhages
	Facial edema and myalgia
	Eosinophilia
	Muscle biopsy
Necator americanus	Hookworm
	Pneumonitis
	Iron deficiency anemia
Strongyloides stercoralis	Threadworm
	Pneumonitis
	Dermatitis
	Eosinophilia
	Autoinfection life cycle
	Larva, *not* eggs, in stool

COMMON LABORATORY VALUES

TEST	CONVENTIONAL UNITS	SI UNITS
Blood, Plasma, Serum		
Alanine aminotransferase (ALT, GPT at 30°C)	8-20 U/L	8-20 U/L
Amylase, serum	25-125 U/L	25-125 U/L
Aspartate aminotransferase (AST, GOT at 30°C)	8-20 U/L	8-20 U/L
Bilirubin, serum (adult): total; direct	0.1-1.0 mg/dL; 0.0-0.3 mg/dL	2-17 μmol/L; 0-5 μmol/L
Calcium, serum (Ca^{2+})	8.4-10.2 mg/dL	2.1-2.8 mmol/L
Cholesterol, serum	Rec: <200 mg/dL	<5.2 mmol/L
Cortisol, serum	8:00 AM: 6-23 μg/dL; 4:00 PM: 3-15 μg/dL 8:00 PM: ≤50% of 8:00 AM	170-630 nmol/L; 80-410 nmol/L Fraction of 8:00 AM: ≤0.50
Creatine kinase, serum	Male: 25-90 U/L	25-90 U/L
	Female: 10-70 U/L	10-70 U/L
Creatinine, serum	0.6-1.2 mg/dL	53-106 μmol/L
Electrolytes, serum		
Sodium (Na^+)	136-145 mEq/L	135-145 mmol/L
Chloride (Cl)	95-105 mEq/L	95-105 mmol/L
Potassium (K^+)	3.5-5.0 mEq/L	3.5-5.0 mmol/L
Bicarbonate (HCO_3^-)	22-28 mEq/L	22-28 mmol/L
Magnesium (Mg^{2+})	1.5-2.0 mEq/L	1.5-2.0 mmol/L
Estriol, total, serum (in pregnancy)		
24-28 wk; 32-36 wk	30-170 ng/mL; 60-280 ng/mL	104-590 nmol/L; 208-970 nmol/L
28-32 wk; 36-40 wk	40-220 ng/mL; 80-350 ng/mL	140-760 nmol/L; 280-1210 nmol/L
Ferritin, serum	Male: 15-200 ng/mL	15-200 μg/L
	Female: 12-150 ng/mL	12-150 μg/L
Follicle-stimulating hormone, serum/plasma (FSH)	Male: 4-25 mIU/mL	4-25 U/L
	Female:	
	Premenopause, 4-30 mIU/mL	4-30 U/L
	Midcycle peak, 10-90 mIU/mL	10-90 U/L
	Postmenopause, 40-250 mIU/mL	40-250 U/L
Gases, arterial blood (room air)		
pH	7.35-7.45	[H^+] 36-44 nmol/L
P_{CO_2}	33-45 mmHg	4.4-5.9 kPa
P_{O_2}	75-105 mmHg	10.0-14.0 kPa
Glucose, serum	Fasting: 70-110 mg/dL	3.8-6.1 mmol/L
	2-hr postprandial: <120 mg/dL	<6.6 mmol/L
Growth hormone-arginine stimulation	Fasting: <5 ng/mL	<5 μg/L
	Provocative stimuli: >7 ng/mL	>7 μg/L
Immunoglobulins, serum		
IgA	76-390 mg/dL	0.76-3.90 g/L

TEST	CONVENTIONAL UNITS	SI UNITS
Blood, Plasma, Serum		
IgE	0-380 IU/mL	0-380 kIU/L
IgG	650-1500 mg/dL	6.5-15 g/L
IgM	40-345 mg/dL	0.4-3.45 g/L
Iron	50-170 µg/dL	9-30 µmol/L
Lactate dehydrogenase, serum	45-90 U/L	45-90 U/L
Luteinizing hormone, serum/ plasma (LH)	Male: 6-23 mIU/mL	6-23 U/L
	Female:	
	Follicular phase, 5-30 mIU/mL	5-30 U/L
	Midcycle, 75-150 mIU/mL	75-150 U/L
	Postmenopause, 30-200 mIU/mL	30-200 U/L
Osmolality, serum	275-295 mOsm/kg	275-295 mOsm/kg
Parathyroid hormone, serum, N-terminal	230-630 pg/mL	230-630 ng/L
Phosphatase (alkaline), serum (p-NPP at 30°C)	20-70 U/L	20-70 U/L
Phosphorus (inorganic), serum	3.0-4.5 mg/dL	1.0-1.5 mmol/L
Prolactin, serum (hPRL)	<20 ng/mL	<20 µg/L
Proteins, serum		
Total (recumbent)	6.0-8.0 g/dL	60-80 g/L
Albumin	3.5-5.5 g/dL	35-55 g/L
Globulin	2.3-3.5 g/dL	23-35 g/L
Thyroid-stimulating hormone, serum or plasma (TSH)	0.5-5.0 µU/mL	0.5-5.0 mU/L
Thyroidal iodine (^{123}I) uptake	8%-30% of administered dose/24 hr	0.08-0.30/24 hr
Thyroxine (T_4), serum	4.5-12 µg/dL	58-154 nmol/L
Triglycerides, serum	35-160 mg/dL	0.4-1.81 mmol/L
Triiodothyronine (T_3), serum (RIA)	115-190 ng/dL	1.8-2.9 nmol/L
Triiodothyronine (T_3) resin uptake	25%-38%	0.25-0.38
Urea nitrogen, serum (BUN)	7-18 mg/dL	1.2-3.0 mmol urea/L
Uric acid, serum	3.0-8.2 mg/dL	0.18-0.48 mmol/L
Cerebrospinal Fluid		
Cell count	0-5 cells/mm³	$0-5 \times 10^6$/L
Chloride	118-132 mEq/L	118-132 mmol/L
Gammaglobulin	3%-12% total proteins	0.03-0.12
Glucose	50-75 mg/dL	2.8-4.2 mmol/L
Pressure	70-180 mm H_2O	70-180 mm H_2O
Proteins, total	<40 mg/dL	<0.40 g/L
Hematology		
Bleeding time (template)	2-7 min	2-7 min
Erythrocyte count	Male: 4.3-5.9 million/mm³	$4.3-5.9 \times 10^{12}$/L
	Female: 3.5-5.5 million/mm³	$3.5-5.5 \times 10^{12}$/L
Erythrocyte sedimentation rate (Westergren)	Male: 0-15 mm/hr	0-15 mm/hr
	Female: 0-20 mm/hr	0-20 mm/hr
Hematocrit (Hct)	Male: 40%-54%	0.40-0.54
	Female: 37%-47%	0.37-0.47
Hemoglobin A_{1C}	≤6%	≤0.06%
Hemoglobin, blood (Hb)	Male: 13.5-17.5 g/dL	2.09-2.71 mmol/L
	Female: 12.0-16.0 g/dL	1.86-2.48 mmol/L
Hemoglobin, plasma	1-4 mg/dL	0.16-0.62 mmol/L
Leukocyte count and differential		
Leukocyte count	4500-11,000/mm³	$4.5-11.0 \times 10^9$/L
Segmented neutrophils	54%-62%	0.54-0.62

Hematology

Bands	3%-5%	0.03-0.05
Eosinophils	1%-3%	0.01-0.03
Basophils	0%-0.75%	0-0.0075
Lymphocytes	25%-33%	0.25-0.33
Monocytes	3%-7%	0.03-0.07
Mean corpuscular hemoglobin (MCH)	25.4-34.6 pg/cell	0.39-0.54 fmol/cell
Mean corpuscular hemoglobin concentration (MCHC)	31%-37% Hb/cell	4.81-5.74 mmol Hb/L
Mean corpuscular volume (MCV)	80-100 μm^3	80-100 fl
Partial thromboplastin time (activated) (aPTT)	25-40 sec	25-40 sec
Platelet count	150,000-400,000/mm³	150-400 $\times 10^9$/L
Prothrombin time (PT)	12-14 sec	12-14 sec
Reticulocyte count	0.5%-1.5% of red cells	0.005-0.015
Thrombin time	<2 sec deviation from control	<2 sec deviation from control
Volume		
Plasma	Male: 25-43 mL/kg	0.025-0.043 L/kg
	Female: 28-45 mL/kg	0.028-0.045 L/kg
Red cell	Male: 20-36 mL/kg	0.020-0.036 L/kg
	Female: 19-31 mL/kg	0.019-0.031 L/kg

Sweat

Chloride	0-35 mmol/L	0-35 mmol/L

Urine

Calcium	100-300 mg/24hr	2.5-7.5 mmol/24 hr
Creatinine clearance	Male: 97-137 mL/min	
	Female: 88-128 mL/min	
Estriol, total (in pregnancy)		
30 wk	6-18 mg/24 hr	21-62 µmol/24 hr
35 wk	9-28 mg/24 hr	31-97 µmol/24 hr
40 wk	13-42 mg/24 hr	45-146 µmol/24 hr
17-Hydroxycorticosteroids	Male: 3.0-9.0 mg/24 hr	8.2-25.0 µmol/24 hr
	Female: 2.0-8.0 mg/24 hr	5.5-22.0 µmol/24 hr
17-Ketosteroids, total	Male: 8-22 mg/24 hr	28-76 µmol/24 hr
	Female: 6-15 mg/24 hr	21-52 µmol/24 hr
Osmolality	50-1400 mOsm/kg	
Oxalate	8-40 µg/mL	90-445 µmol/L
Proteins, total	<150 mg/24 hr	<0.15 g/24 hr

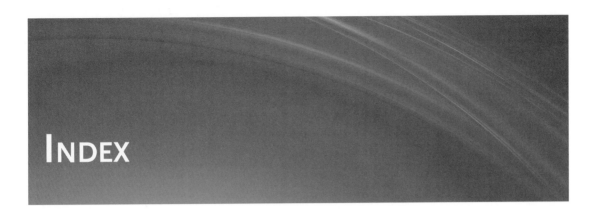

INDEX

Note: Page numbers followed by *b* indicate boxes, *f* indicate figures and *t* indicate tables.

A

ABO blood typing, 41, 42*t*
Actinomyces, 95*t*, 96
Acute hemorrhagic conjunctivitis, 140, 140*b*
Adenoids, 2
Adenoviridae
  diseases of, 130, 130*t*
  identification of, 130
  pathogenesis of, 130
  prevention/treatment of, 131
  transmission of, 131
Adult T cell leukemia/lymphoma (ATLL), 159
Aeromonas, 92, 92*t*
AIDS
  full blown, 157
  indicator diseases of, 158*t*
  -related complex, 157
Alloantigens, 18*b*
Animal pox viruses, 138
Anthrax, 75
Antibacterial immunopathogenesis, 61
  cross-reacting, 61
  inflammation and, 61
Antibacterial responses, 33, 34*f*
Antibacterial vaccines, 68, 68*t*
Antibiotic sensitivity assays, 64
Antibiotics
  bacterial cells and, 56*f*, 59
  peptidoglycan inhibited by, 51
  properties of, 66*t*
  resistance to, 67*b*
Antibody inhibitory tests, 43
Antibody molecules
  antigen reactions with, 27, 41
    agglutination-based assays, 27, 41, 42*t*
    precipitation-based assays, 27, 27*f*, 41, 42*f*
  antigenic determinants on, 24, 25*t*
  B cells and secretion of, 26, 26*b*
  effector mechanisms of, 26
  Fc region functions of, 21, 23*t*
  functional regions of, 21, 22*f*
  terminology of, 22*t*
Antifungal drugs, 168, 168*t*
Antifungal responses, 36
Antigen-presenting cells (APCs), 28, 29*f*
Antigen-recognizing lymphoid cells, 4
Antigens
  antibody molecules, determinants of, 24, 25*t*
  antibody molecules, reactions with, 27, 41
    agglutination-based assays, 27, 41, 42*t*
    precipitation-based assays, 27, 27*f*, 41, 42*f*
  B cell maturation and, 25, 25*f*
  of HBV, 161
  IF/EIA localizing, 42, 42*f*
  immune responses and, 28
  original antigenic sin, 28*b*, 29
  Rh, 30, 32*b*
  super, 61
  TD, B cell stimulation by, 26, 26*b*
  terminology of, 22*t*
  TI, B cell stimulation by, 26

Antimetabolite drugs, 68
Antimicrobial drugs, 65, 65*f*, 66*t*
Antimicrobial responses, 33, 33*t*, 34*b*
Antiparasite responses, 36
Antiparasitic drugs, 175*t*
Antitumor responses, 36
Antiviral drugs, 127
  virus resistance to, 127
  viruses treatable with, 127, 128*t*
Antiviral responses, 33, 35*b*, 35*f*
  components of, 123
  pathologic effects of, 123, 124*t*
Antiviral vaccines, 127
  frequently used, 129*t*
  inactivated, 129
APCs. *See* Antigen-presenting cells
Arenaviridae, 150
Arthropod-associated diseases, 187, 187*t*
Arthus reaction, 32
Aseptic meningitis, 140, 140*b*
Aspergillus fumigatus, 171
Assays. *See specific types*
ATLL. *See* Adult T cell leukemia/lymphoma
Autoimmune responses
  causes of, 36
  disease types in, 37, 37*t*
  HLA and, 38

B

B cells
  antibody molecule secretion and, 26, 26*b*
  antigen-independent maturation of, 25, 25*f*
  TD antigen stimulation of, 26, 26*b*
  TI antigen stimulation of, 26
B19 virus, 132
Bacillus, 75
  B. anthracis
    diseases of, 75
    pathogenesis of, 75
    prevention/treatment of, 75
  B. cereus, food poisoning from, 75
  B. subtilis, 76
Bacitracin, 51
Bacteremia, 58
Bacterial cells. *See also* Endotoxins; Enterobacteriaceae;
      Exotoxins
  adherence of, 56
  antibiotic resistance of, 56*f*, 59
  bacteriophages of, 55
  blood circulation of, 58
  cell envelope, 48, 49*f*
  chromosome of, 54, 55*f*
  colony characteristics of, 64*t*
  division of, 54
  encapsulated, 50, 50*b*, 59, 60*b*
  escape of host attempts at elimination and, 59
  flagella, 50
  genetic transfer of, 55, 56*f*
  genetics of, 54, 54*t*